BRITISH MEDICAL BULLETIN

KU-530-216

Health and the food-chain

Scientific Editors: David I Thurnham & Terry A Roberts

Acknowledgements

The planning committee for this issue of the *British Medical Bulletin* was chaired by Alan Malcolm and also included Richard Gilbert, Terry Roberts, Margaret Ashwell, Michael Morgan and David Thurnham.

The British Council and the Royal Society of Medicine Press are most grateful to them for their help and advice and particularly for the valuable work of the Scientific Editors in completing this issue.

BRITISH MEDICAL BULLETIN

VOLUME 56 NUMBER 1 2000

Health and
the food-chain

Scientific Editors

David I Thurnham
& Terry A Roberts

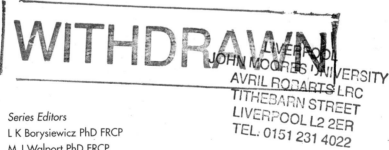

WITHDRAWN

LIVERPOOL
JOHN MOORES UNIVERSITY
AVRIL ROBARTS LRC
TITHEBARN STREET
LIVERPOOL L2 2ER
TEL: 0151 231 4022

Series Editors
L K Borysiewicz PhD FRCP
M J Walport PhD FRCP

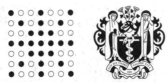

PUBLISHED FOR THE BRITISH COUNCIL BY
THE ROYAL SOCIETY OF MEDICINE PRESS LIMITED

LIVERPOOL JMU LIBRARY

3 1111 01024 0438

ROYAL SOCIETY OF MEDICINE PRESS LIMITED
1 Wimpole Street, London W1M 8AE, UK
207 E. Westminster Road, Lake Forest, IL 60045, USA

© The British Council 2000

Apart from any fair dealing for the purposes of research or private study, or criticism or review, as permitted under the UK Copyright, Designs and Patents Act, 1988, no part of this publication may be reproduced, stored or transmitted, in any form or by any means, without the prior permission in writing of the publishers, or in the case of reprographic reproduction in accordance with the terms of licences issued by the Copyright Licensing Agency in the UK, or in accordance with the terms of licences issued by the appropriate Reproduction Rights Organisation outside the UK. Enquiries concerning reproduction outside the terms stated here should be sent to the publishers at the UK address printed on this page.

British Library Cataloguing in Publication Data
A catalogue record for this book is available from the British Library
ISBN 1–85315–453–9
ISSN 0007–1420

Subscription information *British Medical Bulletin* is published quarterly in January, April, July and October on behalf of the British Council by the Royal Society of Medicine Press Limited. Subscription rates for Volume 56 (2000), including online access, are £154 Europe (including UK), US$265 USA, £158 elsewhere, £73 developing countries. Prices include postage by surface mail within Europe, by air freight and second class post within the USA*, and by various methods of air-speeded delivery to all other countries. Subscription orders and enquiries should be sent to: Publications Subscription Department, Royal Society of Medicine Press Limited, 1 Wimpole Street, London W1M 8AE, UK (Tel +44 (0)20 7290 2928; Fax +44(0)20 7290 2929; Email rsmjournals@roysocmed.ac.uk).
*Periodicals postage paid at Rahway, NJ. US Postmaster: Send address changes to *British Medical Bulletin*, c/o Mercury Airfreight International Ltd, 365 Blair Road, Avenel, NJ 07001, USA.

Single copies and back numbers of issues published from 1996 are available for purchase directly from the distributors: Hoddle Doyle Meadows Limited, Station Road, Linton, Cambs CB1 6UX, UK (Tel +44 (0)1223 893855; Fax +44 (0)1223 893852). Issues published in 1996 and 1997 cost £24.95/US$41 per copy, and issues published from 1998 cost £34.95/US$57 per copy. Please add £2/US$3.50 for postage.

Pre-1996 back numbers: Orders for any title published prior to 1996 should be sent to Jill Kettley, Subscriptions Manager, Harcourt Brace, Foots Cray, Sidcup, Kent DA14 5HP (Tel +44 (0)181 308 5700; Fax +44 (0)181 309 0807).

This journal is indexed, abstracted and/or published online in the following media: Adonis, Biosis, BRS Colleague (full text), Chemical Abstracts, Colleague (Online), Current Contents/ Clinical Medicine, Current Contents/Life Sciences, Elsevier BIOBASE/Current Awareness in Biological Sciences, EMBASE/Excerpta Medica, Index Medicus/Medline, Medical Documentation Service, Reference Update, Research Alert, Science Citation Index, Scisearch, SIIC-Database Argentina, UMI (Microfilms)

Editorial services and typesetting by BA & GM Haddock, Ford, Midlothian, Scotland
Printed in Great Britain by Bell & Bain Ltd, Glasgow, Scotland.

Preface

Our food, our dietary habits and our requirements for some nutrients, are changing rapidly as we enter the 21st century. Energy needs have fallen ahead of our intakes and, as the prevalence of obesity stubbornly increases, we have to accept that food palatability continues to thwart attempts to balance the equation. In the industrialised Western world, people live in times of affluence and few get insufficient food to meet dietary requirements. We take for granted that food will be wholesome and have confidence that the food we obtain from animals will be healthy. Unfortunately, the BSE epidemic indicated how easily changes in animal husbandry could by-pass the controls intended to ensure that only healthy animals entered the food-chain. The controls which are in place today evolved gradually over the last 100 years to meet changing requirements as food processing technology developed and the challenges presented by food preservation, public health and safety needed to be met. We need to be reminded continually that pathogenic microbes still surround us. The same bacteria, viruses and fungi that were around 100 years ago are still present in the environment and so potentially still present in raw agricultural products and untreated water. In addition, improved laboratory methods and sophisticated epidemiological techniques are revealing 'emerging pathogens' previously unrecognised. Care must be taken to avoid altered farming practices replacing one risk that is known and controllable with another that is less apparent, or not recognised. For example, the increasing production of 'organic' foods must not allow a known chemical risk to be replaced with a less apparent biological one. The risk from protozoa and parasites in the industrialised Western world has been brought under control, but the source of food for these countries is now world-wide rather than just our immediate surroundings. Air transport brings exotic fruits to the supermarket shelves from places in the world where parasites abound. Parasites and protozoa are common problems in non-industrialised countries and often transmitted by the faecal-oral route. The reasons for washing raw foods and vigilance in handling food must continue to be taught to each new generation. The success of our food manufacturers in providing us with wholesome and safe food must not lead to complacency in appreciating the risks which can occur. The cumulative effect of small changes in food handling procedures can have disastrous consequences. Nevertheless, much more food is safe than dangerous and, when illness is traced to food, it is usually the consequence of faulty formulation, failure of a process, or gross abuse at the stage of preparation and serving. Most commonly, food is inadequately cooked or reheated coupled with inappropriate storage temperatures.

Food is needed to supply the raw materials for our continued existence. The substances it contains are generally not toxic, or at least the

© The British Council 2000

level of toxicity is below that to which most of us would display a toxic reaction. However, at various points in the food-chain, substances such as vitamins, minerals, antibiotics, pesticides and insecticides may be used for specific purposes and residues may remain in the final product. With a full knowledge of the process, proper quality control can be installed to reduce any risk to human health. However, if this proves unacceptable, for whatever reason, then steps have to be taken to change farming practices as was recently done in the chicken industry with the recommendations to remove growth promoters (antibiotics) from the feed. It is hoped that these changes prove to be beneficial to both men and chickens, but we need to be vigilant they do not give rise to new unforeseen problems. However, exogenously-added substances are only one form of potential food toxin. It has to be realised that plants themselves synthesise a large number of potent substances to protect them against environmental pathogens or threats to their existence. Many of these substances are inactivated by cooking and others we develop tolerance against early in infancy. Nevertheless, mild gastrointestinal problems are not uncommon and are the body's way of providing protection against the occasional overdose of a noxious substance. More severe sensitivities or adverse reactions to specific foods do occur in some people, but generally the true prevalence of such reactions is lower than initial reports indicate. The area of 'food purity' is, however, of public concern and must be seriously considered by those interested in genetically modifying the natural biological resistance of food to pests, and by responsible regulatory bodies and advisory committees. Changes in food composition, in this way, have already been shown to increase skin sensitivity to increased levels of biological toxins.

Over the last 100 years, infantile mortality and early adult death have been dramatically reduced and we all expect to live our three score years and ten. Hence life-styles have changed, particularly so in the last 50 years and public expectations from food are also changing. These days, we are all very much more aware of the chronic diseases facing us in those final years. Magazines, newspapers, television 'soaps' and documentaries make us increasingly aware of the high risk and reduced quality of life which is associated with excess weight, arteriosclerosis, cancers, diabetes, osteoporosis, Alzheimer's and other diseases. At the same time, our dietary habits are believed by many to play a large part in the fate that awaits us. Vegetables and fruits are constantly presented as foods with which there is a lower risk of chronic disease and the authorities tell us we should aim to eat five portions a day. But are there particular ingredients that would provide the magic bullet such as lycopene, β-carotene or vitamin E? Should our foods be enhanced with added nutrients like lycopene, which, it is suggested, may lower the risk of prostate cancer. How should this be done? Extra lycopene can be added to tomato soup without raising public fears of genetic modification, but should we consider enhancing the lycopene in the raw tomato? Are scientists justified in studying plant DNA with a view to 'improving' food products? Can we say, for example, that the lycopene-enriched tomato will be healthier food for human consumption than the current varieties?

The contributors to this issue were asked to discuss particular aspects related to health and the food-chain. Their papers provide a basis for a fuller understanding of the concerns surrounding food safety. Food processing and preservations techniques have advanced to a high level of sophistication over the last century to preserve the nutrient content, to extend shelf-life and minimise the risk of pathogenic microbes and/or their toxins affecting human health. The risks from food poisoning, adulteration and contamination have largely disappeared, but the risk from pathogens is ever present. Vigilance also needs to be maintained as new markets, sometimes with fewer controls, are explored to supply new and exotic tastes. The greatest challenges to face our food authorities, however, may well come from the growing world-wide interest in food biotechnology. Manipulation of genetic structures to maximise food production, produce drought-resistant cereals or β-carotene-containing rice, alter the colour of fruits, increase nutrient levels, delay maturation are all examples of developments already occurring. However, public confidence in authorities' competence to ensure a wholesome, nutritious and safe food supply is currently low following the BSE outbreak. How should debates on food issues be conducted in an atmosphere in which all parties trust each other? What do the authorities understand about public perceptions of food? These are real issues to the consumer and they have to be addressed if the changes currently taking place in world food supplies are to be introduced and managed without conflict and with the full co-operation and understanding of the public at large.

David I Thurnham
Howard Professor of Human Nutrition,
Northern Ireland Centre for Diet and Health,
University of Ulster, Coleraine,
County Londonderry, Northern Ireland

Terry A Roberts
Consultant Food Hygiene & Safety,
Reading, England

Food processing: a century of change

R W Welch and **P C Mitchell**

Northern Ireland Centre for Diet and Health (NICHE), University of Ulster, Coleraine, UK

In 1900, the population was beset with poverty, and infectious and deficiency diseases were common. The first half of the century was blighted by world wars, economic depression and post-war austerity. Nevertheless, a combination of enlightened social policy and the application of medical, nutritional and food science, resulted in substantial improvements in health, such that, by 1950, many hitherto common infectious diseases were under control, and the diet was generally nutritionally adequate. The second half of the century saw increasing economic prosperity, and unprecedented social and scientific advances. The impact on food processing was manifold: nascent technologies such as freezing and chilling were increasingly exploited, and the consumer became the major focus of a food industry that became more sophisticated, embracing automation, computerisation and new developments in, for example, drying, heat processing, controlled and modified atmosphere packaging, ingredients and quality assurance. By 1999, this had led to an industry which provided foods that were not only safe, nutritious and palatable, but which were also increasingly convenient and healthy.

1900–1999 – a century of changes

The 20th century has seen unprecedented political, social, and economic changes, and scientific and technological advances have moved at an ever increasing pace. All these factors have impacted on the food processing industry and influenced the way that food is processed and marketed. Table 1 shows some of the century's milestones, and major developments in food processing through the decades of the century.

A calendar century is essentially an arbitrary unit, but it is notable that the 20th century may be divided into two relatively distinct half centuries. The years 1900–1950, or thereabouts, were characterised by profound political, social and economic upheavals, when ensuring an on-going supply of food to sustain the UK population, preventing or alleviating deficiency diseases, and reducing the incidence of food-borne diseases were the major concerns. The relative economic and political

Correspondence to:
Dr R W Welch, Northern Ireland Centre for Diet and Health (NICHE), University of Ulster, Coleraine BT52 1SA, UK

© The British Council 2000

Table 1 Some political, social, economic and scientific milestones, and developments in food processing 1900–1999

Decade	Milestones	Food developments
1900s		
	Poverty and malnutrition among working classes	First flour bleaching agent
	Infant mortality at around 220 per 1000	Milk pasteurisation
	Existence of vitamins indicated	Drum drying
	Diet–health relationships become clearer	Sanitary can
	Introduction of school meals	Canned baked beans
1910s		
	World War One	Hydrogenation of oils
	Two-thirds of food supply is imported	Higher extraction of flour
	Food shortages and rationing	Post harvest mechanisation
1920s		
	General strike	Vitamins A and D added to margarine
	Stock market crash presages depression	Plate heat exchangers
	Diets of working classes still poor	Tubular blanchers
	Milk promoted for children	Juice extractors
1930s		
	World economic depression	Mechanisation in abattoirs
	Poverty and undernourishment persist	Lacquered can
	Measures to support domestic agriculture	Brine injection technology
	60% of food supply is imported in 1938	Rapid freezing technology
	World War Two commences	Spray drying – instant coffee
	Non-essential imports curtailed	Wrapped, sliced bread
	Measures to control agriculture and food	Milk carton
	2% of homes have refrigerators in 1939	Refrigerated retail cabinets
1940s		
	War-time rationing	Fortification – National loaf
	Consumer food and nutrition education	Preservatives – meat
	National Milk Scheme in 1941	Mass production – chocolate
	World War Two ends	Freeze drying – vegetables
	Establishment of National Health Service	Additives – flour improvers
	Policy to increase agricultural output	HTST[a] milk pasteuriser
1950s		
	Food rationing ends	Dairy herds are 76% TB[b] free
	Food and Drug Act (1955)	Preservatives – baked goods
	Treaty of Rome (1957)	Controlled atmosphere storage
	Consumer spending rises	Aseptic canning
	Concentration of retailing	*Tetra Pak* packaging for milk
	Refrigerators in 8% of homes by 1956	Frozen foods – fish fingers
	First links of cholesterol and heart disease	Tea bag introduced
1960s		
	Computerisation begins	Chorleywood bread process
	Measures to control Salmonella in eggs	Instant mashed potato
	Refrigerators in 23% of homes by 1964	Polyunsaturated margarine
	Trade Description Act (1968)	Meat tenderisation – enzymes
	Intensified competition on price	Ultra-high temperature milk
	Rise of consumerism – residues, irradiation	*Tetra Pak/Brik* packaging (aseptic)
1970s		
	UK accession to EEC[c] in 1973	Growth in convenience food
	Global oil crisis	Automation and computerisation
	Free school milk ceases	Slimming foods
	Fibre-health links popularised	Granary breads
	Freezers in over 40% of homes by 1979	Aseptic filling – pouches

Table 1 (*continued*) Some political, social, economic and scientific milestones, and developments in food processing 1900–1999

1980s

Food Advisory Committee – additives	Advances in plastic packaging
Food Act (1984)	Single cell protein – Quorn
Diet and cardiovascular disease links	Low calorie ingredients
Food Labelling Regulations (1984)	Nutritional labelling
Food scare – Salmonella	Chilled prepared foods
Consumer concerns about diet and health	Monounsaturated margarine
Bar codes introduced	Modified atmosphere packaging
Consumer led market place	Aseptic foods – particulates

1990s

Food Safety Act (1990)	Increasing company specialisation
Food scares – allergens, BSE[d], GMOs[e]	Fat substitutes – Simplesse
Reform of CAP[f]	Limited use of irradiation
Health of the Nation published	Minimal processing
Ageing population	Functional foods
Consumer concern about environment	Growth in organic foods
Retailing and processing globalisation	Genetically modified foods

[a] High-temperature, short-time
[b] Tuberculosis
[c] European Economic Community
[d] Bovine spongiform encephalopathy
[e] Genetically modified organisms
[f] Common Agricultural Policy
Data from sources in the references cited.

stability, and the increasing prosperity of the latter half of the century resulted in changes in emphasis. By 1999, food was no longer in short supply, with the consumer expecting the continuing availability of a wide range of foods with good palatability and increased convenience in terms of storage and preparation. The focus had changed from deficiencies and food-borne diseases to the potential of foods to prevent or alleviate chronic diseases, such as cancers, heart disease, diabetes, and associated conditions such as obesity and hypertension. As the consumers' awareness of the role of food in health has increased, so have concerns about the safety of the new technologies which are being introduced throughout the food-chain.

Food processing – an historical context

Almost all foodstuffs are derived from natural products – from plants and animals. The purpose of the earliest food processing methods was to render these products safe to eat, and to present them in a range of palatable forms. Another important purpose was to preserve food, and thus enable storage or transport. Often these objectives were combined.

For example milk, which provides a nutritious food, deteriorates very rapidly unless processed, and a wide range of traditional methods were developed which both extended the shelf-life, and yielded a range of palatable products such as cheeses, yoghurt and butter. These traditional methods brought about complex transformations involving the use of fermentations, and changes in the structure of the food. It is a tribute to earlier agriculturally based communities that such methods were developed without an understanding of the underlying science and technology.

The aims of modern processing are manifold, and include the prolongation of shelf-life, ensuring safety, improving palatability, increasing variety, improving nutritional value and increasing convenience. There is a large, and increasing number of technologies available and, as is outlined below, combined technologies are often applied. Throughout the 20th century, the development and application of these technologies has been enhanced and informed by the advances in science and engineering. However, the utilisation of the technologies has depended on the prevailing economic and social conditions and, increasingly towards the end of the century, on the attitudes and beliefs of the consumer concerning these technologies and their perceived implications.

Food processes – definition, commercial context, scope

In this article, food processing is defined as any procedure undergone by food commodities after they have left the primary producer, and before they reach the consumer, who may themselves further cook or process the food. Food processes take many forms which vary greatly in the degree of complexity of the technologies employed. At the simplest level, food processing may involve no more than controlled storage such as refrigeration. At more complex levels, commodities may be processed to yield ingredients which are later combined to yield foodstuffs as varied as canned baked beans in tomato sauce, frozen baked products, or chilled ready meals.

Although small companies play a role, often in the production of niche products, food processing has become increasingly undertaken by large enterprises which have progressively mechanised, automated, specialised and internationalised throughout the 20th century. The major aim of the commercial food processor has been to run a viable and profitable enterprise. In order to achieve this, the processor has had to conform to increasingly stringent legal standards, and to the standards laid down by large retailers who dominated the food market at the end of the 20th century. Public health and related consumer needs have been central to these standards.

It is beyond the scope of this paper to review all the changes that have occurred in the food-chain during the past 100 years. Past and on-going changes in areas such as biotechnology and food safety are reviewed in subsequent papers. Taking a UK perspective, the focus here is on changes in post-harvest processing, and on the way in which the exploitation of technological advances in the processing of selected commodities has enabled the food industry to respond to the changing social, economic and political conditions of the century in order to satisfy the changing needs and expectations of the population.

The food-chain in 1900 and 1999, an overview

Basic steps in the food-chain for 1900 and for 1999 are shown in Figure 1. In 1900, the food raw materials, which are mostly the products of plant and animal husbandry and fishing were consumed as 'fresh' produce, processed into foodstuffs, or into ingredients for processing.

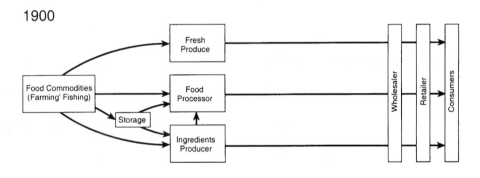

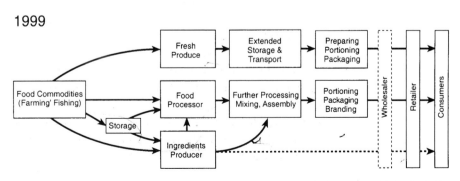

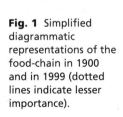

Fig. 1 Simplified diagrammatic representations of the food-chain in 1900 and in 1999 (dotted lines indicate lesser importance).

Some raw materials or ingredients were stored prior to processing. In 1900, these fresh and processed foods, and the food ingredients were essentially commodities, going on to wholesale markets and thence to retailers and the consumer, with little packaging or branding. By 1999, the food-chain had become much more complex. Fresh produce is subjected to extended storage and to prolonged transport, and may be prepared, portioned and packaged before supply to the market. Processed foods and ingredients are subjected to further processing to yield a range of even more complex foodstuffs designed for specific market niches. Conversely the supply of ingredients to the consumer had declined (Fig. 1). These changes have resulted in very large increases in both the range of products available, and in the ease with which these products can be made ready for consumption by the consumer. In 1900, there were national grocery chains which had been developed by entrepreneurs such as Julius Drew, Thomas Lipton and John James Sainsbury; their stores, like those of the numerous independent food retailers, for the most part portioned and packaged the commodities supplied through wholesalers[1]. By 1999, the supermarket chains, buying directly from primary producers and processors, dominated the market, and the role of the wholesaler had declined. Furthermore, by 1999, an increasingly complex regulatory and legal framework had evolved with the aim of improving and ensuring the safety and probity of the food-chain for the consumer.

Developments in food processing during the 20th century

Many of the food processes in use in 1999 were developments of processes extant in 1900. This section outlines these developments, and the range of new processes developed since 1900. Changes in the processing of specific foodstuffs are outlined in the next section.

Drying

Drying (dehydration) preserves food by reducing the water activity, thus inhibiting the activity of micro-organisms and enzymes. Drying not only prolongs storage life, but it also reduces bulk which facilitates storage and transport. Traditionally, drying was applied to both animal and vegetable products and relied primarily on the action of the sun and wind. However, a wide range of commercial driers suitable for both solid and liquid foods have been developed[2]. For example, the drum roller drying of milk was introduced in the first decade of the century.

The dried product was easily reconstituted and represented a significant advance on the products from earlier crude evaporation techniques. Further advances in the first half of the century include spray drying which was used for milk, and for other liquids including coffee, to give the first instant coffee powder. The utilisation of these procedures under partial vacuum yielded dried products with less heat damage, and which were consequently of higher quality. Heat damage, which can occur in both drying and heat processing, includes the development of unpleasant aromas and colours, the loss of nutrients, a decrease in solubility for liquid foods, and undesirable structural changes in solid foods[2]. Dried milk and dried egg were imported in substantial quantities during the Second World War and helped to provide an adequate diet.

Freeze drying involves freezing followed by the sublimation of the ice under reduced pressure. This technique, pioneered in the 1940s and popularised in the 1960s, can be applied to prepared foods and to ingredients such as vegetables, fruit and meat[2,3]. There is no heat damage, and the sensory, structural and nutritional characteristics of the foods are well maintained with the result that freeze-dried products combine good quality with convenience[2,3]. The variety of dried products increased until the 1970s when other processes gave the consumer access to other convenience products of even higher quality.

Heat processing

Heat processes inactivate enzymes, reduce or eliminate microbial contamination, and may also bring about desirable changes in palatability. As with drying, heat damage can also occur. However, advances during the 20th century have enabled the consumer to capitalise on the advantages while minimising the disadvantages.

Canning is a heat process introduced in the early 19th century[4], and is applicable to a wide range of foodstuffs[2,5,6]. However, the underlying principles of sterilisation and air exclusion were not appreciated until after the work of Pasteur. The sanitary can with improved sterilisation efficiency was introduced in the 1900s. The canned baked bean also made its first appearance in this decade. However, this nutritious and convenient foodstuff did not gain general popularity until the 1940s. Improved cans with internal lacquering were developed in the 1930s, and large quantities of canned foodstuffs were imported during the Second World War. Aseptic canning, whereby the food is sterilised before being put into a sterile can was introduced in the 1950s. Aseptic canning enables the food to be sterilised by heating to high temperatures and for a shorter time than would be used in conventional canning which is usually carried out at 115–120°C[7]. Aseptic processing (also known as ultra-high temperature or UHT) results in less heat damage and gives better quality products[2,5,6,8]. New packaging materials for aseptic processing were introduced in the 1970s and included plastic retortable pouches in which foods could be sealed and heat sterilised[2,6-8]. Although canning declined somewhat in the 1980s with the introduction of other processes, the safety, long ambient shelf-life and convenience of canned foods has ensured that their popularity has continued to the end of the 20th century. Pasteurisation is a milder heat treatment designed to eliminate vegetative pathogens, such as *Salmonellae*, often combined with refrigerated storage, which is applicable to many foodstuffs. Milk pasteurisation is described below. A number of other processes such as blanching, baking and frying which also involve the use of heat have been increasingly refined throughout the 20th century[2].

Freezing and chilling

Freezing inhibits enzymic action and microbial growth. However, slow freezing of the water in foodstuffs results in the formation of large ice crystals and osmotic imbalances which damage the structure of the food and lead to unacceptable products on thawing[2]. In the 1930s, rapid freezing was shown to substantially mitigate this damage and this consequently enabled the development of the market in frozen foods, which has now extended from commodities such as fish and vegetables to fully prepared convenience foods[2,6,9,10]. On the other hand, chilling (or refrigeration) only reduces the activity of enzymes and micro-organisms; chilling does not extend storage life as much as freezing, but the structure of the food remains intact[2,10-13]. Although the potential of freezing and chilling had long been appreciated, it was not until the latter half of the 20th century that technologies became sufficiently available to permit their extensive use. Freezing and chilling equipment is not only needed for processing, but also for transport, retail display and storage in the home. Before the Second World War, the only products subjected to below ambient temperatures for storage and transport were fish, which used ice, and ice cream which used solid carbon dioxide (dry ice) to maintain the low temperatures required[14]. The first refrigerated cabinets appeared in retail outlets in 1939, but only 2% of homes had refrigerators, and fewer had freezers. As prosperity increased in the 1950s, so did the supply of frozen foods, with peas and fish fingers among the first available. Vehicles that did not have to rely on ice or dry ice became available in the 1960s and the increasing availability of freezers and refrigeration units for storage in retail premises and the home enabled a rapid expansion in the market for frozen and chilled foods[14].

The application of low temperature technologies is a major change in food processing in the 20th century. The majority of the so-called 'fresh' fruit and vegetables on sale by 1999 was the culmination of the 'cold chain' by which freshly harvested crops are stored and transported to the retailer[14]. Coupled with the sourcing of supplies from around the world, this has enabled the year round availability of once seasonal crops, and the introduction of exotic 'fresh' foods. Chilling is also used extensively for prepared foods including cooked meats, sandwiches and complete dishes and meals.

Controlled and modified atmospheres

The use of controlled atmospheres (CA) or modified atmospheres (MA) to extend the storage life of foods is a late 20th century development. The atmospheres used vary, but generally carbon dioxide is increased and oxygen is reduced; this reduces respiratory and other enzymic changes in unprocessed foods such as fruit, vegetables and meat, and will also limit oxidative changes[2]. In MA, a single change is made to the atmosphere. In CA storage, the atmosphere is modified, and the modification is maintained by monitoring and making appropriate adjustments. Bulk MA and CA storage were introduced in the 1950s. Following that, MA was introduced for individual packages. The availability of packaging materials that allow the selective exchange of gases enabled CA to be used in individual packages from the 1980s. The use of combined technologies is increasing, and MA and CA are generally combined with chilling[12,15].

Radiation

Various parts of the electromagnetic spectrum are of use in food processing. UV light can be used to help maintain sterility in food processing plants. Ionising radiation (irradiation) can be used for various purposes including inhibition of sprouting, disinfestation, prolonging shelf-life, and for total sterilisation[16,17]. Although first proposed as a method of food preservation in the 1920s, food irradiation met with substantial consumer opposition in many countries (see also chapter by Gould), and was only approved for a limited range of foods in certain countries (*e.g.* the UK has given clearance of all foods up to treatments of 10 kGy) during the 1990s. Microwave radiation is useful for heating, but cost precludes its widespread use within the food processing industry[2]. However, by 1996–7, the presence of microwave ovens in over 75% of homes enabled the consumer to take advantage of the convenience offered by ready-prepared chilled and frozen foodstuffs[18].

Other advances

A number of other important advances in food processing technology have been made in the 20th century, and examples are given below. Extrusion is used for a wide range of products including pastas, texturised vegetable protein and ready-to-eat breakfast cereals[21]. Developments in microbiology and biotechnology have resulted in advances in fermentation technologies valuable in the production of cheese, butter, yoghurt and beer, and food ingredients such as enzymes and gums. Low temperature and high pressure technologies have enabled the use of supercritical fluids, such as liquid carbon dioxide, for the extraction of caffeine from coffee beans and cholesterol from eggs[20]. Extremely high pressures have been shown to extend the shelf-life of foods such as fruit juices with minimal effects on the sensory qualities[21]. The increasing demand by consumers for 'fresh' foods with increased shelf-life has led to the development of minimal processing techniques. Such techniques often use a combination of technologies, such as CA and chilling or MA, irradiation and chilling[22].

New ingredients

Wheat flour and sugar were the main ingredients in the food supply chain in 1900; while these remained important in 1999, the range and applications of ingredients had expanded substantially. Technological innovations throughout the century have produced new ingredients, including refined starches, gums, fats, proteins and sweeteners with well-defined functionalities and applications[23]. For example new sweeteners, including aspartame and acesulfame-K, were introduced in the 1980s as consumer interest in 'slimming' foods intensified[24]. However, the production of low-calorie soft drinks required not only the substitution of sugar by an artificial sweetener, but also the replacement of the texture or 'mouth-feel' provided by the sugar. A range of food gums are used for this purpose. Food gums are also used as stabilisers to improve the sensory and storage characteristics of a wide range of normal and low-calorie foodstuffs as diverse as frozen prepared products, salad dressings, low-fat spreads, ready prepared sauces and ice cream. A wide range of other additives have also become available and are used under controlled conditions to improve the sensory and keeping qualities of many processed foods[25]. A number of fat replacers have been developed and evaluated for safety and efficacy, and became available in the 1990s. These include the protein-based Simplesse, and the sucrose polyester, Olestra[24,26].

Mechanisation, automation, standardisation and safety

Food processing has seen prodigious advances in mechanisation and automation throughout the 20th century. The utilisation of the advances in engineering and in computer and information technology has turned a labour-intensive industry into a capital-intensive industry. Mechanisation of fruit and vegetable processing started in the 1910s[27]. Mechanisation of primary processing of meat and poultry, and the brine injection technology for meat, were introduced in the 1930s[28]. The ongoing computerised automation started in the 1960s when the first automated bakery was opened[28]. With the rise in automated processing and in the promotion of branded foodstuffs came an increased need for quality control and the standardisation of products. This has led to increasingly sophisticated management procedures for all forms of food processing. However, food safety remains a priority. Any food processor who fails to maintain consumer product safety risks serious, even terminal, financial losses. The major hazard in most food processing operations is microbial contamination, and effective design, operation and control is essential to minimising risk. Starting in the late 1950s, management and operating procedures including cleaning-in-place[29], and hazard analysis critical control point (HACCP) have been developed and implemented [29-32]. However, the marketplace is dynamic and unpredictable, and to remain viable the food processor has to respond adequately to consumer issues such as potential food allergies, or the use of genetically modified raw materials.

Food processing 1900–1999: examples of change

The implementation of scientific and technological advances in response to economic opportunities and consumer demand has led to substantial changes in all areas of food processing. Changes in the processing of two staples, bread and milk, are briefly described, and changes in other sectors are outlined. The implications for health are considered in the next section.

Bread

The quality of bread in 1900 reflected changes in the latter part of the 19th century. The displacement of stone-grinding mills by roller mills which commenced in 1877, was complete by 1890. With this change, the extraction rate (the percentage of the whole grain retained in the flour) fell from 75–80% to 70–73%, and the germ was lost. However, sensory qualities were good and the nutritional significance of this change was not realised[4]. The First World War resulted in food shortages and rationing. In order to increase the amount of bread flour available, legislation was introduced to increase the extraction rate to 76% in 1916, 81% in 1917 and to 91% in 1918 and admixtures of coarse grains, potato flour and soya were also permitted. Bread was grey and of reduced palatability, but this strategy was undoubtedly preferable to the introduction of rationing[4]. Between 1918 and the outbreak of the Second World War in 1939, extraction rates fell to about 70% which gave the millers an optimum yield of white flour[33]. Shortages in the Second World War again led to changes in bread processing. However, the new discoveries in nutritional and cereal science were thoughtfully applied. Bread flour was enriched with thiamin (vitamin B1) in 1940. This ceased in 1942 when 85% extraction National Flour was introduced. National Flour was milled to contain the maximum possible levels of thiamin, riboflavin, niacin and protein and the minimum possible levels of bran, and was enriched with calcium to combat potential deficiencies due to decreased intakes of calcium from cheese and milk[33]. In 1945, the extraction of National Flour was decreased to 80%. However, in 1946, post-war austerity necessitated the introduction of bread rationing and extraction rates were raised briefly to 90% before decreasing to 85%. Bread rationing ended in 1948, extraction rates fell to 82% in 1950 and National Flour ceased in 1953. However, since then, flours with extraction rates below 82% have been enriched with thiamin, niacin, calcium and iron to ensure minimum levels of these nutrients. The first wrapped sliced bread which had been introduced in the 1930s, was re-introduced in the 1950s and gained in popularity throughout the 1960s and 1970s. Most of this bread was made by the Chorleywood bread process developed in the 1960s. In this process, the previous lengthy bulk fermentation is replaced by an input of intense mechanical energy using special mixers which develop the dough matrix in a few minutes. Fat is added (0.7%), and somewhat increased levels of yeast and water are used, with ascorbic acid (100 mg/kg) as an improver. Gluten is the visco-elastic protein in wheat responsible for the establishment of the dough matrix. During the 1970s, commercial processes were developed for the separation of gluten from wheat without loss of functionality[34]. This freeze-dried material is known as vital gluten. Since the accession of the UK to the European Union, imports of American and other high quality bread wheats have been curtailed and thus vital gluten is often added to bread flours made from home-grown wheats. The increased demand for convenience, and for freshly baked breads in the 1980s and 1990s led to the development of part-baked frozen bread products. These are baked off in the home, or in bakeries often located within supermarkets.

Milk

Milk is potentially a highly nutritious and wholesome foodstuff. However, the shelf-life of unprocessed milk is short, it is easily adulterated, and it may carry a number of infectious diseases. Throughout the 19th century, the quality of milk was very poor, particularly in the industrialised cities. In 1850, most milk in London was contaminated with blood or pus, cattle were poorly housed and disease-ridden, and adulteration was commonplace[4]. Brucellosis and bovine tuberculosis were common and often transmitted to those drinking unpasteurised milk. Pasteurisation was first introduced in the 1900s, since it increased shelf-life by reducing the level of spoilage organisms. However, it was soon appreciated that pasteurisation destroyed most of the pathogens associated with milk and, despite opposition from some farmers and consumers, its use has been increased to the point where the sale of non-pasteurised milk has been prohibited in Scotland on public health grounds. The major change in pasteurisation since 1900 has been from a batch process using lower temperatures for a longer time (63.5°C for 30 min) to a high-temperature, short-time (HTST) process (71.7°C for 15 s)[35]. The HTST process uses more efficient, flow-through equipment; it also reduces prolonged heat exposure and the concomitant undesirable sensory and nutritional changes. These changes are even more pronounced on sterilisation, and it was not until the introduction of ultra-high temperature (UHT) treatment that sterilised milk was successful as a consumer product. UHT uses temperatures of 135–150°C for 1–4 s using flow through heat exchangers as for pasteurisation. Homogenisation is essential for the stability of UHT milk[36]. Homogenisation involves the reduction in the size of the fat globules so that a cream layer does not form, and it is also applied to whole milk and to the reduced fat milks that have been introduced. Developments in aseptic packaging have also been important to the success of UHT milk; in this process, the sterile milk is packaged into sterile plastic or laminated containers[35].

Some other important changes in food processing

Many other important changes in food processing occurred in the 20th century. Advances in meat and poultry processing include the production of re-formed, low-fat and convenience products[34–39]. In the spreadable fats' market, the development of hydrogenated fat margarine in the 1910s was followed by their enrichment with vitamins A and D in the 1920s[27]. In the latter half of the century, a wide range of spreadable fats became available, including low-fat products, products high in polyunsaturated or monounsaturated fats and, latterly, functional food products with novel cholesterol-lowering ingredients[40]. Yoghurt, which in 1900 was an exotic curiosity, acquired fruit flavourings in the 1950s. Since then, a range of flavours, low-fat and no-fat varieties have been developed; a number of brands are available which contain probiotic bacteria, which are claimed to confer a number of health benefits[41].

Health implications of changes in food processing

It is pertinent here to consider the degree of understanding of disease aetiology, and of the complex relationships between diet and disease processes. In 1900, infectious and dietary deficiency diseases were still poorly understood. Tuberculosis and other infectious diseases were common causes of morbidity and mortality. The role and significance of the micronutrients had yet to be discovered. General malnutrition and scurvy were common, rickets was almost universal among the children of the working poor, and anaemia was common among working women[4,42]. It has been estimated, with hindsight, that the roller milled flour, whose introduction was complete by 1890, had only about 50% of the iron, and 33% thiamin and niacin, of that found in the stone-ground flour which it had displaced. This change almost certainly accounts for the fact that the working classes, for whom bread was the main source of sustenance, were more malnourished in 1900 than at any time since Tudor times[4,42]. Malnutrition also increases susceptibility to infectious diseases. In 1900, lack of hygiene meant that many foodstuffs were sources of pathogens. This was particularly true for milk and milk products, which are potential sources not only of tuberculosis, but also brucellosis, typhoid, diphtheria, salmonellosis and streptococcal infections[25,36]. The increasing appreciation that heat processing, and in particular pasteurisation, will destroy pathogens in milk, and the increasing use of pasteurisation and other measures led to a rapid decline in milk-borne diseases in the first half of the century.

Economic factors are also important. In 1930, there was economic depression and, although the causes of deficiencies and infectious diseases were more fully understood, the health of the working classes was little better than in 1900[4]. Nevertheless, by 1939, the advances in nutritional, medical and food sciences were being consolidated and adopted; despite stringent food rationing, the general health of the population increased during the Second World War when diets became generally adequate[43]. Food rationing continued after the war until 1954, but this was contemporary with the establishment of the National Health Service, and the continued provision of nutritional supplements, such as cod liver oil and concentrated orange juice, to the young and to pregnant women. Antibiotics and immunisation also led to the control of the serious infectious diseases. The austerity of the post-war years gave way to the social and economic changes which commenced in the late 1960s. Women had access to the contraceptive pill, and also began to work outside the home in increasing numbers. Economic prosperity increased, food was readily available, and the variety of foodstuffs increased. The common life-threatening and disabling infectious and deficiency diseases were a thing of the past. The dominance of the consumer was emerging, and the food processors spurred on by the expanding supermarket chains, were driven to address the life-style and convenience demands of these consumers. The chronic conditions of heart disease, cancers and diabetes emerged as the major causes of morbidity and mortality. Nutritional and epidemiological research implicated diet as a major factor in the aetiology of these diseases, and a number of foodstuffs and diet components were suggested as causative. These included over-consumption of fat, in particular saturated fat, over-consumption of refined carbohydrate, and under-consumption of dietary fibre[44–47]. Although the mechanisms of action of these diet components in the aetiology of these diseases was, and remains, unclear, dietary guidelines recommended changes to correct these perceived imbalances[48,49]. In response to consumer demand, the food processors produced a range of new products. These included food with increased polyunsaturated fats, and low and reduced fat foods, reduced sugar foods, and foods with high fibre levels. At the end of the century, attention is being increasingly focused on food which can confer specific health benefits, so-called functional foods, whose further development may help the population to attain even greater health in the twenty-first century[41].

Plus la change....

'A population beset by a range of diseases, apparently caused or exacerbated by dietary factors, but whose aetiologies are poorly understood. Consumers concerned about the safety of the food they eat.'

Although the diseases and the public anxieties may have changed, these statements held true for the UK in both 1900 and 1999. The population in 1900 was smitten by deficiency and infectious diseases; by 1999, it was afflicted by chronic diseases, by cancers, heart disease and diabetes and attendant conditions. In 1900, the population was concerned about the effects of adulteration, and the use of potentially harmful additives.

By 1999, the concerns were manifold, additives were still an issue, added to which were concerns about issues such as the use of genetically modified food species, the presence of chemical residues from farming or processing, the possible presence of pathogens and allergens, and the ethical and environmental implications of a food-chain which linked ever more efficient production with increasingly centralised and standardised processing systems. Despite these parallels, there have been enormous improvements in the general health, well-being and life expectancy of the majority of the population, and developments in food processing have contributed substantially to these improvements.

References

1   Mathias P. *Retailing Revolution*. London: Longmans, 1967
2   Fellows PJ. *Food Processing Technology, Principles and Practice*. Chichester: Ellis Horwood, 1988
3   Anderson K. Other preservation methods. In: Arthey D, Dennis C (Eds) *Vegetable Processing*. London: Blackie, 1991; 154–85
4   Drummond JC, Wilbraham A. *The Englishman's Food*. London: Jonathan Cape, 1957
5   Hersom A. Thermal processing. In: Arthey D, Dennis C (Eds) *Vegetable Processing*. London: Blackie, 1991; 69–101
6   Burrows G. Production of thermally processed and frozen fruit. In: Arthey D, Ashurst PR (Eds) *Fruit Processing*. London: Blackie, 1996; 135–64
7   Holdsworth SD. *Aseptic Processing and Packaging of Food Products*. London: Elsevier, 1992
8   Bettison J. Packaging. In: Arthey D, Dennis C (Eds) *Vegetable Processing*. London: Blackie, 1991; 186–229
9   Reid D. Freezing. In: Arthey D, Dennis C (Eds) *Vegetable Processing*. London: Blackie, 1991; 102–22
10 Veerkamp CH. Chilling, freezing and thawing. In: Mead GC (Ed) *Processing of Poultry*. London: Elsevier, 1989; 103–25
11 Brown MH, Gould GW. Processing. In: Dennis C, Stringer M (Eds) *Chilled Foods, A Comprehensive Guide*. Chichester: Ellis Horwood, 1992; 112–46
12 Beattie B, Wade N. Storage, ripening and handling of fruit. In: Arthey D, Ashurst PR (Eds) *Fruit Processing*. London: Blackie, 1996; 40–69
13 Brimelow C, Vadehra D. Chilling. In: Arthey D, Dennis C (Eds) *Vegetable Processing*. London: Blackie, 1991; 123–53
14 Young M. The cold storage chain. In: Dellino CVJ (Ed) *Cold and Chilled Storage Technology*, 2nd edn. London: Blackie, 1997; 1–52
15 Day BFP. Chilled food packaging. In: Dennis C, Stringer M (Eds) *Chilled Foods, A Comprehensive Guide*. Chichester: Ellis Horwood, 1992; 147–63
16 World Health Organization. *High Dose Irradiation of Food Irradiated with Doses above 10 kGy*. WHO Technical Report, Series No. 890. Report of a joint FAO/IAEA/WHO Study Group (September 1997). Geneva: WHO, 1999
17 Kaferstein FK, Moy GG. Public health aspects of food irradiation. *J Public Health Policy* 1993; **14**: 149–63
18 Government Statistical Service. *Standard of Living*, available at http://www.statistics.gov.uk/stats/ukinfigs/stand.htm (accessed on 28 July 1999)
19 Kent NL, Evers, AD. *Technology of Cereals*, 4th edn. Oxford: Pergamon, 1994
20 Grandison AS, Lewis MJ (Eds) *Separation Processes in the Food and Biotechnology Industries, Principles and Applications*. Cambridge: Woodhead, 1996
21 Ledward DA, Johnston DE, Earnshaw RG, Hasting APM (Eds) *High Pressure Processing of Foods*. Nottingham: University Press, 1995

22 Singh RP, Oliveira AR (Eds) *Minimal Processing of Foods and Process Optimisation*, Boca Raton: CRC, 1994

23 Earle MD. Innovation in the food industry. *Trends Food Sci Technol* 1997; **8**: 166–75

24 Keuning R. Food ingredients for the 90s. In: Birch GG, Campbell-Platt G, Lindley MG (Eds) *Food for the 90s*. Barking: Elsevier, 1990; 115–33

25 Georgala DL. Modern food processing. In: Cottrell R (Ed) *Food Processing*. Carnforth: Parthenon, 1987; 15–38

26 Artz WE, Hansen, SL. Other fat substitutes. In: Akoh CC, Swanson BG (Eds) *Carbohydrate Polyesters as Fat Substitutes*. New York: Marcel Dekker, 1994; 197–236

27 Gould WA. *Fundamentals of Food Processing and Technology*. Timonium: CTI, 1997

28 Anon. Sixty years of food history, *Food Processing* 1991; **60**: 22–98

29 Jowitt R (Ed) *Hygienic Design and Operation of a Food Plant*. Chichester: Ellis Horwood, 1980

30 Anon. *Food and Drink, Good Manufacturing Practice, A Guide to its Responsible Management*, 4th edn. London: Institute of Food Science and Technology, 1998

31 International Commission on Microbiological Specifications for Foods (ICMSF). *Application of the Hazard Analysis Critical Control Point (HACCP) System to ensure Microbiological Safety and Quality*. Oxford: Blackwell, 1988

32 Mortimer S, Wallace C. *HACCP – A Practical Approach*. London: Chapman & Hall, 1994

33 Kent NL. *Technology of Cereals*. Oxford: Pergamon, 1970

34 McDermott, EE. The properties of commercial glutens, *Cereal Foods World* 1985; **30**: 169–71

35 Harding F. Processed milk. In: Harding OF (Ed) *Milk Quality*. London: Blackie, 1995; 112–32

36 Varnam AH, Sutherland JP. *Milk and Milk Products. Technology, Chemistry and Microbiology*. London: Chapman & Hall, 1994

37 Mandigo RW, Eilert SJ. Strategies for reduced-fat processed meats. In: Hafs HD, Zimbelman RG (Eds) *Low-fat Meats, Design Strategies and Human Implications*. San Diego: Academic, 1994; 145–66

38 Baker RC, Bruce CA. Further processing of poultry. In: Mead GC (Ed) *Processing of Poultry*. London: Elsevier, 1989; 251–82

39 Huffman DL, Cordray JC. Formulations for restructured red meat products. In: Pearson AM, Dutson TR (Eds) *Advances in Meat Research, vol 3, Restructured Meat and Poultry Products*. New York: Avi, 1987; 383–403

40 Hallikainen MA, Uusitupa MIJ. Effects of 2 low-fat stanol ester-containing margarines on serum cholesterol concentrations as part of a low-fat diet in hypercholesterolemic subjects. *Am J Clin Nutr* 1999; **69**: 403–10

41 Sadler MJ, Saltmarsh M (Eds). *Functional Foods, the Consumer, the Products, the Evidence*. Cambridge: Royal Society of Chemistry, 1998

42 Rowntree, BS. *Poverty, A Study of Town Life*, 1922 edn. New York: Howard Fertig, 1971

43 Anon. Food processing, a nutritional perspective. In: Cottrell R (Ed) *Food Processing*. Carnforth: Parthenon, 1987; 189–224

44 Department of Health and Social Security. *Diet and Coronary Heart Disease*. Report on health and social subjects, 7. London: HMSO, 1974

45 Department of Health and Social Security. *Diet and Cardiovascular Disease*. London: HMSO, 1984

46 Department of Health. *Nutritional Aspects of Cardiovascular Disease*. Report of the Cardiovascular Review Group of the Committee on Medical Aspects of Food Policy. Report on health and social subjects 46. London: HMSO, 1994

47 Department of Health. *Nutritional Aspects of the Development of Cancer*. Report of the Working Group on Diet and Cancer of the Committee on Medical Aspects of Food Policy. Report on health and social subjects 48. London: HMSO, 1998

48 Department of Health. *Dietary Reference Values for Food Energy and Nutrients in the United Kingdom*. Report on health and social subjects, 41. Committee on Medical Aspects of Food Policy. London: HMSO, 1991

49 Department of Health. *The Health of the Nation, A Strategy for Health in England*. London: HMSO, 1992

Nutrient requirements and optimisation of intakes

Judith Buttriss

British Nutrition Foundation, London, UK

In 1991, dietary reference values were published in the UK. These refer to nutrients and provide the basis for dietary advice. To complement this, practical food-based guidance on how to plan a healthy and balanced diet has been developed. Interest continues in how best to establish guidance which helps individuals modify their diets so as to better match the dietary targets established as a means of promoting health and avoiding disease.

Furthermore, in recent years, interest has grown in the potential to optimise nutrition and so promote health and well-being, rather than just avoiding deficiency. This has been accompanied by an awareness that many foods, particularly plant foods, contain substances that may have health promoting properties but are not, as yet, regarded as conventional nutrients.

It has been recognised for some time that, for health and the normal functioning of the body, humans need to consume foods and drinks that are sources of energy (calories) and which together provide protein and contain a specific range of vitamins, minerals and trace elements. However, awareness is now growing of the provision by foods, especially plant foods, of a wide variety of substances that are yet to be recognised as nutrients as such, but which may confer health-promoting properties. These phytochemicals are represented in nature by various groups of structures that together include 3000–4000 individual compounds, and which possess a number of different properties. For example, they may have antioxidant characteristics which are believed to allow them to protect the body against the harmful effects of products produced as a result of oxidation. In the past 10 years, there has been considerable growth in research interest in optimal nutrition, which has developed from a focus on nutrient protection in relation to free radical induced cellular damage. This rapidly growing body of research is currently the focus of a British Nutrition Foundation task force, due to report in 2001.

An optimal diet has been defined as one that maximises health and longevity and, therefore, prevents nutrient deficiencies, reduces risks of diet-related chronic diseases, and is composed of foods that are safe and palatable[1]. Throughout the course of human history, societies have

Correspondence to:
Dr Judith Buttriss, Science Director, British Nutrition Foundation, High Holborn House, 52–54 High Holborn, London WC1V 6RQ, UK

© The British Council 2000

developed a considerable range of dietary patterns that took advantage of the food plants and animals available to them, as a result of local climate, geography and trade. It follows that the diets of those communities that survived must have provided sufficient energy and nutrients to support growth and reproduction, but whether they adequately promoted adult health is more difficult to determine. Evidence of the sharp increases in human life expectancy observed in this century suggests this to have been unlikely[1].

Requirements for a specific nutrient differ from one individual to another. In particular, they vary with age, gender and life-stage (*e.g.* pregnancy, lactation). Furthermore, the composition and nature of the diet as a whole may affect the efficiency with which nutrients are absorbed and/or utilised[2].

Classically, an individual's requirement for a nutrient has been the amount required to prevent clinical signs of deficiency. Whilst this remains an important facet of the process that is undertaken in the definition of the nutrient needs of populations, it is now acknowledged that allowance needs to be made for individual variation and for losses of the nutrient that might occur during storage or processing the particular foods that make a major contribution to its intake. It has also been suggested that levels of intake considerably higher than those that arise as a result of the above considerations, may have particular beneficial or therapeutic effects. However, equally, it is acknowledged that some nutrients can be toxic if consumed in large quantities, for example selenium[2].

Dietary Reference Values – what are they?

In the UK, the most recent published review of advice on dietary intakes of energy and nutrients is contained in *Dietary Reference Values for Food Energy and Nutrients*, which is a report from the Committee on Medical Aspects of Food Policy (COMA), an advisory group to Government[2]. This report broke new ground in that, instead of publishing single figures for the vitamin and mineral needs of each population sub-group, it published a range of figures, known as Dietary Reference Values. A similar approach has subsequently been adopted in North America[3]. This range is based on the Estimated Average Requirement (EAR) for the population group in question, and incorporates the Reference Nutrient Intake (RNI), calculated to meet the needs of 97.5% of the population sub-group to which it relates, and the Lower Reference Nutrient Intake (LRNI), calculated to be sufficient for only 2.5% of the population sub-group[2]. In practice, the RNI, which replaces the old Recommended Daily (or dietary) Amount (RDA) is used

Table 1 Reference Nutrient Intakes for vitamins

Age	Thiamin mg/day	Riboflavin mg/day	Niacin (nicotinic acid equivalent) mg/day	Vitamin B6 # mg/day	Vitamin B12 µg/day	Folate µg/day	Vitamin C mg/d	Vitamin A µg/day	Vitamin D µg/day
0–3 months	0.2	0.4	3	0.2	0.3	50	25	350	8.5
4–6 months	0.2	0.4	3	0.2	0.3	50	25	350	8.5
7–9 months	0.2	0.4	4	0.3	0.4	50	25	350	7
10–12 months	0.3	0.4	5	0.4	0.4	50	25	350	7
1–3 years	0.5	0.6	8	0.7	0.5	70	30	400	7
4–6 years	0.7	0.8	11	0.9	0.8	100	30	500	–
7–10 years	0.7	1.0	12	1.0	1.0	150	30	500	–
Males									
11–14 years	0.9	1.2	15	1.2	1.2	200	35	600	–
15–18 years	1.1	1.3	18	1.5	1.5	200	40	700	–
19–50 years	1.0	1.3	17	1.4	1.5	200	40	700	–
50+ years	0.9	1.3	16	1.4	1.5	200	40	700	**
Females									
11–14 years	0.7	1.1	12	1.0	1.2	200	35	600	–
15–18 years	0.8	1.1	14	1.2	1.5	200	40	600	–
19–50 years	0.8	1.1	13	1.2	1.5	200	40	600	–
50+ years	0.8	1.1	12	1.2	1.5	200	40	600	–
Pregnancy	+0.1***	+0.3	*	*	*	+100	+10	+100	10
Lactation									
0–4 months	+0.2	+0.5	+2	*	+0.5	+60	+30	+350	10
4+ months	+0.2	+0.5	+2	*	+0.5	+60	+30	+350	10

*No increment; **after age 65 years the RNI is 10 µg/day for men and women; ***for last trimester only; #based on protein providing 14.7% of EAR for energy.
Data from Department of Health[2]; crown copyright reproduced with the permission of the Controller of Her Majesty's Stationery Office.

as a point of reference against which to assess the average intakes of subgroups of the population and the LRNI is used to assess the suitability of intakes that fall at the lower end of the spectrum. However, it is important to recognise that all these values apply to **populations,** and not to the needs of **individuals.** They are yardsticks to be used in determining the adequacy of the diets of **groups** of people. However, some assumptions can be made, which err on the side of caution and which allow the values to be used in the assessment of individual patients' diets.

1 If an individual is routinely consuming the RNI for a particular nutrient, it can be assumed that his or her diet provides adequate amounts (or more than adequate amounts) of that nutrient. However, if intake is regularly below the RNI, it cannot necessarily be assumed that the diet is inadequate as that person may have a lower requirement than average for that particular nutrient.

2   If an individual is consistently consuming less than the LRNI for a nutrient, it can be assumed that his or her diet is deficient in that particular nutrient, although this does not imply that the person is clinically ill.

3   The DRVs refer to the needs of healthy people and it can not be assumed that the needs of those who are ill are identical. In some instances, their individual needs may be greater for some nutrients.

Reference values exist for energy, fat, non-starch polysaccharides (dietary fibre), sugars, starch, protein, vitamin A, thiamin, riboflavin, niacin (and tryptophan), vitamin B6, vitamin B12, folate, vitamin C, vitamin D, calcium, magnesium, phosphorus, sodium, potassium, chloride, iron, zinc, copper, selenium, and iodine[2]. Reference Nutrient Intakes (RNIs) for vitamins and minerals are shown in Tables 1 and 2, respectively.

Although, the RNIs should not be regarded as targets to be above, in most cases, if the RNI is exceeded 2–3-fold as a result of a high dietary

Table 2 Reference Nutrient Intakes for minerals

Age	Calcium mg/day	Phosphorus[a] mg/day	Magnesium mg/day	Sodium[b] mg/day	Potassium[c] mg/day	Chloride[d] mg/day	Iron mg/day	Zinc mg/day	Copper mg/day	Selenium µg/d	Iodine µg/d
0–3 months	525	400	55	210	800	320	1.7	4.0	0.2	10	50
4–6 months	525	400	60	280	850	400	4.3	4.0	0.3	13	60
7–9 months	525	400	75	320	700	500	7.8	5.0	0.3	10	60
10–12 months	525	400	80	350	700	500	7.8	5.0	0.3	10	60
1–3 years	350	270	85	500	800	800	6.9	5.0	0.4	15	70
4–6 years	450	350	120	700	1100	1100	6.1	6.5	0.6	20	100
7–10 years	550	450	200	1200	2000	1800	8.7	7.0	0.7	30	110
Males											
11–14 years	1000	775	280	1600	3100	2500	11.3	9.0	0.8	45	130
15–18 years	1000	775	300	1600	3500	2500	11.3	9.5	1.0	70	140
19–50 years	700	550	300	1600	3500	2500	8.7	9.5	1.2	75	140
50+ years	700	550	300	1600	3500	2500	8.7	9.5	1.2	75	140
Females											
11–14 years	800	625	280	1600	3100	2500	14.8[e]	9.0	0.8	45	130
15–18 years	800	625	300	1600	3500	2500	14.8[e]	7.0	1.0	60	140
19–50 years	700	550	270	1600	3500	2500	14.8[e]	7.0	1.2	60	140
50+ years	700	550	270	1600	3500	2500	8.7	7.0	1.2	60	140
Pregnancy	*	*	*	*	*	*	*	*	*	*	*
Lactation											
0–4 months	+550	+440	+50	*	*	*	*	+6.0	+0.3	+15	*
4+ months	+550	+440	+50	*	*	*	*	+2.5	+0.3	+15	*

*No increment; [a]phosphorus RNI is set equal to calcium in molar terms; [b]1 mmol sodium = 23 mg; [c]1 mmol potassium = 39 mg; [d]corresponds to sodium 1 mmol = 35.5 mg; [e]insufficient for women with high menstrual losses where the most practical way of meeting iron requirements is to take iron supplements.
Data from Department of Health[2]; crown copyright reproduced with the permission of the Controller of Her Majesty's Stationery Office.

Table 3 Estimated Average Requirements (EARs) for energy

Age	EARs MJ/day (kcal/day)	
	Males	Females
0–3 months	2.28 (545)	2.16 (515)
4–6 months	2.89 (690)	2.69 (645)
7–9 months	3.44 (825)	3.20 (765)
10–12 months	3.85 (920)	3.61 (865)
1–3 years	5.15 (1230)	4.86 (1165)
4–6 years	7.16 (1715)	6.46 (1545)
7–10 years	8.24 (1970)	7.28 (1740)
11–14 years	9.27 (2220)	7.92 (1845)
15–18 years	11.51 (2755)	8.83 (2110)
19–50 years	10.60 (2550)	8.10 (1940)
51–59 years	10.60 (2550)	8.00 (1990)
60–64 years	9.93 (2380)	7.99 (1900)
65–74 years	9.71 (2330)	7.96 (1900)
75+ years	8.77 (2100)	7.61 (1810)
Pregnancy		+0.80* (200)
Lactation		
1 month		+1.90 (450)
2 months		+2.20 (530)
3 months		+2.40 (570)
4–6 months (Group 1)		+2.00 (480)
4–6 months (Group 2)		+2.40 (570)
> 6 months (Group 1)		+1.00 (240)
> 6 months (Group 2)		+2.30 (550)

*Last trimester only.
Data from Department of Health[2]; crown copyright reproduced with the permission of the Controller of Her Majesty's Stationery Office.

intake, this will not pose a problem for most people. However, there are exceptions to this, *e.g.* sodium. The RNI for sodium is 1.6 g/day, which is equivalent to about 4 g NaCl/day. This amount is estimated to meet most people's needs for sodium and yet the current average intake is about 9 g NaCl/day. In 1994, COMA recommended a decrease to 6 g/day, a reduction of about a third. Achieving this specific recommendation, alongside all the others that exist, can be particularly difficult.

Only Estimated Average Requirements (EARs) exist for energy (calories) (Table 3) because it is important that individuals match their energy intake to their requirement in order to avoid losing or gaining weight; for most other nutrients there is a wide range of tolerance[2]. Having said this, an increasing number of individuals are consuming more energy than they need.

Energy intakes have been falling over a number of years, presumably as a result of the lower energy requirements associated with a more sedentary life-style, and are currently below the EAR. Despite this, the proportion of men and women who are overweight reached 62% and

Table 4 Dietary Reference Values for fat and carbohydrate for adults as a percentage of daily total energy intake (percentage of food energy)

	Individual minimum	Population average	Individual maximum
Saturated fatty acids		10 (11)	
Cis-polyunsaturated fatty acids		6 (6.5)	10
n-3	0.2		
n-6	1.0		
Cis-mono-unsaturated fatty acids		12 (13)	
Trans fatty acids		2 (2)	
Total fatty acids		30 (32.5)	
TOTAL FAT		33 (35)	
Non-milk extrinsic sugars	0	10 (11)	
Intrinsic and milk sugars and starch		37 (39)	
TOTAL CARBOHYDRATE		47 (50)	
NON-STARCH POLYSACCHARIDE (g/day)	12	18	24

The average percentage contribution to total energy does not total 100% because figures for protein and alcohol are excluded. Protein intakes average 15% of total energy which is above the RNI. It is recognised that many individuals will derive some energy from alcohol, and this has been assumed to average 5% approximating to current intakes. However, the Panel allowed that some groups might not drink alcohol and that, for some purposes, nutrient intakes as a proportion of food energy (without alcohol) might be useful. Therefore, average figures are given as percentages both of total energy and, in brackets, of food energy.
Data from Department of Health[2]; crown copyright reproduced with the permission of the Controller of Her Majesty's Stationery Office.

53%, respectively, in 1997, having been 39% and 32%, respectively, in 1980[3,5]. Included within this figure is a prevalence of obesity of 17% in men and 20% in women[4]. By contrast, in 1980, 6% of men and 8% of women were obese[5]. This trend is an indication of an increasing public health problem that needs urgent attention[6].

For fat, sugars and starches, because there is no absolute requirement for any of these individually, it was not possible to derive a range of reference figures. Instead, the COMA Panel[2] made pragmatic judgements based on the changes from current intakes that would be expected to result in specific changes in physiological and/or health outcomes, particularly in relation to coronary heart disease (see Table 4). Almost 10 years later, a reduction in deaths from coronary heart disease and cancer remain national targets in the UK[7].

Since publication of the Dietary Reference Values (DRV) report, COMA has advised the need to adjust the ratio of n-3 and n-6 fatty acids in the diet in favour of the former[8]. COMA suggests this could be achieved by increasing fish consumption to two servings per week, one of which is oil-rich fish, which might be expected to achieve a weekly

Table 5 Safe intakes for nutrients for which insufficient information exists to set DRVs

Nutrient			Safe intakes
Vitamins			
	Pantothenic acid		
		Adults	3–7 mg/day
		Infants	1.7 mg/day
	Biotin		10–200 µg/day
	Vitamin E		
		Men	Above 4 mg/day
		Women	Above 3 mg/day
		Infants	0.4 mg/g polyunsaturated fatty acids
	Vitamin K		
		Adults	1 µg/kg/day
		Infants	10 µg/day
Minerals			
	Manganese		
		Adults	1.4 mg (26 µmol)/day
		Infants and children	16 µg (0.3 µmol)/day
	Molybdenum		
		Adults	50– 400 µg/day
		Infants, children and adolescents	0.5–1.5 µg/kg/day
	Chromium		
		Adults	25 µg (0.5 µmol)/day
		Children and adolescents	0.1–1.0 µg (2–20 µmol)/kg/day
	Fluoride (for infants only)		0.05 mg (3 µmol)/kg/day

Data from Department of Health[2]; crown copyright reproduced with the permission of the Controller of Her Majesty's Stationery Office.

intake of very long chain n–3 fatty acids of 1.5 g/week. More details are available in a BNF publication on this subject[9].

Insufficient evidence was considered to be available to set DRVs for pantothenic acid, biotin, vitamin E, vitamin K, molybdenum, manganese, chromium and fluoride; instead, safe intakes were published (Table 5). A safe intake is a range of intakes sufficient to meet the needs of almost all individuals, but not high enough to cause undesirable effects[2].

All of the DVRs are intended to be met, on average, over a period of days, rather than on a single day, and can be used in many ways. They are used by dietitians as a yardstick in the assessment of the adequacy of the diets of individuals. But expertise and caution is needed when using the values for this purpose. DRVs give a general guide to whether or not an individual's diet is likely to be nutritionally adequate. However, it is very difficult, even with considerable experience, to get a precise estimate of an individual's food intake and it is not possible to accurately predict a person's requirement for nutrients.

The values are also used to interpret the dietary data collected in national surveys, to establish whether the national diet is adequate in

Table 6 Proportion of subjects in the survey of British adults, by age, whose intakes fell below the LRNI values for various nutrients

Nutrient	Age 16–18 years		Age 19–50 years		Age 51–64 years	
	LRNI	%	LRNI	%	LRNI	%
Calcium (mg)	480	27	400	10	400	5
Iron (mg)	8	33	8	26	8	1
Magnesium (mg)	190	39	150	13	150	9
Potassium (mg)	2000	30	2000	27	2000	23
Zinc (mg)	4	6	4	4	4	2
Iodine (μg)	70	4	70	3	70	3
Vitamin A (μg)	250	7	250	3	250	2
Riboflavin (mg)	0.8	9	0.8	8	0.8	5
Vitamin C (mg)	10	0	10	1	10	1
Folate (μg)	100	4	100	4	100	3
Vitamin B12 (μg)	1.0	4	1.0	1	1.0	1

Data taken from Ministry of Agriculture, Fisheries and Food[10].

respect to the provision of various nutrients for a range of age groups. Data from the survey of British adults can be used to demonstrate this point[10]. Table 6 shows the LRNI values for a number of vitamins and minerals measured in the survey. Using these figures, the survey reveals that a considerable proportion of women, especially the youngest age group, had intakes of micronutrients that can be considered inadequate. The proportion of men achieving low intakes was considerably lower, probably because men tend to eat more food in general and so are more likely to achieve micronutrient needs.

Similarly, data from the recently published survey of people over the age of 65 years shows that a substantial proportion have intakes of some micronutrients that fall below the LRNI[11]. This large national survey

Table 7 Average intakes of a range of vitamins, expressed as %RNI, in subjects aged over 65 years.

	Free-living		Living in institutions	
	Men	Women	Men	Women
Vitamin A	168	161	151	160
Thiamin	166	148	149	142
Riboflavin	134	130	138	147
Niacin	200	206	170	194
Vitamin B6	168	160	154	158
Vitamin B12	404	298	329	304
Folate	135	103	117	99
Vitamin C	167	152	124	119
Vitamin D	41	29	38	33

Data from Finch et al[11].

Table 8 Average intakes of a range of minerals, expressed as %RNI, in subjects aged over 65 years

	Free-living		Living in institutions	
	Men	Women	Men	Women
Iron	127	99	111	94
Calcium	119	99	136	123
Phosphorus	225	180	218	192
Magnesium	85	73	72	70
Sodium	168	128	170	138
Potassium	78	63	69	61
Zinc	93	98	88	101
Iodine	134	106	138	125

Data from Finch et al[11].

included subjects living in their own homes as well as people living in various types of residential institutions. Tables 7 and 8 show the average intakes of a range of vitamins and minerals as a proportion of the RNIs, the amounts believed to cover the needs of 97.5% of the population group to which they apply. Vitamin D intakes were particularly low and this can become clinically important if mobility and exposure to sunlight are reduced. The average folate intake (in institutionalised women) was close to the RNI. For the minerals (Table 8), average intakes of potassium and magnesium were well below the RNIs, zinc was close to the RNI and the average iron intakes of both groups of women were also close to the RNI, as were average calcium intakes in free-living women.

It is also interesting to note that, with one or two exceptions, the intakes of vitamins and minerals in the institutionalised participants were lower than those of free-living participants (though they were generally above the RNI). However, for several nutrients, namely calcium, riboflavin and vitamin A, those in institutions fared better. These three nutrients are provided by milk, and milk intake was higher in institutions than in the free-living subjects.

Although the average intakes of most nutrients were well above the RNI, a small proportion of subjects had intakes below the LRNI (the quantity sufficient for only 2.5% of the population). There is no LRNI for vitamin D; however, virtually all the subjects had intakes below the RNI (Table 9). A substantial proportion of subjects had intakes of magnesium and potassium below the LRNI (Table 10). The data in Tables 7–10 represent the picture for the group as a whole, but for those nutrients marked with an asterisk, there was evidence that the situation worsened in the older age groups.

Use of the dietary reference values in this way is immensely valuable in determining public health nutrition issues that need to be tackled within a particular population sub-group.

Table 9 Proportion of subjects over 65 years with vitamin intakes from food below the LRNI (%)

	Free-living		Living in institutions	
	Men	Women	Men	Women
Vitamin A	5	4	1	1
Thiamin	> 0.5	> 0.5	1	> 0.5
Riboflavin*	5	10	3	3
Niacin	> 0.5	> 0.5	> 0.5	> 0.5
Vitamin B6*	2	3	1	2
Vitamin B12	> 0.5	1	nil	nil
Folate*	1	6	4	5
Vitamin C*	2	2	1	nil
Vitamin D	97% below RNI		99% below RNI	

*Increases with age.
Data from Finch et al[11].

Bioavailability

Although a particular food may provide considerable amounts of a particular nutrient, it does not always follow that the nutrient will be available for absorption and utilisation. The efficiency with which a nutrient is used by the body is known as its bioavailability. For some nutrients (amino acids, fatty acids and other lipids, starch and sugar), bioavailability is high (90% or more). But for others, especially some minerals, bioavailability is low and poorly predicted. This is an important concept that needs to be taken into account in the calculation of DRVs for nutrients, especially those with variable bioavailabilities[2]. For example, the absorption of iron present in the form of haem iron (*e.g.* as in meat) is considerably greater than the absorption of iron, present as ferric iron,

Table 10 Proportion of subjects over 65 years with mineral intakes from food below the LRNI (%)

	Free-living		Living in institutions	
	Men	Women	Men	Women
Iron*	1	6	5	6
Calcium	5	9	1	> 0.5
Magnesium*	21	23	39	22
Sodium	nil	nil	nil	nil
Potassium*	17	39	28	42
Zinc*	8	5	13	4
Iodine	2	6	1	1

*Increases with age.
Data from Finch et al[11].

from cereals and vegetables (non-haem iron). Similarly, calcium is relatively well absorbed from milk and some vegetables, *e.g.* broccoli, but very poorly absorbed from spinach. Although spinach contains plenty of calcium, this is very poorly absorbed because it remains bound within the plant's structure.

Factors that influence bioavailability include:

1   The chemical form of the nutrient, *e.g.* haem iron is better utilised than inorganic iron

2   Antagonistic ligands, *e.g.* phosphates, phytate, polyphenols, oxalates, factors in wheat bran. These bind the nutrient and reduce its availability for absorption.

3   Facilitatory ligands, *e.g.* ascorbic acid (aids iron absorption), some sugars, amino acids, carboxylic acids. These improve absorption.

4   Competitive interaction, *e.g.* copper versus iron versus zinc versus cadmium.

5   Bacterial fermentation in the colon can influence availability of products resulting from the fermentation of dietary fibre.

6   Changes in mucosal structure and function.

7   Anabolic requirement, *e.g.* utilisation (and proportional absorption) of some nutrients is increased in response to growth, pregnancy or lactation.

8   Systemic factors, such as infection, stress and catabolism.

9   Homeostatic setting for nutrient determined by previous (recent) dietary supply, *e.g.* iron.

Food labelling

Reference values for selected vitamins and minerals are increasingly used on food labels. In this context, they are described as RDAs and the quantities to which they are refer are usually different to the RNIs established in the UK. This is because the RDAs used in food labelling are part of European food legislation and reflect the variation in opinion across Europe as to the precise value to use. Also, there is only one figure for each nutrient, derived from figures for adults, rather than a range of figures that vary with age, sex and physiological status. The labelling RDAs, like the RNIs, are estimates of the amounts sufficient to meet the needs of groups rather than individuals. To aid consumers' understanding of how a particular food might fit into a balanced diet, the Institute of

Grocery Distribution has published guidelines derived from the DRVs. These concern fat and energy (calorie) intake and recommend the use on packaging of bench marks against which the fat or energy content per serving of a food can be compared[12].

Optimising nutritional status

The traditional view has been that once intake is sufficient to ensure that an individual is not deficient in a particular nutrient and that sufficient stores exist to ward off any transient increase in demand, then there is little point in increasing intake of the nutrient any further. This view is being challenged in a number of ways. One of the best known examples is that of folate. There is now firm evidence that the risk of a woman having a baby affected by spina bifida or other form of neural tube defect (NTD) is influenced by her folate/folic acid intake[13,14]. Women who have babies affected by NTDs are not necessarily folate deficient, using traditional criteria, but the higher their folate status is, within the physiological range, the less likely they are to have an NTD affected baby[15]. For this reason, folic acid supplements (400 µg/day) are now recommended for all women of childbearing age[16]; yet the RNI is only 200 µg.

Similarly, there is growing evidence that plasma levels of homocysteine, a predictor of risk for cardiovascular disease[17,18], can be reduced by intakes of folic acid that are just a little above current RNIs[19,20]. The evidence does not imply the need for megadoses in either example, the effects were seen at intakes of folate at the top of the range associated with a healthy diet.

Intense attention is being focused on the possible beneficial effects of a whole host of substances found in plants. It is now well recognised that a high consumption of fruit and vegetables is protective against conditions such as heart disease and some forms of cancer[8,21]. However, the nature of the protective effect is yet to be fully elucidated. Although some of the substances present in such foods are already recognised as nutrients, *e.g.* vitamins C and E, carotenoids and minerals such as potassium, it may well be that in the future other factors such as specific flavonoids, *e.g.* phytoestrogens, flavanols and flavones, will be added to the list of recognised 'nutrients'.

Translation of nutrient requirements into dietary guidelines

There is general agreement that there is a need to pop pop recommendations on nutrient intake (e.g. 35% energy from fat) into food-based dietary guidelines. The recent FAO/WHO[22] report on the preparation of food-based dietary guidelines identifies two key principles that should apply. The first is that dietary guidelines should be based on an existing public health problem rather than a difference between prevailing nutrient intake and some recommended ideal nutrient intake. The second principle is that food-based dietary guidelines should be developed in a cultural context, which implies that they should be derived from prevailing patterns of food intake rather than some epidemiologically based ideal. Within these guiding principles, the translation of nutrient recommendations into food-based dietary guidelines should be flexible to accommodate different levels of knowledge of prevailing food and nutrient intakes of the target group.

In Britain, expert scientific advice has been pop popd into eight general dietary guidelines: (i) enjoy your food; (ii) eat a variety of different foods; (iii) eat the right amount to be a healthy weight; (iv) eat plenty of foods rich in starch and fibre; (v) eat plenty of fruit and vegetables; (vi) do not eat too many foods that contain a lot of fat; (vii) do not have sugary foods and drinks too often; and (viii) if you drink alcohol, drink sensibly.

These form the core of the population-targeted dietary advice in the UK and are supported by a food selection guide, depicting a plate, showing the types and proportions of foods needed for a balanced and healthy diet[23]. The categories represented on the 'plate' used as the basis of the food selection guide are: fruit and vegetables (33%); bread, other cereals and potatoes (33%); milk and dairy foods (15%); meat, fish and alternatives (12%); foods containing fat, foods containing sugar (8%).

To help set dietary guidelines, data from national surveys such as the Dietary and Nutritional Survey of British Adults[12,24] can be used to identify statistically significant differences between sub-groups of the study population that met, or failed to meet, population nutritional goals for intakes of total fat, saturates and dietary fibre.

Using this technique, it was found that several patterns of eating habits, including greater consumption of starchy foods (particularly wholemeal varieties), greater consumption of fruit and the substitution of reduced fat milk for whole milk, were shared by the sub-groups that met each of the nutritional goals targeted in the study[23].

It should be noted that a major problem in examining food intake data to devise food-based dietary guidelines is that of selective under-reporting. Most dietary surveys encounter under-reporting of energy, but we know very little about which foods tend to be under-reported or whether it is frequency of intake or serving size that is under-reported.

The approach recommended by FAO/WHO[22] has been used as the basis for exploring various options for food-based dietary guidelines in Ireland[25]. Four particular approaches have been used to explore the impact of various strategies on the potential to increase the fibre intake of Irish women. The first approach looked at whether it might be possible to get more women to eat a particular food category recognised as being a good source of fibre. The second and third focused on consumers of particular foods and asked whether the frequency of intake could be increased and whether serving size could be increased. The final strategy explored whether, within a given food category, nutrient intake could be increased by switching to a comparable alternative. It became apparent that whereas it might be possible to increase the proportion of women consuming breakfast cereals and pulses, it would not be realistic to expect this to happen with the rest of the foods identified as good sources of fibre, *e.g.* potatoes, because most women were already eating them. However, it was also apparent that it might be feasible to increase the frequency of consumption of fruit and pulses. Also, for bread and breakfast cereals, a change to higher fibre versions might prove acceptable and successful.

Using these strategies, they considered the impact on fibre intake of prevailing patterns compared with three different levels of possible change. Based on their analysis, it is apparent that it would not be feasible to increase fibre intake via potatoes, but achievement of this might be possible by promoting wholemeal bread and high fibre breakfast cereals as appropriate alternatives to lower fibre versions. Other strategies would be to increase daily fruit intake and weekly intake of pulses.

Gibney[25] suggests that this approach can be systematically applied to each nutrient and micronutrient and, through some appropriate modelling, be applied to the diet as a whole. Used in conjunction with other strategies, such as food patterns associated with high and low fibre intakes (as described above), it is more likely that a set of attainable and culturally acceptable guidelines on food intake will be the outcome.

Key points for clinical practice

- A set of dietary reference values exists for energy and nutrients. These relate to the needs of groups of healthy people and are designed to be met, on average, over a period of days.

- They are also of use to dietitians as a yardstick for the assessment of individuals' diets. But experience and caution is required if they are used in this way.

- If an individual is routinely consuming the RNI for a particular nutrient, it can be assumed that his or her diet provides adequate amounts. If an individual is consistently consuming less than the

LRNI, it can be assumed that his or her diet is deficient in that nutrient, although it does not imply the person is clinically ill.

- Although a particular food may provide considerable amounts of a particular nutrient, it does not always follow that the nutrient will be available for absorption and utilisation.

- The traditional view that there is no point in increasing intake of a nutrient above the amount needed to maintain moderate stores or adequate plasma levels is being challenged. One of the best known examples of this is folate.

References

1 Nestle M. Animal *v.* plant foods in human diets and health: is the historical record equivocal? *Proc Nutr Soc* 1999; **58**: 211–8

2 Department of Health. *Dietary Reference Values for Food Energy and Nutrients* Report of the Panel on Dietary Reference Values of the Committee on Medical Aspects of Food Policy. Report on Health and Social Subjects 41. London: HMSO, 1991

3 Institute of Medicine. *Dietary Reference Intakes: Calcium, Phosphorus, Magnesium, Vitamin D and Fluoride.* Washington DC: National Academy Press, 1997

4 Department of Health. *Health Survey for England, Adults Reference Tables '97.* London: Department of Health, 1999; 15–6

5 Knight I. *The Heights and Weights of Adults in Great Britain.* London: HMSO, 1984

6 British Nutrition Foundation. *Obesity: Report of the British Nutrition Foundation Task Force.* Oxford: Blackwell, 1999

7 Department of Health. *Saving Lives: Our Healthier Nation.* London: HMSO, 1999

8 Department of Health. *Nutritional Aspects of Cardiovascular Disease.* Report of the Cardiovascular Review Group, Committee on Medical Aspects of Food Policy. Report on Health and Social Subjects 46. London: HMSO, 1994

9 British Nutrition Foundation. *n-3 Fatty Acids and Health.* London: BNF, 1999

10 Ministry of Agriculture, Fisheries and Food. *The Dietary and Nutritional Survey of British Adults: Further Analysis.* London, HMSO, 1994.

11 Finch S, Doyle W, Lowe C *et al. National Diet and Nutrition Survey: People Aged 65 Years and Older,* vol 1: Report of the diet and nutrition survey. London, The Stationery Office, 1998

12 Institute of Grocery Distribution. *Communication and Labelling Guidelines for Genetically Modified Foods: Conclusions of a Four-year Research Programme.* Watford: IGD, 1997

13 MRC Vitamin Study Group. Prevention of neural tube defects: results of the Medical Research Council Vitamin Study. *Lancet* 1991; **338**: 131–7

14 Wald N. CIBA Foundation Symposium 181. London: Wiley, 1994

15 Daly LE, Kirke PM, Molloy A, Weir DG, Scott JM. Folate levels and neural tube defects: implications for prevention. *JAMA* 1995; **274**: 1698–702

16 Department of Health. *Folic acid and the Prevention of Neural Tube Defects, Report from Expert Advisory Group.* Lancashire: Health Publication Unit, 1992

17 Daly L, Robinson K, Tan, KS, Graham IM. Hyperhomocysteinaemia: a metabolic risk factor for coronary heart disease determined by both genetic and environmental influences? *Q J Med* 1993; **86**: 685–9

18 Wald NJ, Watt HC, Law MR, Weir DG, McPartlin J, Scott JM. Homocysteine and ischaemic heart disease: results of a prospective study with implications regarding prevention. *Arch Intern Med* 1998; **158**: 862–7

19 Schorah CJ, Devitt H, Lucock M, Dowell AC. The responsiveness of plasma homocysteine to small increases in dietary folic acid: a primary care study. *Eur J Clin Nutr* 1998; **52**: 407–11

20 Homocysteine Lowering Trialists Collaboration. Lowering blood homocysteine with a folic acid based supplement: meta-analysis of randomised trials. *BMJ* 1998; **316**: 894–8

21 Department of Health. *Nutritional Aspects of the Development of Cancer.* Report of the Working Group on Diet and Cancer of the Committee on Medical aspects of Food and Nutrition Policy. London: The Stationery Office, 1998

22 FAO/WHO *Preparation of Food Based Dietary Guidelines.* Geneva: WHO, 1998

23 Wearne SJ, Day MJL. Clues for the development of food-based dietary guidelines: how are dietary targets being achieved by UK consumers? *Br J Nutr* 1999; **81**: S119–26

24 Gregory J, Foster K, Tyler H, Wiseman M. *The Dietary and Nutritional Survey of British Adults.* London: HMSO, 1990

25 Gibney MJ. Development of food-based dietary guidelines: a case-study of fibre intake in Irish women. *Br J Nutr* 1999; **81**: S151–2

Adverse reactions and intolerance to foods

T J David

Department of Child Health, University of Manchester, Manchester, UK

Food allergy is a form of adverse reaction to food in which the cause is an immunological response to a food. Common food triggers are eggs, cow's milk, peanuts and fish. Food allergy is most common in young infants, most of whom grow out of the allergy by the age of 5 years. The exception is allergy to peanuts, which is life-long. The term food intolerance does not imply any specific type of mechanism, and is defined as a reproducible adverse reaction to a specific food or food ingredient. Mechanisms for food intolerance comprise immunological reactions (*i.e.* food allergy), enzyme defects, pharmacological effects, irritant effects, and toxic reactions. Despite the popular phobia of food additives and food processing, and the obsession for so-called natural foods, the greatest dangers come from naturally occurring foods and food ingredients.

Over the years, a large number of disorders have been attributed to reactions to foods. The uncritical and over-enthusiastic nature of many claims, plus the anecdotal evidence upon which they were based, have generally discredited the whole subject. The introduction of double-blind provocation tests has placed studies on a more scientific footing, but they are impractical in routine management. The lack of objective and reproducible diagnostic laboratory tests which could eliminate bias has ensured that controversy about food intolerance continues.

After defining the key terms, this review describes immunological followed by non-immunological reactions to foods.

Definitions

Correspondence to:
Prof. T J David, University Department of Child Health, Booth Hall Children's Hospital, Charlestown Road, Blackley, Manchester M9 7AA, UK

The word allergy is frequently misused, and applied indiscriminately to any adverse reaction, regardless of the mechanism.

An **allergic response** is a reproducible adverse reaction to a substance mediated by an immunological response. The substance provoking the reaction may have been ingested, injected, inhaled or merely have come into contact with the skin or mucous membranes.

Food allergy is a form of adverse reaction to food in which the cause is an immunological response to a food.

© The British Council 2000

Food intolerance does not imply any specific type of mechanism, and is simply defined as a reproducible adverse reaction to a specific food or food ingredient.

Food aversion comprises food avoidance, where the subject avoids a food for psychological reasons such as distaste or a desire to lose weight, and psychological intolerance (see below).

Psychological intolerance is an unpleasant bodily reaction caused by emotions associated with the food rather than the food itself. Psychological intolerance will normally be observable when a food is given under open conditions, but will not occur when the food is given in an unrecognisable form. Psychological intolerance may be reproduced by suggesting (falsely) that the food has been administered.

The term anaphylaxis or anaphylactic shock is taken to mean a severe and potentially life-threatening reaction of rapid onset, with circulatory collapse. The term anaphylaxis has also been used to describe any allergic reaction, however mild, that results from specific IgE antibodies, but such usage fails to distinguish between a trivial reaction (*e.g.* a sneeze) from a dangerous event.

Food allergy – immunological reactions to food

Mechanisms of food allergy

Understanding of the mechanisms of food allergy is poor, and in many cases the precise mechanism is obscure.

Sensitisation
Possible factors which contribute to immunological sensitisation leading to food intolerance are listed in Table 1.

Immunological and molecular mechanisms
Despite the gastrointestinal barrier, small amounts of immunologically intact proteins enter the circulation. Normal individuals, although capable of mounting a rapid and potent response against foreign substances, develop tolerance to ingested food antigens[1]. The means by which tolerance develops is poorly understood.

Heat treatment
Heat treatment renders certain (but not all) foods less likely to provoke an allergic reaction in a subject who is allergic[2]. In cow's milk, whey proteins are easily denatured by heat but casein is highly resistant. Heat renders a large number of fruits and vegetables less likely to provoke

Table 1 Possible factors which contribute to sensitisation to foods

Factor	Comments
Genetic predisposition	Food allergy is commonly familial, and commonly co-exists with atopic disease, suggesting the importance of genetic factors
Immaturity of the immune system or the gastrointestinal mucosal barrier in newborn infants	Studies to see if food allergy or atopic disease can be prevented by interventions during pregnancy or lactation are based on the idea that there is a critical period during which sensitisation can occur
Dosage of antigen	It is possible that high dosage leads to the development of tolerance, and low dosage leads to sensitisation. This might explain the development of allergy to traces of foods that reach an infant through mother's breast milk
Certain food antigens are especially likely to lead to sensitisation, for example egg, cow's milk, fish and peanut	We do not know why, for example, peanuts and fish are more capable of inducing allergic reactions than lamb or cauliflower. The molecular acrobatics that make one antigen an allergen and another antigen a non-allergen are not known
A triggering event, for example a viral infection	There is a suggestion that food allergy may develop in a previously non-allergic subject after a viral infection such as infectious mononucleosis (glandular fever)
Alteration in the permeability of the gastrointestinal tract, permitting abnormal antigen access	It is possible that acute viral gastroenteritis may damage the small intestinal mucosa, allowing abnormal absorption of food proteins, leading to sensitisation

adverse reactions in subjects who are intolerant. Thus, for example, it is not uncommon to see children who are allergic to raw potatoes or fresh pineapple, but almost all such children can tolerate cooked potatoes or tinned pineapples[2].

Prevalence of food allergy

Reports of food allergy from individuals or parents of children are notoriously unreliable. It is common for parents to believe that foods are responsible for a variety of childhood symptoms. Double blind provocation tests in children with histories of reactions to food only confirm the story in one-third of all cases[3]. In the case of purely behavioural symptoms, in one study the proportion that could be reproduced under blind conditions was zero[4]. Adults' beliefs about their own symptoms are just as unreliable[5,6].

The parents of 866 children from Finland were asked to provide a detailed history of food allergy, and for certain foods the diagnosis was further investigated by elimination and open challenge at home[7]. Food allergy was reported in 19% by the age of 1 year, 22% by 2 years, 27% by 3 years, and 8% by 6 years. In a prospective study of 480 children in the US up to their third birthday, 16% were reported to have had reactions to fruit or fruit juice and 28% to other food[8]. However, open challenge confirmed reactions in only 12% of the former and 8% of the latter.

Prospective studies indicate that about 2.5% of infants experience allergic reactions to cow's milk[1,9]. Allergic reactions to egg occur in about 1.3% of children[10], and to peanut in about 0.5% of children in the UK and US[1]. The prevalence of food allergy in adults is believed to be less than in children, but a recent national survey in the US suggested that peanut and tree nut allergy together affect 1.3% of adults. If one adds to this the estimated frequency of shellfish allergy (approximately 0.5%) it appears likely that 2% of the adult population in the US is affected by food allergy[1].

Natural history of food allergy

The natural history of food allergy is poorly documented. It is well known that a high proportion of children with food intolerance in the first year of life lose their intolerance in time[11]. The proportion of children to which this happens varies with the food and probably with type of symptoms which are produced. Thus it is common for allergy to cow's milk or egg to spontaneously disappear with time[2,11], whereas peanut allergy is usually life-long. In the North American study referred to above, it was found that the offending food or fruit was back in the diet after only 9 months in half the cases, and virtually all the offending foods were back in the diet by the third birthday[8]. In a population based study from Norway, two-thirds of reactions to foods in children had disappeared within 6 months[12]. A further study of 9 children with very severe adverse reactions to food showed that, despite the severity, 3 were later able to tolerate normal amounts of the offending food and a further 4 became able to tolerate small amounts[13].

In adults with food allergy, the problem is far more likely to be life-long. Nevertheless, some adults do become tolerant to foods to which they were allergic. In one adult follow-up study, approximately one-third of adults were found to lose their allergy after maintaining an elimination diet for 1 year[14].

Clinical features

The clinical features of an allergic reaction include urticaria (nettle rash), angioedema, rhinitis (sneezing, nasal discharge, blocked nose), worsening of pre-existing atopic eczema, asthma (wheezing, coughing, tightness of

Table 2 Cross reaction between foods of different species, and between foods and other antigens

Food item(s)	Cross reactions
Milk from cows, goats, sheep and horses	The marked antigenic similarity between the proteins in the milk of cows, goats, sheep and horses means that almost all subjects who are allergic to cow's milk protein are allergic to the milks of these other animals
Bird eggs	The eggs from turkeys, duck, goose and seagull all contain ovalbumin, ovomucoid and ovotransferrin, the major allergens in hens' eggs
Legumes (beans, peas, soya, lentils, peanuts, liquorice, carob and gum arabic)	Cross-reactivity is uncommon
Seafood	The taxonomic diversity (fish, molluscs, crustaceans) explains why complete cross-reactivity for all seafood is uncommon
Cross reactions between inhaled pollen and ingested food allergens	An example is the association between allergy to birch tree pollen combined with allergy to apple, carrot, celery, potato, orange and tomato

the chest, shortness of breath), vomiting, abdominal pain, diarrhoea, and anaphylactic shock.

Cross reactions

This term refers to: (i) cross-reaction between different food species; and (ii) cross-reactions between foods and non-food items. Most studies of cross-reactivity are based on skin prick and IgE antibody test results which are of little relevance to clinical sensitivity. The position is summarised in Table 2.

Timing of allergic reaction and delayed reactions

Most allergic reactions to foods occur within minutes of ingestion of the food; but sometimes a reaction may be delayed. For example, in cow's milk protein allergy, three types of reaction are recognised[15]. In the 'early skin reaction' group, symptoms begin to develop within 45 min of cow's milk challenge. In the 'early gut reaction' group, symptoms begin to develop between 45 min and 20 h after cow's milk challenge. In the 'late reaction' group, symptoms begin to develop about 20 h after cow's milk protein challenge.

Quantity of food required for allergic reaction

The quantity of food required to produce an allergic reaction varies. Some patients with cow's milk protein allergy, for example, are highly sensitive and develop anaphylaxis after ingestion of less than 1 µg of casein, β-lactoglobulin or α-lactalbumin. In contrast, there are children and adults who only react adversely to 200 ml or more[16]. There is a relationship between the quantity of milk required and the time of onset of symptoms. In one study, the median reaction onset time in those who reacted to 100 ml milk challenges was 2 h, but the median reaction onset time in those who required larger amounts of milk to elicit reactions was 24 h[16].

Other factors required for an allergic reaction to occur

In some individuals, adverse reactions only occur when ingestion of a trigger food is combined with some other factor.

Food-dependant exercise-induced anaphylaxis
In this unusual condition, attacks only occur when the exercise follows within a couple of hours of the ingestion of specific foods such as celery, shellfish, squid, peaches or wheat[2].

Effect of disease activity
It is a common, but poorly understood, observation that children with eczema and food allergy can often tolerate some or all food triggers when the skin disease clears (usually when the child is on holiday in a sunny country).

Drug-dependant food allergy
There are individuals who only react to specific foods while taking a drug. The best recognised examples of this are individuals who only react to foods while taking salicylate (aspirin).

Diagnosis of food allergy

The diagnosis of food allergy is usually made from the history (*see* Table 3), supported by information about the response to the avoidance of specific food triggers. In practice, there are some common diagnostic difficulties.

Lack of simple reliable tests
The skin prick test and the radio-allergosorbent (RAST) blood test both detect specific IgE antibodies to individual antigens. These tests are easy

LIVERPOOL JOHN MOORES UNIVERSITY
LEARNING SERVICES

Table 3 Points to be noted when obtaining a history of reactions to foods

Points from history	Comments
Speed of onset	The quicker the onset of the allergic reaction, the more reliable is the history
Exclude co-incidences	If an individual becomes unwell (*e.g.* starts wheezing) an hour after eating a specific food, the wheezing could be caused by the food, or it could just be a co-incidence. The more times that such a sequence has been observed, the more likely it is that there is a cause and effect relationship
Seek evidence of internal consistency	(1) Have the same symptoms occurred on occasions when the trigger food was not taken? (2) Have there been occasions when the suspect food was taken without there being any adverse effects?
Need to probe a label of 'allergy'	It is common for people to believe they are allergic to something (1) Misdiagnosis based on flimsy evidence such as allergy test results (2) Misinterpretation of sequence of events such as attributing an allergic reaction to sesame seeds coated on a bun; in an infant, such reactions are more likely to be due an allergic reaction to the egg glaze that has been used as an adhesive for the seed coating

to perform, but difficult or impossible to interpret (see Table 4). They still have a place in research studies, but are of little use in clinical practice[2]. The difficulties in interpretation of skin prick tests are summarised in Table 4. Depending upon the criteria used for positivity, there is a fair degree of correlation between RAST test and skin prick test results. Thus the clinical interpretation of RAST test results is subject to most of the same pitfalls as the interpretation of skin prick testing. Additional problems with RAST tests are the cost, and the fact that a very high level of total circulating IgE (*e.g.* in children with severe atopic eczema) may cause a false positive result.

The results of these tests cannot be taken alone, and standard textbooks of allergy acknowledge that 'the proper interpretation of results requires a thorough knowledge of the history and physical findings'. The problems in clinical practice are, for example, whether an individual with symptoms suggestive of food intolerance will benefit from attempts to avoid certain foods or food additives. However, skin prick test results are unreliable predictors of response to such measures.

Skin prick tests and RAST tests mainly detect IgE antibody. However, many adverse reactions to food are not IgE mediated, in which case these tests can be expected to be negative. Taking cow's milk protein intolerance as an example, patients with quick reactions often have positive skin prick tests to cow's milk protein, but those with delayed reactions usually have negative skin prick tests[15].

Table 4 Practical difficulties in the interpretation of skin prick test results

- False positive tests: a positive skin prick test may be present in subjects with no clinical evidence of allergy – sometimes described as 'asymptomatic hypersensitivity' or 'subclinical sensitisation'. Positive results may persist after a child has grown out of a food allergy

- False negative tests: skin prick tests are negative in some subjects with genuine food allergies. False negative results are a special problem in infants and toddlers

- Lack of agreed definition about what constitutes a positive reaction

- Size of the skin reaction depends to some extent on the potency of the extract

- Antihistamines and related drugs (*e.g.* tricyclic antidepressants) suppress, for days, weeks or even months, the histamine-induced weal and flare response of a skin test

- Poor correlation between the results of provocation tests (*e.g.* double-blind food challenges) and skin prick tests. For example, in one study, of 31 children with a strongly positive (weal > 3 mm in diameter) skin prick test to peanut, only 16 (56%) had symptoms when peanuts were administered

- Commercial food extracts (sometimes heat treated) and fresh or frozen raw extracts may give different results (more positives with raw foods), reflecting the fact that some patients are allergic to certain foods only when taken in a raw state. In others the reverse is the case

Inability to predict outcome

In many clinical situations (*e.g.* a child with severe eczema), the subject wants to know whether there will be any benefit from food avoidance (*e.g.* not drinking cow's milk or not eating apples). Even if there were valid tests for the diagnosis of food intolerance, the outcome of avoidance measures depends on a number of other variables. Allergen avoidance may succeed for a number of quite unrelated reasons, such as: (i) the patient was intolerant to the item; (ii) co-incidental improvement; or (iii) placebo response.

Table 5 Reasons why a trial of avoidance of a specific food may fail to help

- The subject is not allergic to the food

- The period of elimination was too short. For example, where a child has an enteropathy (damage to the small intestine) due to food allergy, it may take a week or more for improvement in symptoms to occur

- The food has been incompletely avoided, as in a subject supposed to be on a cow's milk protein free diet who still continues to receive food which contains cow's milk proteins such as, for example, casein or whey

- The subject is allergic to other items which have not been avoided, such as a child with cow's milk protein allergy who fails to improve when given a soya based milk to which there is also an allergy

- Co-existing or intercurrent disease, for example gastroenteritis in a child with loose stools who is trying a cow's milk-free diet

- The patient's symptoms are trivial and have been exaggerated, or alternatively do not exist at all and have either been imagined or fabricated

Even if an individual is allergic to a food, a trial of food avoidance may fail to help for a number of reasons (see Table 5).

Provocation tests

The aim of a food challenge is to study the consequences of food or food additive ingestion. An **open challenge** is where the subject and the observer know the identity of the administered material. In a **single-blind challenge** the observer but not the patient or family know the identity of the test material. In a **double blind challenge**, neither the subject nor the observer know the identity of the administered material. Provocation tests are helpful either to confirm a history or diagnosis, to see if a subject has grown out of a food intolerance, and as a research procedure.

Open food challenges are the simplest approach, but open food challenges run the risk of bias influencing parents', patients' or doctors' observations. Often this is unimportant. Where belief in food intolerance may be disproportionate, and there is no substitute for a double-blind placebo-controlled challenge. For example, in Britain, parents widely believe that there is an association between reactions to food additives and bad behaviour, but in one series, double-blind challenges with tartrazine and benzoic acid were negative in all 24 children with a clear parental description of adverse reaction[4].

The double-blind placebo-controlled challenge is regarded as the state-of-the-art technique to confirm or refute histories of adverse reactions to

Table 6 Limitations and difficulties with double-blind placebo-controlled challenges

Problem	Comment
Effect of dose	In some, microgram quantities are sufficient to provoke symptoms. In others, much larger quantities of food are required
Concealing foods can be difficult	Standard capsules which contain up to 500 mg of food are suitable for validation of immediate reactions to tiny quantities of food, but concealing much larger quantities of certain foods (especially those with a strong smell, flavour or colour) can be very difficult
Route of administration	Reactions to food occurring within the mouth will be missed if the challenge by-passes the oral route, for example by administration of foods in a capsule or via a nasogastric tube
Capsule problems	Capsules are unsuitable for use in children who cannot swallow large capsules, a major limitation as most cases of suspected food allergy are in infants and toddler It is unsatisfactory to allow patients or parents to break open capsules and swallow the contents mixed into food or drink, as the colour (e.g. tartrazine) or smell (e.g. fish) will be difficult or impossible to conceal and the challenge will no longer be blind
Danger of anaphylaxis	There is a danger of producing anaphylactic shock, even if anaphylactic shock had not occurred on previous exposure to the food. For example, in Goldman's classic study of cow's milk protein intolerance, anaphylactic shock had been noted prior to cow's milk challenge in 5 children, but another 3 out of 89 children developed anaphylactic shock as a new symptom after cow's milk challenge[16]
Additive effect of triggers	Although some patients react repeatedly to challenges with single foods, it is possible (but unproven) that some patients only react adversely when multiple allergens are given together. Also, there are some subjects who only react in the presence of a non-food trigger, such as exercise or taking aspirin

foods[17,18]. However, the technique is subject to a number of potential limitations, not all of which can be overcome (see Table 6).

Mechanisms of food intolerance

The principal mechanisms resulting in food intolerance and the pathophysiology (where this is understood) are discussed below.

Food allergy

As described in the earlier part of this review, the term allergy implies a definite immunological mechanism. This could be antibody mediated, cell mediated, or due to circulating immune complexes.

Enzyme defects

Inborn errors of metabolism due to enzyme defects may affect the digestion and absorption of carbohydrate, fat or protein. In some subjects the enzyme defect is primarily gastrointestinal, causing defects in digestion or absorption. An example is lactase deficiency, described below. In other subjects, the enzyme defect is systemic. An example is the rare disorders of hereditary fructose intolerance, also described below.

Lactase deficiency

In this condition, there is a reduced or absent concentration of the enzyme lactase in the small intestinal mucosa[19,20]. Affected subjects are unable to break down ingested lactose, which is the main sugar found in milk. If unabsorbed, lactose passes into the large intestine. One consequence is an osmotic diarrhoea. Another is that some of the unabsorbed lactose is broken down by intestinal bacteria, accompanied by the production of gas and organic acids. The clinical symptoms that result comprise loose stools, flatus, and perianal soreness and excoriation.

The diagnosis of lactase deficiency is made most simply by observing disappearance of symptoms when lactose is withdrawn from the diet, and re-appearance of symptoms when lactose is re-introduced. The diagnosis can be confirmed by the breath hydrogen test. In this test, the subject swallows a dose of lactose. Breath is collected every 30 min and the hydrogen content is measured. In the normal individual, the sugar is absorbed and hydrogen is not produced. In the intolerant individual, the sugar is not absorbed, hydrogen is produced, and a steep rise in hydrogen concentration is found in the exhaled air.

The management of lactose intolerance is to avoid foods that contain lactose, mainly cow's milk and its products.

In infants and young children, lactase deficiency is usually a transient problem occurring after an episode of viral gastroenteritis, but it can be a feature of any disease (such as coeliac disease) which causes damage to the intestinal mucosa. Levels of lactase tend to fall during mid to later childhood, and in a number of populations (*e.g.* Africa, Mexico, Greenland Eskimo) a high proportion of adults have very little lactase activity. This adult deficiency is believed to have a genetic basis.

Hereditary fructose intolerance

This condition is inherited as an autosomal recessive. Deficiency of the liver enzyme fructose 1,6-bisphosphate aldolase results in the accumulation of fructose-1-phosphate in liver cells, and acts as a competitive inhibitor for phosphorylase. The resulting inhibition of the conversion of glycogen to glucose leads to hypoglycaemia[21].

Affected infants are symptom-free as long as their diet is limited to human milk. Once patients receive a milk formula, or any food that contains fructose, they develop hypoglycaemia. There may also be jaundice, an enlarged liver, and sometimes progressive liver disease. Treatment requires the complete elimination of fructose from the diet. The need to avoid many types of confectionery leads to one advantage, a reduction in dental caries.

Pharmacological mechanisms

Pharmacological substances present in food can be responsible for adverse reactions to the food. Some examples are given below.

Caffeine

The stimulant effects of 60 mg caffeine in a cup of tea or 100 mg caffeine in a cup of coffee are well recognised, as is the diuretic effect. Less well known is that those who regularly consume large quantities of caffeine can suffer a number of other side effects, including heartburn, nausea, vomiting, diarrhoea, intestinal colic, tachycardia, arrythmia, sweating, tremor, anxiety and sleeplessness.

Sodium nitrite

Sodium nitrite is an antioxidant used as an anti-bacterial agent, and in quantities of 20 mg or more it can cause dilatation of blood vessels causing flushing and headache[22], and urticaria[23].

Tyramine, histamine and other vasoactive amines

Vasoactive amines, such as tyramine, serotonin, tryptamine, phenyl-ethylamine and histamine, are the normal constituents of many foods, which include tuna, pickled herring, sardines, anchovy fillets, bananas, cheese, yeast extracts (such as Marmite), chocolate, wine, spinach, tomato and sausages. Vasoactive amines arise mainly from the decarboxylation of amino acids, but they may also develop during normal food cooking and during the storage of food. The largest amount of histamine and tyramine are found in fermented foods such as cheese, alcoholic drinks, sausage, sauerkraut and tinned fish[24,25]. Badly stored food such as mackerel and tuna can contain large amounts of histamine

Adverse effects can occur as the result of:

1   An abnormally high intake: for example a high intake of histamine or tyramine, due to either a high content in food or because of synthesis of these substances in the gut as the result of action by bacteria.

2   Pharmacological substances in food which interfere with the enzymatic breakdown of vasoactive amines.

3   Release from mast cells of histamine and other mediators of inflammation, triggered by eating certain foods such as strawberries, shellfish and alcohol.

The effects of large doses of tyramine, histamine and other vasoactive amines are extremely variable. Histamine causes flushing, constriction of smooth muscle in the intestine and the bronchi, increased heart rate, headache, fall in blood pressure and asthma. Tyramine causes constriction of blood vessels, stimulates the release of noradrenaline, and can also cause the release of histamine and prostaglandins from mast cells. Dietary tyramine is known to induce hypertension and headache in patients who are taking monoamine oxidase inhibitor drugs. This effect has been shown to be due to inhibition, by these drugs, of intestinal and hepatic metabolism of tyramine, so that the amine accumulates.

There is uncertainty about tyramine as a trigger of migraine[2]. Most attempts to induce migraine by tyramine challenge in children and adults have been unsuccessful. In addition, a controlled study of exclusion of dietary vasoactive amines in children with migraine failed to demonstrate benefit[26]. In this study, patients were randomly allocated to either a high fibre diet low in dietary amines or a high fibre diet alone. Both groups showed a highly significant decrease in the number of headaches, emphasising the need for a control diet in studies designed to show that dietary manipulation improves symptoms.

Of the foods reported to be common triggers of attacks of migraine, only cheese is rich in tyramine. Chocolate is low in this and other vasoactive amines, and red wine usually contains no more tyramine than white wine. Alcoholic drinks, particularly red wine, are commonly

Table 7 Naturally occurring toxins in foods

Substance	Comments
Protease inhibitors	Widely distributed throughout the plant kingdom, particularly in legumes, but to a lesser extent in cereal grains and tubers. Heat labile
Lectins	Present in most legumes and cereals. Some lectins, such as ricin from the castor bean, are extremely toxic. Others, such as those in the soya bean, are non-toxic. Heat labile, *e.g.* inadequate cooking of red kidney beans can cause severe gastrointestinal upset, with vomiting and diarrhoea
Lathyrogens	Lathyrism is a paralytic disease that is associated with the consumption of chickling pea or vetch, *Lathyrus sativus*. The causative factor is an amino acid derivative, β-N-oxalyl-α,β-diaminopropionic acid, a metabolic antagonist of glutamic acid
Mimosine	An amino acid that comprises 1–4% of the dry weight of the legume *Leucaena leucocephala*. Consumption of the leaves, pods and seeds leads to hair loss
Djenkolic acid	The djenkol bean (from Sumatra) is a seed of the leguminous tree, *Pithecolobium lobatum*. Consumption leads to renal failure
Goitrogens	Present in cabbage, turnip, broccoli, cauliflower, brussel sprouts, kale, rape seed and mustard seed
Cyanogens	The most common plants that contain glycosides from which hydrogen cyanide may be released by enzymatic hydrolysis are lima beans (*Phaseolus lunatus*), sorghum, cassava, linseed meal, black-eyed pea (*Vigna sinensis*), garden pea (*Pisum sativum*), kidney bean (*Phaseolus vulgaris*), Bengal gram (*Cicer arietinum*) and red gram (*Cajanus cajans*)
Vicine and convicine	These are β-glucosides that are present in broad beans (*Vicia faba*). When consumed by individuals with deficiency of the enzyme glucose-6-phosphate dehydrogenase, these substances precipitate haemolytic anaemia (favism)
Cycasin	Cycad seeds or nuts are obtained from *Cycad circinalis*, a tropical palm-like tree. The toxic ingredient methyl-azoxymethanol, the aglycone of cycasin, is released on hydrolysis of cycasin by intestinal bacteria
Pyrrolizidine derivatives	Pyrrolizidine alkaloids are found in a wide variety of plant species. Poisoning has resulted from the consumption of contaminated cereal and grain crops, and possibly also from milk from cows that have consumed pyrrolizidine containing plants
Lupin alkaloid	Milk from animals that have eaten plants from the lupin family, notably *Lupinus latifolius*, may contain quinolizidine alkaloids such as anagyrine, which are teratogenic in animals and possibly also man

reported to provoke attacks of migraine. Whether these attacks are due to alcohol itself or some other compound is unclear.

11β-hydroxysteroid dehydrogenase and liquorice
Liquorice contains an enzyme that inhibits 11β-hydroxysteroid dehydrogenase, resulting in sodium and water retention, hypertension, hypokalaemia, and suppression of the renin-aldosterone system[27].

Irritant mechanisms for food intolerance

Certain foods have a direct irritant effect on the mucous membranes of the mouth or gut, such as the irritant effect of coffee or curry. In some individuals, food intolerance only occurs in the presence of a co-existing medical disorder. For example, the ingestion of spicy food, coffee or orange juice provoke oesophageal pain in some patients with reflux oesophagitis.

Specific drug–food combinations

One example of drug-induced food intolerance is potentiation of the pressor effects of tyramine-containing foods (*e.g.* cheese, yeast extracts and fermented soya bean products) by monoamine oxidase inhibitor drugs. Another is the effect of taking alcohol in patients with alcohol dependence during treatment with disulfiram (Antabuse). The reaction, which can occur within 10 min of alcohol and may last several hours, consists of flushing and nausea.

Toxic mechanisms

Nature has endowed plants with the capacity to synthesise substances that are toxic, and thus serve to protect them from predators whether they be fungi, insects, animals or humans[28]. Many plant foods contain naturally occurring toxins which protect the plant from predators such as fungi, insects or animals. Some examples are given in Table 7. There are numerous other examples of toxic substances present in food-stuffs. These include solanidine in potatoes, cyanide in tapioca, mycotoxins in mushrooms and cereal grains, and phototoxic furocoumarins in angelica, parsley, dill and celeriac, which in sufficient quantities can give rise to a wide variety of toxic reactions.

Food storage

Chemical changes in food during storage can produce substances which cause food intolerance. One example is the production of histamine in badly stored mackerel. Another example is intolerance to ripe or stored tomatoes in subjects who can safely eat green tomatoes, where ripening of the fruit produces a new active glycoprotein. Contamination of food by antigens such as storage mites or microbial spores may give rise to adverse effects, particularly asthma and eczema. Contamination of food by micro-organisms may result in adverse effects. For example, celery, parsnip and parsley may become infected with the fungus *Sclerotinia scleriotiorum* ('pink rot'), resulting in the production of the photosensitising chemicals psoralen, 5-methoxypsoralen and 8-methoxypsoralen.

Conclusions

Food arouses not only the appetite but also the emotions. The current phobia of food additives and food processing, and the obsession for so-called natural or health food arises largely out of misinformation and ignorance. Obsession with so-called natural or health food ignores the wide range of naturally occurring toxins in foods. For example, a survey of 'crunchy' peanut butter showed that 11 out of 59 samples from health food producers contained over 100 µg/kg of aflatoxins, over 10 times the proposed maximum permitted level for total aflatoxins[29]. Only one of the 26 samples from other producers contained aflatoxins in excess of 10 µg/kg, and none contained more than 50 µg/kg. By far the greatest danger comes from allergy to naturally occurring allergens present in foods such as peanut, fish, egg and cow's milk. At present, the only practical management is specific food avoidance.

Key points for clinical practice

- Food allergy is a form of adverse reaction to food in which the cause is an immunological response to a food. The word allergy is frequently misused, and applied indiscriminately to any adverse reaction, regardless of the mechanism.

- Heat treatment renders certain (but not all) foods less likely to provoke an allergic reaction in a subject who is allergic.

- Reports of food allergy or intolerance from individuals or parents of children are notoriously unreliable, and when tested by double-blind placebo-controlled challenge not all reports of reactions can be verified.

- A high proportion of children with food intolerance in the first year of life lose their intolerance in time. The notable exception is allergy to peanut, which is life-long.

- Most allergic reactions to foods occur within minutes of ingestion of the food.

- The quantity of food required to produce an allergic reaction varies. Some patients are highly sensitive and develop reactions after ingestion of less than 1 µg of a food trigger. In contrast, there are children and adults who, for example, only react adversely to 200 ml or more of cow's milk.

- The diagnosis of food allergy is usually made from the history, supported by information about the response to the avoidance of specific food triggers.

- There is a lack of clinically useful simple diagnostic tests for food allergy. Skin prick tests and radio-allergosorbent tests, both of which detect specific IgE antibodies, are unreliable because of a large number of false positive and false negative reactions.

- Intolerance to food can result from enzyme defects. Examples are lactase deficiency and hereditary fructose intolerance.

- Pharmacological substances present in food such as caffeine, sodium nitrite or vasoactive amines such as histamine and tyramine, may be responsible for some adverse reactions to food.

- Food intolerance can also result from a direct irritant effect, for example from spicy food, or from toxins present in food

References

1 Sampson HA. Food allergy. Part 1: immunopathogenesis and clinical disorders. *J Allergy Clin Immunol* 1999; **103**: 717–28
2 David TJ. *Food and Food Additive Intolerance in Childhood*. Oxford: Blackwell, 1993
3 May CD, Bock SA. A modern clinical approach to food hypersensitivity. *Allergy* 1978; **33**: 166–88
4 David TJ. Reactions to dietary tartrazine. *Arch Dis Child* 1987; **62**: 119–22
5 Bentley SJ, Pearson DJ, Rix KJB. Food hypersensitivity in irritable bowel syndrome. *Lancet* 1983; ii: 295–7
6 Young E, Patel S, Stoneham M, Rona R, Wilkinson JD. The prevalence of reaction to food additives in a survey population. *J R Coll Physicians Lond* 1987; **21**: 241–7
7 Kajosaari M. Food allergy in Finnish children aged 1 to 6 years. *Acta Paediatr Scand* 1982; **71**: 815–9
8 Bock SA. Prospective appraisal of complaints of adverse reactions to foods in children during the first three years of life. *Pediatrics* 1987; **79**: 683–8
9 Host A, Halken S. A prospective study of cow milk allergy in Danish infants during the first 3 years of life. Clinical course in relation to clinical and immunological type of hypersensitivity reaction. *Allergy* 1990; **45**: 587–96
10. Nickel R, Kulig M, Forster J *et al*. Sensitization to hen's egg at the age of twelve months is predictive for allergic sensitization to common indoor and outdoor allergens at the age of three years. *J Allergy Clin Immunol* 1997; **99**: 613–7
11 Sampson HA. Food allergy. Part 2: Diagnosis and management. *J Allergy Clin Immunol* 1999; **103**: 981–9
12 Eggesbo M, Halvorsen R, Tambs K, Botten G. Prevalence of parentally perceived adverse reactions to food in young children. *Pediatr Allergy Immunol* 1999; **10**: 122–32
13 Bock SA. Natural history of severe reactions to foods in young children. *J Pediatr* 1985; **107**: 676–80
14 Pastorello EA, Stocchi L, Pravettoni V *et al*. Role of the elimination diet in adults with food allergy. *J Allergy Clin Immunol* 1989; **84**: 475–83
15 Hill DJ, Ford RPK, Shelton MJ, Hosking CS. A study of 100 infants and young children with cow's milk allergy. *Clin Rev Allergy* 1984; **2**: 125–42

16 Goldman AS, Anderson DW, Sellers WA, Saperstein S, Kniker WT, Halpern SR. Milk allergy. I. Oral challenge with milk and isolated milk proteins in allergic children. *Pediatrics* 1963; **32**: 425–43

17 Bernstein M, Day JH, Welsh A. Double-blind food challenge in the diagnosis of food sensitivity in the adult. *J Allergy Clin Immunol* 1982; **70**: 205–10

18 Bock SA, Sampson HA, Atkins FM *et al*. Double-blind, placebo-controlled food challenge as an office procedure: a manual. *J Allergy Clin Immunol* 1988; **82**: 986–97

19 Johnson JD, Kretchmer N, Simoons FJ. Lactose malabsorption: its biology and history. *Adv Pediatr* 1974; **21**: 197–237

20 Lebenthal E, Rossi TM. Lactose malabsorption and intolerance. In: Lebenthal E (Ed) *Textbook of Gastroenterology and Nutrition in Infancy*. New York: Raven, 1981; 673–88

21 Gitzelman R, Steinmann B, Van den Berghe G. Disorders of fructose metabolism. In: Scriver CR, Beaudet AL, Sly WS, Valle D (Eds) *The Metabolic and Molecular Bases of Inherited Disease*, 7th edn. New York: McGraw-Hill, 1995; 905–34

22 Henderson WR, Raskin NH. 'Hog-dog' headache: individual susceptibility to nitrite. *Lancet* 1972; **ii**: 1162–3

23 Moneret-Vautrin DA, Einhorn C, Tisserand J. Le role du nitrite de sodium dans les urticaires histaminiques d'origine alimentaire. *Ann Nutr Alim* 1980; **34**: 1125–32

24 Malone MH, Metcalfe DD. Histamine in foods: its possible role in non-allergic adverse reactions to ingestants. *N E R Allergy Proc* 1986; **7**: 241–5

25 Taylor SL, Leatherwood M, Lieber ER. A survey of histamine levels in sausages. *J Food Protect* 1978; **41**: 634–7

26 Salfield SAW, Wardley BL, Houlsby WT *et al*. Controlled study of exclusion of dietary vasoactive amines in migraine. *Arch Dis Child* 1987; **62**: 458–60

27 Edwards CRW. Lessons from licorice. *N Engl J Med* 1991; **325**: 1242–3

28 Leiner IE. *Toxic Constituents of Plant Foodstuffs*. New York: Academic Press, 1980

29 Ministry of Agriculture, Fisheries and Food. *Mycotoxins*. The 18th report of the Steering Group on Food Surveillance. The working party on naturally occurring toxicants in food: sub-group on mycotoxins. London: HMSO, 1987

Animal health and food safety

A M Johnston

Department of Farm Animal and Equine Medicine and Surgery, Royal Veterinary College, University of London, Hatfield, Hertfordshire, UK

Foods of animal origin have an important role in a balanced diet and must be safe for human consumption. Equally important is the need for the food to be perceived as safe by the consumer. Safe food of animal origin must be free from animal pathogens that infect man and from contamination by residues. While intensive farming practices have been linked with the rise in foodborne illness in humans, it is interesting to note that the rise has continued even when there has been a shift to less intensive farm production systems. While the production of meat, milk and eggs, regardless of new technology or changes in production methods, cannot be expected to achieve zero bacterial risk, there is the need to reduce the risk and, where possible, eliminate it at the 'on the farm stage'. The current use of the terms 'farm-to-table', 'stable-to-table' and 'plough-to-plate' clearly identifies the farm as one part of the production chain which must be considered in terms of food safety.

Micro-organisms are widely present in animals and in their environment. With animals, disease is inevitable; perfectly healthy animals can also be carriers and may be asymptotic excretors of pathogens. The diseases of animals which affect the safety of food are predominantly those that cause enteric disorders. The prevalence of pathogens on the farm, or on a unit within a farm, depends on many factors, not least being the type of husbandry, the environmental pressure on that farm and the standard of stockmanship. There are organisms which are pathogenic to man but do not cause clinical illness in the animals, such as *Escherichia coli* O157, and others which are excreted in large numbers before there is evidence of the animal being unwell or following apparent recovery from an illness.

Correspondence to:
Prof. A M Johnston.
Department of Farm
Animal and Equine
Medicine and Surgery,
Royal Veterinary College,
University of London,
Hawkshead Lane, North
Mymms, Hatfield,
Hertfordshire
AL9 7TA, UK

Hazard analysis critical control point and livestock

Whenever food production and processing is mentioned in relation to food safety the use of the hazard analysis critical control point (HACCP) system is suggested. HACCP identifies and evaluates hazards and enables

© The British Council 2000

decisions on whether control, absolute or in part, can be applied to limit the hazards, and determines the methods for monitoring and controlling the process. The use of HACCP has become rather 'all things to all in the food industry', and perhaps even to different Governments but there is good reason for using HACCP principles behind the farm gate. In livestock production, there are a number of points where controls can be applied.

The first is with the birth of the animal, or at hatching in the case of poultry, and extends through all stages of animal production and includes the foodstuffs fed to the animals. The aim should be to have the young born fit and healthy with good levels of maternal immunity. In addition to the appropriate use of available vaccines in the neonate, vaccines can be given to the pregnant dam, such as the bovine combined rotavirus and K99 *E. coli* vaccine for calf scours, to protect the young in the first 2–3 weeks of life. Animals and birds are usually kept in groups, either outside in fields or housed for all or part of the year. The access to the housed accommodation or to the pasture may be voluntary or controlled according to the farming system in place. Whichever system is used, the animals must be kept in the very best conditions, with the aim being able to prevent disease in individual animals or the whole herd or flock. The type of husbandry directly impacts on this, as the most certain way to reduce or remove the risk of introducing disease organisms to animal(s) is to use biosecure housing. This, of course, is contrary to the trend towards extensive systems where there is the inevitable exposure to wild-life vectors of a number of important pathogens. The use of systems of production which have biosecure housing does allow a policy of 'all in, all out', followed by thorough cleaning and disinfection of the house before restocking, to be used. The original method was to apply this practice to each house as it was emptied of animals or birds. More recently, this practice has been extended to involve all animal accommodation on the site, which is emptied of livestock then all cleaned and disinfected before any unit on that site is restocked.

In addition to keeping animals healthy, a critical part of the husbandry is also to make sure they are kept visibly clean. It is of particular importance, to reduce the possibility of contamination of the food, for milking animals and for animals destined for slaughter not have dirty outer coats. A major influence on the cleanliness of the animals is the type of housing, the material used as bedding and the underfoot conditions if the animals are kept outside. There are a variety of housing systems in practice, including straw or deep litter yards, cow cubicles with straw, sand, rubber mats or even water-beds as bedding, and sheds with slatted floors, or a combination of these. Straw bedding is a much-favoured system for comfort and cleanliness, but is only satisfactory if the existing bedding is regularly replaced with clean straw. In some parts of the country, straw may not be available locally, which requires the transport of straw from the arable counties. A major factor in the effectiveness of any system in keeping the animals clean is the standard of the management. Failure to attend to detail will lead to an increase in environmental organisms and inevitably also pathogens. The stockman, therefore, has a crucial role to play both from the animal health and public health perspectives.

Food-stuffs which are fed to animals must be free from both pathogens and undesirable residues. The role of animal feed in food safety has been highlighted both in relation to salmonella, in particular *Salmonella enteritidis* phage type 4 in poultry[1,2], bovine spongiform encephalopathy in cattle (BSE)[3], and, more recently, dioxins in animal feeds in Belgium. Animal feeds are produced from both home-grown and imported ingredients most frequently as a compounded, nutritionally balanced, ration from commercial feed mills. The farmer may well prepare the feeds on the farm using either home-grown or purchased forage and cereals. The ingredients for animal feeds may carry pathogens. The process of producing some forms of compounded feed, such as pelleted feed, requires a heat treatment stage which is effective against bacterial pathogens; however, subsequent handling stages may allow recontamination. The farm does have a role to play in making sure the feed is stored in a manner which prevents contamination from external influences such as wild life on the farm.

The bringing on to the farm of new animals, whether as replacement breeding stock or animals to be fattened for slaughter, is frequently a way by which diseases are introduced. In most cases, the major impact will be from diseases which affect animals but frequently can include zoonotic organisms. It is of the utmost importance that incoming animals are kept separate from those already on the farm for the necessary period of quarantine and, where possible, come from a farm with a known health history.

Growth promotion techniques

There is also pressure on the industry to use production methods that will deliver the slaughter animal at a predetermined weight, with the required carcass conformation, in the shortest time and at the lowest possible cost. This has lead to the use of growth promotion techniques, including sub-therapeutic levels of antibiotics in the feed and steroid hormones during the growing phase. The use of substances having a thyrostatic, oestrogenic or gestagenic effect for growth promotion purposes has been prohibited within the EU, or for products to be imported into the EU, since January

1989. The counter argument to justify the use of steroid hormones is that they are naturally occurring substances and, if the withdrawal periods are followed, there is no risk to human health. This issue was reviewed by the Scientific Veterinary Committee on Matters Relating to Public Health in 1999. They considered that the scientific evidence necessary to make a balanced scientific judgement is lacking but it is known that one, 17β-oestradiol, is a complete carcinogen and, as such, is able to initiate and promote cancer. The Committee considered that there was sufficient uncertainty in terms of consumer public health that the ban on their use in the EU should continue[4].

The use of antibiotics, without veterinary prescription, for the purposes of increasing growth in food animal production, started in the early 1950s. Following an outbreak of food poisoning due to multi-drug resistant salmonella, an Expert Committee chaired by Professor Swann, reviewed the use of antibiotics in agriculture. Their report in 1969[5] resulted in significant changes in the use of antibiotics, including their use for growth promotion purposes. More recently, there has again been considerable concern about the use of antibiotics, especially for growth promotion purposes, in animals, and specifically about food being a vector of antibiotic resistance from animals to humans. This has led to a number of reports from groups of experts, nationally and internationally, considering the use of antibiotics in animals, in man and for plant protection purposes[6,7]. There is agreement that there should be prudent use of antibiotics in veterinary and human medicine, but little justification for the uncontrolled use of antibiotics at sub-therapeutic levels to promote growth. The major concern is if there is evidence of medical equivalence for the antibiotic, either where the same drug is used in man and in animals, or if there is known antibiotic resistance. Of major concern is where there is a possible impact on the effectiveness of important antibiotics used in human medicine, especially when the antibiotic is one of last choice for life-threatening infections. The growth promotion debate will undoubtedly continue, but already there is evidence of sectors of the industry stopping the use of antibiotic growth promoters as part of their production systems. It is easy to say that there should be no use of these products just to sustain cheap food production systems and make animals grow faster. However, some of the very same 'antibiotic growth promoters' also control disease in the animals and stopping their use would require a greater use of therapeutic antibiotics. There is a balance, which can be achieved between the two schools of thought, which requires the husbandry systems to be changed to reduce the need for use of antibiotics in any form. The issue of consumption of residues in food of animal origin is also important and there are established testing programmes for residues in meat and milk and a requirement only to use drugs which are licensed for use in food producing species within EU Member States.

Disease in animals

Disease in animals is inevitable on farms, no matter how good the husbandry. In terms of food safety, one option for control would be to eradicate specific agents if they are identified on the farm. This, however, depends first on being able to identify the agent in the herd or flock. In addition to there being an accurate 'test' available, there is the need to decide if eradication is really necessary, for animal health and human health reasons, or for both. The biological way forward of disease control using vaccines promises to be an important alternative to the need for use of antibiotics. While it has always been important to use available vaccines in the appropriate manner, with the increasing efficacy, and at the same time specificity, of modern vaccines, precise diagnosis becomes a must. There is, therefore, a future for the veterinary clinician on the farm as a means by which there can be improvements to the health status of the food production animals following proper assessment of all relevant factors including the provision of a farm veterinary health plan. The success of any scheme for any farm or unit requires, as a minimum: (i) surveillance of possible diseases or risks; (ii) management structure in place to avoid the need to react; (iii) active supervision at all levels, and (iii) investigation of all possible, or actual, problems or variations from the normal.

Of all the foods produced on UK farms, milk has for many years been a good example of what can be achieved in terms of consumer health protection by a combination of legislative control with financial incentive, or penalty, according to the quality of the milk produced. This has now been extended by producer schemes from the milk companies and major retailers which include routine audits of all aspects of on farm production. Milk in the UK is produced from cows, sheep and goats, although there is provision in the legislation for the production of buffalo milk. Although the presence of some bacteria in milk is inevitable, either directly from the udder or by contamination during milking, the systems currently in use aim to minimise the possibility of contamination during the milking process. One of the more clearly defined parts of the farming operation to which the HACCP concept can be applied is in the production of milk. Over the years, the critical points in milking have been clearly identified and the working practices necessary to ensure clean milk production established. A major problem in the dairy industry is mastitis, either clinical or subclinical. Mastitis-causing organisms can broadly be divided into contagious bacteria and environmental bacteria as shown in Table 1. Contagious bacteria are predominantly associated with the cow's udder and tend to be spread from cow to cow during milking. Environmental organisms are always present in the discharges from the alimentary or reproductive tracts and survive and multiply in the bedding[8].

Table 1 Organisms commonly causing mastitis

Contagious bacteria	Streptococcus agalactiae
	Streptococcus dysgalactiae
	Staphylococcus aureus
Environmental bacteria	Escherichia coli
	Coliforms
	Streptococcus uberis
	Corynebacterium pyrogenes

Other organisms such as *Listeria monocytogenes*[9], *Streptococcus zooepidemicus*[10], *Salmonella typhimurium* DT 104[11] and 49a[12] and *Salmonella enteritidis*[13] have, on rare occasions, been attributed to cases of mastitis. While most cases of mastitis in sheep are caused by Gram-positive cocci[14], a proportion of cases are due to Gram-negative bacteria, predominantly *Pasteurella haemolytica*[15], with occasional cases due to *Pseudomonas aeruginosa*[16]. While Gram-positive organisms are found in goat's milk, bacteriological problems are related to poor hygiene during production. In all species it is also possible to find Q fever (*Coxiella burnetti*) and *Brucella* organisms in the milk. Mastitis is usually divided, on the basis of clinical signs, into three broad categories. Acute mastitis is sudden in onset and tends to be severe, and chronic mastitis causes a considerable loss of milk forming tissue – both are easily recognisable by the farmer. Subclinical mastitis, which is not detected by the usual visual signs, is detected by an increase in the somatic cell count (SCC). The somatic cell count in milk is the measurement most commonly used as an indicator of udder health. Normal milk has a SCC of less than 200,000/ml and elevation is an indication of inflammation of the udder. To encourage good hygienic milk production and good udder health, the price paid for cows' milk varies with the SCC and the total bacterial count (TBC) and there is a financial penalty for elevated counts. In addition, there is a maximum of 400,000/ml for SCC, set by the EU, for milk. The TBC has now been replaced by the Bactoscan which is said to provide a better measure of bacterial loading of a milk sample as it takes account of both live and dead bacterial cells. The intramammary route for the administration of antimicrobial drugs is a convenient route for treating infections of the quarter of the udder affected and for the administration of long-acting preparations at the end of the lactation. Dry cow therapy is designed to remove infections present then in the udder and to prevent new infections during the dry period. The udder is naturally resistant to Gram-negative organisms but, in addition to specially targeting *Staph. aureus* and *Strep. uberis,* the preparation should be effective against any *E. coli* present in the udder.

Table 2 Food poisoning organisms associated with meat dishes

Clostridium perfringens
Salmonellae
Verotoxigenic Escherichia coli
Campylobacter
Yersinia enterocolitica
Listeria monocytogenes
Aeromonas hydrophilia
Staphylococcus aureus

Meat can be contaminated with a large variety of pathogens and spoilage bacteria. The organisms associated with the majority of food poisoning associated with meat dishes[17] are given in Table 2. These organisms can be found in the alimentary tract of healthy animals and in the case of *E. coli* O157, while it has prevalence in the ruminant of at least 10% with a seasonal variation in excretion rates[18], it is not a recognised cause of disease in animals.

Meat, in the unskinned and uneviscerated healthy animal or bird, can be regarded as sterile[19]. The removal of the outer coat and the act of evisceration are points in the slaughter of animals when contamination can occur. The exception is when there is an invasive organism, such as *Salmonella,* in some organ or lymph node. A major control point is the conversion of the live animal to meat in a hygienic manner by the careful removal of the outer coat and the entire alimentary tract without contamination or spillage of gut contents. Live poultry carry large numbers of many different micro-organisms on the skin, among feathers as well as in the alimentary tract. When birds are being transferred from the farm to the processing plant there is an increase in shedding and spread of faecal material with an increase in *E. coli* on the breast surface. During processing, a high percentage of the organisms will be removed but the very nature of poultry processing, where the birds are passed through a scalding tank before defeathering, leads to cross contamination. The changes in the skin from the scald process also favour entrapment of bacteria. In order to reduce the risk of gut rupture during evisceration, the feed is removed a number of hours before transport. This practice also reduces the excretion rate of *Salmonella* by the birds arriving at the slaughter plant. However, recent work has shown that fasting prior to transport may lead to an increase in the *Salmonella* levels in the crop, an organ also likely to burst during mechanical evisceration[20]. Current slaughter practice keeps the carcass whole, which makes evisceration without rupture of the viscera more difficult.

One of the food safety controls for many has been *post mortem* inspection of meat in the abattoir. The use of a physical meat inspection in slaughter animals has been questioned with good evidence that there is increased spread of zoonotic organisms by the actions carried out during the meat inspection process. Pathogenic bacteria, such as *Salmonella* and *Campylobacter* species, can be present in the lymph nodes, digestive tracts and on the surface of symptomless carrier animals[21] and have been shown to be spread by actions of the meat inspection team. Gross lesions such as parasitic cysts and kidney conditions can be missed by current inspection techniques[22-24] especially in high-throughput abattoirs[25]. Traditional meat inspection will not reveal the presence of zoonotic agents such as *Salmonella*, *Campylobacter* and *Yersinia* species, *Trichinella spiralis* and *Toxoplasma gondii*[23,26,27].

Production and health information from the poultry unit has been used for a number of years to target the level of *post mortem* meat inspection necessary for each batch of broilers delivered to the slaughter plant. There is a strong possibility that all inspection systems will change to one based on an analysis of risk. An important part of any new system will be the monitoring of salmonella on the farms of origin. Studies of the type by Edwards *et al*[28] and Fries *et al*[29] are required to provide the basis for any alternative system of integrated meat inspection. Such studies might give the background for designing a truly targeted organoleptic *post mortem* inspection system that yields a net benefit to consumer health protection.

One of the big food scares followed the announcement by Edwina Currie in 1989 about *Salmonella* in eggs. There then followed a dramatic drop in egg sales. A whole raft of measures were put in place by Government to control *S. enteritidis* and *S. typhimurium*, which included slaughter arrangements for infected flocks. The recommendations contained in the Richmond Committee Report[1] dealt specifically with poultry industry and made a number of recommendations relating to housing, husbandry and animal feed. A code of practice was published by MAFF in 1996 which provides guidance on good hygiene principles and practice on the production site, at the grading and packing station and during distribution and storage. The British Egg Industry Council operates a Code of Practice for Lion Quality eggs. This has been revised to include a requirement by the flocks to use vaccination for *S. enteritidis*. These measures collectively appear to be reducing the incidence of *S. enteritidis* in the laying flocks in the UK.

Future assurance to consumers

A cornerstone of future assurance to consumers, the EU and the rest of the world will be that proper supervision and checks are being carried out on the farm with adequate records being maintained. To provide this assurance, the aim must be a minimum of 100% compliance with current legislation with evidence available that this level of compliance is being maintained. There has been, in recent years, an increase in the number of farm assured schemes and the direct influence by the major retailers on agricultural practices through their producer schemes. These farm quality assurance programs stress the importance of a strong working relationship between producers and their veterinarians and emphasise that efficient management practices are a way on the farm of improving the safety of the food supply. One major problem is that when HACCP is said to be used it is usually as part of the farm Quality Assurance scheme when in reality it is frequently 'safety' equals 'welfare' and there is little consideration of true food safety issues. There is a real need for the whole area to be properly established so that any HACCP or risk assessment/management approach is set up to **manage** and not to **react**.

The reputation of the stakeholders – the farming industry, and the professions must not be compromised in any way, for whatever reason. However, the consumer must recognise that there is a cost to all the improvements to the on-farm situation in the UK. The same high standards must also apply to foods of animal origin imported from countries where the controls, both food safety and welfare, will not be as rigorous as in the UK and reflected in the lower cost of the product.

The role of food from non-traditional species must also be considered in the future. World supplies of animal derived protein are limited and, in some parts of the world, under considerable pressure. It is possible to harvest more from the wild, provided care is taken while drawing on wild life reserves. Already game farming and fish farming, in particular, have changed the availability of different types of meat.

Often the concerns about the whole food-chain are associated with food scares and presented as a perceived worry about food-related issues that has little, if anything, to do with reason for the food scare. On the other hand, if the controls placed on the industry are so stringent, there will be such an increase in cost of production that the result will be increased imports of produce from countries where the standards of husbandry and slaughter are less than here in the UK.

It is also most important, when considering the need for legislation, to recognise the differences between disease in respect of animal health or human health. At present, there are, however, no specific statutory food safety controls applicable to on-farm production. It is very easy to say that more control is necessary on the farm, and even increase the legislative controls on farming; however, legislation is not always the answer, especially if there is no audit of compliance. Equally, in the EU and world-wide market place, there is little point in disadvantaging UK agriculture such that it is priced out of the market and the food is imported from farming systems of lesser standards both in terms of welfare and of food safety, but cheaper. An example could be the banning of sow stalls, on welfare grounds, in the UK, with a significant extra cost on the UK pig producer, which has not been applied to any other country. Equally of concern at this time are the increasing reports of animal medicines available illegally, even by mail order, with suggestions that they are 'on the internet'. They must be very tempting to farmers at this time of economic crisis in farming, not least when they are advertised at less cost than the veterinary surgeon can purchase the same drug.

The food-producing industry has increasingly become a target for consumers campaigning for changes in animal welfare and husbandry systems, as well as their expressions of concern for the environment. These concerns about the food animal production systems and the methods by which the product is harvested, including how animals and birds are slaughtered to produce meat, are very relevant to the whole subject of veterinary public health.

It is often forgotten that farming is a commercial enterprise but one which involves animals. As such, it should be an efficient operation producing clean food, to be consumed directly or incorporated in other foodstuffs, with the highest standards of animal husbandry, yet making a reasonable return on the farmer's investment.

References

1   Committee on the Safety of Food (Chairman Sir Mark Richmond). *The Microbiological Safety of Food*, Part I. London: HMSO, 1990; 45–58

2   Ministry of Agriculture Fisheries and Food. *The Report of the Expert Group on Animal Feedingstuffs* (The Lamming Report). London: HMSO 1992; 2

3   Johnston AM. *Bovine Spongiform Encephalopathy*. CPD Veterinary Medicine, vol 1. London: Rila Publications, 1998; 26–9

4   Opinion of the Scientific Committee on Veterinary Measures Relating to Public Health. *Assessment of potential risks to human health from hormone residues in bovine meat and meat products*. Brussels: European Commission, 30 April 1999 [also on www.europa.eu.int/comm/dg24/health/sc/scv/outcome_en.html]

5   *Report of the Joint Committee on the Use of Antibiotics in Animal Husbandry and Veterinary Medicine*. Chairman Professor M Swann. London: HMSO, 1969

6   *Advisory Committee on the Microbiological Safety of Food. Report on Microbial Antibiotic Resistance in Relation to Food Safety*. London: The Stationery Office, 1999

7   *Opinion of the Scientific Steering Committee on Antimicrobial Resistance*. Brussels: European Commission Directorate-General XXIV,, 28 May 1999 [also on www.europa.eu.int/comm/dg24/health/sc/ssc/outcome_en.html]

8   Berry EA. Mastitis incidence in straw yards and cubicles. *Vet Rec* 1998; **142**: 517–8

9   Sharp MW. Bovine mastitis and *Listeria monocytogenes*. *Vet Rec* 1989;.**125**: 512–3

10 Edwards AT, Roulson M, Ironside MJ. A milkborne outbreak of serious infection due to *Streptococcus zooepidemicus* (Lancefield group C). *Epidemiol Infect* 1988; **101**: 43–51

11 Sharp MW, Rawson BC. Persistent *Salmonella typhimurium* DT 104 infection in a dairy herd. *Vet Rec* 1992; **131**: 375–6

12 Giles N, Hopper, SA, Wray C. Persistence of *S. typhimurium* in a large dairy herd. *Epidemiol Infect* 1989; **103**: 235

13 Wood J, Chalmers G, Fenton R *et al. Salmonella enteritidis* from the udder of a cow. *Can Vet J* 1989; **30**: 833

14 Watson DL, Franklin NA, Davies B *et al.* Survey of intramammary infections in ewes on the New England Tableland of New South Wales. *Aust Vet J* 1990; **67**: 6–8

15 Jones JET. Mastitis in sheep. In: Owen JR, Axford RFE (Eds) *Breeding for Disease Resistance in Farm Animals.* Wallingford: CAB International 1991; 412–23

16 Las Heras A, Dominguez L, Lopez M *et al.* Outbreak of acute ovine mastitis associated with *Pseudomonas aeruginosa* infection. *Vet Rec* 1999; **145**: 111–2

17 Foegeding PM, Roberts T, Bennett JM *et al. Foodborne Pathogens: Risks and Consequences,* Task Force Report no 122. Ames, Iowa: Council for Agricultural Science and Technology (CAST) 1994

18 Chapman PA, Siddons CA, Wright DJ *et al.* Cattle as a source of verocytotoxin-producing *Escherichia coli* O157 infections in man. *Epidemiol Infect* 1993; **111**: 439–47

19 Gill CO. Intrinsic bacteria in meat. *J Appl Bacteriol* 1976; **47**: 367–78

20 Corrier DE, Byrd BM, Hargis ME *et al.* Presence of *Salmonella* in crop and caeca of broiler chickens before and after preslaughter feed withdrawal. *Poult Sci* 1999; **78**: 45–9

21 Peel B, Simmons GC. Factors in the spread of *Salmonella* in the meatworks with special reference to contamination of knives. *Aust Vet J* 1978; **54**, 106–10

22 Samuel JL, O'Boyle DA, Mathers WJ, Frost AJ. Isolation of salmonella from mesenteric lymph nodes of healthy cattle at slaughter. *Res Vet Sci* 1979; **28**: 238–41

23 Hathaway SC, McKenzie AI. Postmortem meat inspection programs; separating science and tradition. *J Food Protect* 1991; **54**: 471–5

24 Berends BR, Snijders JMA, van Logtestijn JG. Efficacy of current meat inspection procedures and some proposed revisions with respect to microbiological safety: a critical review. *Vet Rec* 1993; **133**: 411–5

25 Madie P. Do we still need meat inspection? *Vet Cont Ed* 1992; **145**: 7–85

26 Hathaway S, McKenzie I, Royal WA. Cost effective meat inspection programs; separating science and tradition. *J Food Protect* 1987; **120**, 78

27 Hathaway SC, Pullen MM, McKenzie AI. A model for risk assessment of organoleptic post mortem meat inspection procedures for meat and poultry. *J Am Vet Med Assoc* 1988; **192**: 960–6

28 Edwards DS, Christiansen KH, Johnston AM, Mead GC. Determination of farm-level risk factors for abnormalities observed during post mortem meat inspection of lambs: a feasibility study. *Epidemiol Infect* 1999; **123**: 109–19

29 Fries R, Bandick A, Dahms S, Kobe A, Sommerer M, Weiss H. *Field experiments with a meat inspection system for fattening pigs in Germany.* World Congress on Food Hygiene, August 29th 1997, Den Haag, The Netherlands, 9–14

Genetically modified crops: methodology, benefits, regulation and public concerns

Nigel G Halford and **Peter R Shewry**

IACR-Long Ashton Research Station, Department of Agricultural Sciences, University of Bristol, Bristol, UK

The genetic modification of crop plants from the methodology involved in their production through to the current debate on their use in agriculture are reviewed. Techniques for plant transformation by *Agrobacterium tumefaciens* and particle bombardment, and for the selection of transgenic plants using marker genes are described. The benefits of currently available genetically modified (GM) crops in reducing waste and agrochemical use in agriculture, and the potential of the technology for further crop improvement in the future are discussed. The legal requirements for containment of novel GM crops and the roles of relevant regulatory bodies in ensuring that GM crops and food are safe are summarized. Some of the major concerns of the general public regarding GM crops and food: segregation of GM and non-GM crops and cross-pollination between GM crops and wild species, the use of antibiotic resistance marker genes, the prevention of new allergens being introduced in to the food chain and the relative safety of GM and non-GM foods are considered. Finally, the current debate on the use of GM crops in agriculture and the need for the government, scientists and industry to persevere with the technology in the face of widespread hostility is studied.

What is genetic modification?

Correspondence to:
Dr Nigel G Halford, IACR-Long Ashton Research Station, Department of Agricultural Sciences, University of Bristol, Long Ashton, Bristol BS41 9AF, UK

Plant genetic modification (also known as genetic engineering) may be defined as the manipulation of plant development, structure or composition by the insertion of specific DNA sequences. These sequences may be derived from the same species or even variety of plant. This may be done with the aim of altering the levels or patterns of expression of specific endogenous genes, in other words to make them more or less active or to alter when and where in the plant they are 'switched' on or off. Alternatively, the aim may be to change the biological (*i.e.* regulatory or catalytic) properties of the proteins that they encode. However, in many cases, the genes are derived from other species, which may be plants,

© The British Council 2000

animals or microbes, and the aim is to introduce novel biological properties or activities.

Farmers and plant-breeders have been changing the genes of crop plants for thousands of years. However, genetic modification differs from conventional plant breeding in the precision of gene transfer. Conventional breeding is based on the crossing of genotypes containing literally tens of thousands of expressed genes and the selection of progeny that combine the best features of the two parents. In some cases the progeny may contain almost equal numbers of genes from each parent. In others, an attempt may be made to incorporate a single gene from parent *a* into parent *b* by production of a hybrid followed by repeated backcrossing with parent *b* and selection of a desired trait over many generations. However, even after repeated backcrossing, it is inevitable that many undesired genes will also be transferred, and it is almost impossible to identify all of these and their products.

Conventional breeding is limited by fertility barriers that allow only plants of the same, or closely related, species to be crossed. However, 'wide crossing' with more distantly related species can be achieved if 'embryo rescue' is used to culture and regenerate embryos that would normally abort. Similarly, mutagenesis with chemical or physical mutagens can be used to induce new variation in the species of interest. Both wide crossing and mutation breeding can result in the expression in crop plants of many novel or modified genes, the effects of which cannot be assessed readily. However, both approaches are considered to be 'conventional', with no requirement for detailed assessment of the plants produced before they are introduced into the food-chain.

DNA delivery and selection of transgenic plants

Plant transformation can be divided broadly into two stages: DNA delivery and plant selection and regeneration. Two methods are widely used to deliver DNA into plant cells. The first[1] exploits nature's own genetic engineer, the naturally occurring soil bacterium *Agrobacterium tumefaciens,* which infects wounds on some plants to form a tumourous growth called a 'crown gall'. The tumour formations (Fig. 1A) result from integration of a DNA fragment (the T-DNA) from the *Agrobacterium* into the plant genome. As well as inducing tumour growth, genes present in the T-DNA cause the tumourous cells to produce compounds on which the bacteria feed. The T-DNA is present in a plasmid (the Ti or tumour-inducing plasmid), a closed circle of extra-chromosomal DNA, rather than the bacterial chromosome. This means that it can be isolated and manipulated to remove the genes that would be inserted into a plant by wild *Agrobacterium* and replace them with novel genes. After infection of plant material with the modified *Agrobacterium*, whole plants can be regenerated from the resulting genetically modified tumour-like cell clumps (callus) by application of plant hormones.

The second widely used method is particle bombardment, in which the DNA is coated onto the surface of microscopic gold particles which are then shot into plant cells using a burst of helium gas. Some of the DNA is washed off the particles and becomes integrated into the plant genome (Fig. 1C,D). As with the first method, whole plants can be regenerated from genetically modified cells by careful culturing and the application of plant hormones. This method, which has acquired the unfortunate name of biolistics, has been particularly successful in the production of genetically modified cereals[2].

A current limitation to plant genetic modification is that only some of the cells in the target tissue are genetically modified, irrespective of the method of transfer. It is, therefore, necessary to kill all of the cells that are not modified and this requires that the gene of interest be accompanied by at least one other gene that acts as a selectable marker. In practice, this is usually a gene which makes the transformed cells resistant to an antibiotic (*e.g.* kanamycin; Fig. 1B) or herbicide (*e.g.* phosphinothricin, the active ingredient of Basta; Fig. 1C) which is toxic to untransformed cells. The use of antibiotic resistance genes is discussed further below, but the presence of a selectable marker gene is currently the minimum requirement for plant transformation. A scoreable marker gene may also be present to allow the transformed cells to be visualised, and the bacterial *UidA* (gus; Fig. 1D) or the jellyfish green fluorescent protein (GFP) genes[3,4] may be used for this. However, the presence of these genes is not essential and it is accepted that they should be avoided when producing transgenic plants for food or animal feed.

Benefits of GM crops currently in commercial production and future prospects

The UK is a world leader in this technology, but at present the growing of genetically modified (GM) crops is limited to a few selected test sites. In comparison, 49 million acres of GM crops were planted in the US alone in 1998. However, three imported products from GM crops grown commercially elsewhere in the world have been approved for food use in the UK: slow-ripening tomatoes; soya that is tolerant of a broad-range herbicide (weedkiller) called glyphosate; and insect-resistant maize.

The tomatoes are used to make tomato paste, reducing waste and processing costs, and 2 million tins of clearly labelled GM tomato paste have been sold in the UK since its introduction in 1996. It has a clear consumer benefit in that it is cheaper than its non-GM competitors and of a thicker consistency. Glyphosate-tolerant crops enable farmers to use a

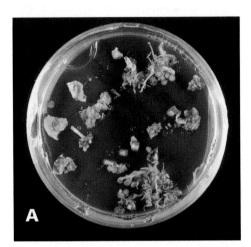

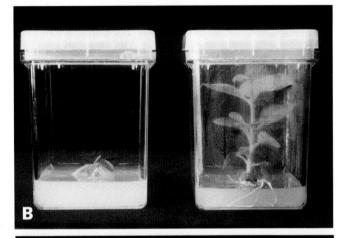

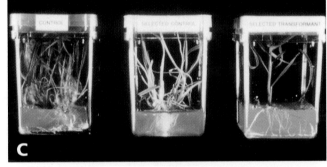

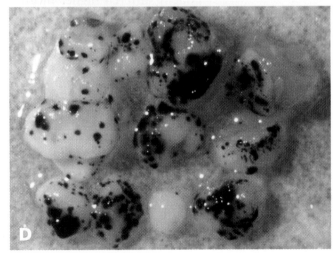

Fig. 1 Introduction of foreign DNA into plant tissue and the selection of genetically modified plants. (**A**) Undifferentiated (tumourous) potato callus tissue produced by infection of leaf discs with *Agrobacterium tumefaciens*. Some of the tissue is producing shoots in response to the application of a plant shoot-inducing hormone. (Picture courtesy of Patrick Purcell.). (**B**) Selection of transgenic plants containing an antibiotic resistance marker gene. The genetically modified tobacco plant (right) is thriving in the presence of kanamycin, whereas the unmodified control (left) is bleaching and dying. (**C**) Selection of transgenic plants containing a herbicide-tolerance marker gene. Unmodified wheat plants are shown in the absence (left) and presence (middle) of the herbicide Basta. A genetically modified wheat plant growing in the presence of the herbicide is shown on the right. (Picture courtesy of Pilar Barcelo.). (**D**) Wheat embryos showing expression of the scoreable marker gene *UidA* (gus) after its introduction by particle bombardment. The genetically modified cells make an enzyme that produces a blue product from a substrate present in the medium. (Picture courtesy of Sophie Laurie)

single, safe, rapidly-degrading herbicide instead of a battery of more expensive, more poisonous and more persistent herbicides, reducing total herbicide use by almost half in some cases[5]. They also allow farmers to use no-till agriculture, leaving the soil and weed cover undisturbed over winter, greatly reducing soil erosion and loss of groundwater, as well as providing habitats for insects and birds. Herbicide tolerant soya made up half of the US and 70% of the Argentine crop in 1998, and is popular with farmers throughout the Americas. However, the lack of a clear benefit to the consumer and the widespread, erroneous belief that use of herbicide tolerant varieties would lead to an increase in the amounts of herbicide being applied has made consumer acceptance difficult to achieve in the UK.

The maize approved for food use in the UK contains a gene (commonly called the bt gene) from a bacterium, *Bacillus thuringiensis*. The protein produced by this gene is toxic to some insects, mainly caterpillars, and the bacteria themselves have been used as an insecticide by organic farmers for decades. Variants of the bt gene have been introduced into several crops grown in the US[6], including cotton, sugar beet and potato, as well as maize. The effect of its use in cotton has perhaps been the most striking. Conventional cotton is very susceptible to insect damage and one quarter of US insecticide production is used on this one crop, including 'hard', persistent and completely unselective insecticides such as organophosphates. GM cotton on average requires 15% of the insecticide used on conventional cotton and in some areas of the US in 1996–1998 was not sprayed with insecticide at all. The bt protein does not affect bees or many other benign insects, and has no toxicity to mammals, birds or fish.

A recent study found that caterpillars of the monarch butterfly (which is not a pest species) that were forced under laboratory conditions to eat large quantities of pollen from bt maize (they would not normally eat pollen) suffered higher mortality levels than caterpillars that were not fed the pollen[7]. However, it should be remembered that spraying caterpillars and other insects with pesticide, which equates with the regimen used in the field for almost all non-GM maize, kills them all outright. Use of 'hard' pesticides, such as organophosphates, has been reduced greatly or eradicated altogether with the introduction of GM varieties.

These crops represent the first generation of GM plants in agriculture, but there are many other targets for crop biotechnology. These include other agronomic traits, such as virus resistance[8] and new quality attributes such as nutritional value, including levels of vitamins and other micro-nutrients, such as iron, iodine and folate, as well as colour and flavour. Crops will soon be available that contain modified oils[9], either tailored to meet the specific requirements of processors, or with pharmaceutical[10] or other industrial uses, such as the production of biodegradable plastics. The use of genetic modification to improve the bread-making quality of UK wheat varieties (UK and European wheats are poor in this respect) is already well advanced[11] and wheat, potato and maize are also being modified to produce starch for industrial uses. Other non-food targets include pharmaceuticals, fragrances, pigments and safe, cheap, edible vaccines[12]. The latter have already reached the human testing stage for vaccines against diarrhoea *Escherichia coli* and hepatitis B, and is obviously most relevant to those areas of the world where drugs, clean needles and syringes are not readily available.

Containment, safety assessment and the role of regulatory authorities

While recognising that GM technology is already benefiting agriculture elsewhere in the world and that the potential benefits of the technology in the UK justify supporting and investing in it, the government, scientists and industry are aware that, as with all new technologies that impact upon the environment and consumer, it should be introduced carefully. For this reason, any organization that seeks to use genetic modification, even in contained conditions, must first obtain approval from the Health and Safety Executive (HSE)[13,14]. A successful application requires that the facilities meet certain standards to ensure that GM organisms are contained, that procedures are in place for sterilization of GM material, and that there is sufficient experience in handling potentially hazardous biological material amongst the staff. Typically GM plants are kept in a greenhouse with filtered negative air pressure ventilation, sealed drains and a chlorination treatment system for drainage water.

There is also a legal requirement for the organization to assess, before beginning a GM project, whether the plants that will be produced could represent a risk to humans, other plants or the environment, including the chances and consequences of cross-pollination with other plants. The HSE inspects organizations regularly to ensure that this assessment process is being carried out satisfactorily.

Before any GM plants can be planted outside of a containment facility in the UK, permission has to be granted by the Department for the Environment, Transport and Regions (DETR)[15,16]. Applications are considered by the Advisory Committee for Release into the Environment (ACRE), an independent committee of experts who consider a similar set of questions on the safety of GM crops to those detailed above, on a case-by-case basis. As well as a detailed risk assessment, the Committee has available the data on the genetic stability and performance of the crop, obtained under contained conditions, usually over several years prior to release.

Assessment of the safety of GM foods is undertaken in the UK by the Advisory Committee on Novel Foods and Processes (ACNFP), another independent committee of experts, with members from universities and research institutes. Any GM food, no matter where it is produced, must be approved by this Committee before it is permitted to enter the UK food-chain. ACNFP requires that information be provided on the composition of materials, effects of production, stability, nutritional characteristics and the likelihood of genetic transfer. It has been argued that GM foods should be subjected to the same testing and approval procedures as medicines (*i.e.* clinical trials). The Government's view, which we share, is that this is impractical and that the methods recommended by the World Health Organization[17,18] are adequate to ensure that any possibility of an adverse effect on human health from a GM food can be detected.

Public concerns

Segregation of GM and non-GM crops and the environmental impact of cross-pollination between GM crops and wild species

Unless GM food is accepted universally, which seems unlikely in the foreseeable future, it is important that alternatives remain available to allow consumers to exercise choice. For imported food-stuffs, UK suppliers will have to contract farmers overseas to grow non-GM varieties. This means paying a guaranteed price to a farmer to use old-fashioned varieties and high chemical inputs. The additional cost will be passed on to the consumer and non-GM soya is already 40% more expensive than the GM alternative. For crops grown in the UK, the main issue will be segregation of GM and non-GM crops and food. Segregation could break down through accidental mixing of GM and non-GM seed for planting, by cross-pollination between GM and non-GM crops (which is less of a problem for inbreeding species such as wheat) or by mixing of the product between the farm gate and the consumer. Some inadvertent mixing is almost inevitable and the production of certifiably GM-free food is, therefore, likely to be expensive. Clearly, a farmer who had paid for expensive GM seed in order to produce a high-value product would wish to avoid pollination from a nearby non-GM crop, and segregation is likely to be a subject of considerable dispute.

The potential environmental impact of cross-pollination with wild species has to be assessed case-by-case, taking into account the species and genes involved. Wheat, maize and potato, for example, do not cross with any wild species in the UK (although forced crosses can be made between potato and black nightshade in the laboratory). Sugar beet crosses with wild and weed beet, but this poses little threat to agriculture. Indeed, the only major crop in which cross-pollination could be a problem is oilseed rape. This will cross with other cultivated and wild *Brassicas*, including Chinese cabbage, Brussels sprouts, Indian mustard, hoary mustard, wild radish and charlock. The extent of such crossings in agricultural systems is the subject of continuing research, but it does not necessarily mean that GM oilseed rape represents a threat, as this will also depend on whether the gene involved could confer a competitive advantage on a plant that acquired it. The issue of cross-pollination with wild species is reviewed in more detail by Raybould[19].

Antibiotic resistance marker genes

Another topic that has generated much debate, some of it wildly overblown, is the use of antibiotic resistance genes as selectable markers. The use of marker genes to select cells that have been modified with genes of interest is discussed above, and antibiotic resistance genes have been extremely valuable in the development of GM technology. Many scientific bodies around the world, including the World Health Organization and regulatory committees set up by the European Union and several national governments have considered the safety of antibiotic genes in food and have concluded that those that are being used do not represent a health threat. The British Medical Association, however, has expressed reservations[20], and the ACNFP has called for the development of alternative marker systems[21].

The main reason for believing that antibiotic resistance genes in GM crops do not represent a health threat is that they already occur in natural microbial populations, indeed they are widespread amongst soil bacteria[22]. Those that are used most frequently confer resistance to antibiotics that are not used at all in oral medical formulations, such as kanamycin and neomycin, although one notable exception to this is the insect-resistant GM maize of Novartis, which contains a gene for resistance to ampicillin. Further re-assurance can be taken from the fact that horizontal transfer of a gene from ingested plant material to bacteria has never been demonstrated, and there is no indication that it has ever occurred during evolution. The probability that it could occur is, therefore, considered to be so low that it is not relevant when compared with the natural occurrence of antibiotic resistance genes. Antibiotic resistant strains of pathogenic bacteria do represent a health threat, but they arise naturally and thrive because of the sloppy management of antibiotics in human and animal medicine, not because of the use of antibiotic resistance marker genes in biotechnology.

Allergenicity

It has been suggested that consumption of GM foods could lead to increases in toxicity and allergenicity. This is particularly relevant to the use of protective proteins to confer resistance to pests and pathogens as these can reasonably be expected to also show some toxicity to humans. In addition, there was a widely reported case where a methionine-rich 2S albumin storage protein from Brazil nut was expressed in soybean in order to increase the methionine content for animal feed[23]. The protein was subsequently shown to be an allergen, as are a number of related 2S albumins from other species. The plant breeding programme was, therefore, discontinued as it would be difficult to guarantee that the GM soya would not enter the human food chain. This case certainly illustrates the potential for introducing allergens and toxins by genetic modification. However, the fact that the problem was identified before commercial material was produced, and appropriate action taken, demonstrates the high level of awareness of such problems in the plant

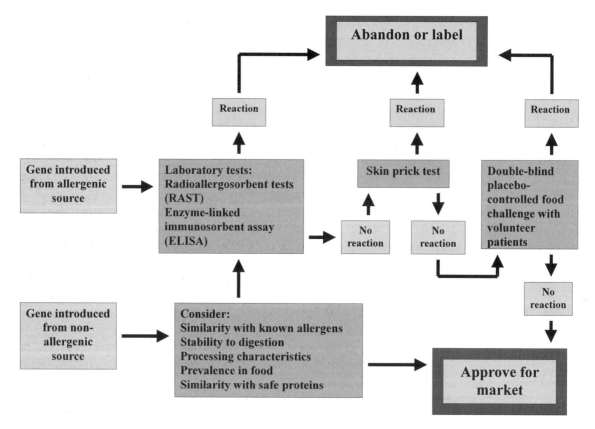

Fig. 2 Flow diagram showing the assessment and testing of possible allergenicity in GM foods. Redrawn from Astwood *et al*[24], with the publisher's permission.

biotechnology industry and the effectiveness of 'in house' screening programmes. A typical procedure used to test for the presence of food allergens in transgenic plants is summarized in Figure 2, while the application of this procedure to the GM soybeans containing the Brazil nut 2S albumin is described by Nordlee et al[23]. The biotechnology industry takes the view that release of new allergenic products into the food chain is entirely avoidable[24] and the legal requirements for feeding trials provide an additional, effective safety net. Consequently, GM foods may well prove to be safer than those produced by conventional plant breeding, as discussed below.

Relative safety of GM foods compared with 'traditional' foods

The major arable and horticultural crops grown and consumed in Western Europe have been developed using conventional breeding methods, often over centuries or even millennia. Consequently, they are assumed by the consumer to be safe and wholesome. However, most, if not all, of these crops contain compounds that are potentially toxic or allergenic. In most cases, these compounds have probably evolved to provide protection against animal predators or pathogenic micro-organisms and it is, therefore, not surprising that they are also toxic to humans. Furthermore, they are particularly abundant in seeds and tubers, whose rich reserves of proteins, starch and oil are particularly attractive to pests and pathogens. Well-known examples are glyco-alkaloids in potatoes, cyanogenic glycosides in linseed, glucosinolates in *Brassica* oilseeds and proteinase inhibitors in soybean and other legume seeds. It is very doubtful whether these, or many other generally accepted foods, would be approved for food use were the toxins introduced by genetic modification. Similarly, the introduction of new types and varieties of food crops produced by conventional breeding requires no specific testing for the presence of allergens and toxins, although genes may have been introduced from exotic varieties or related wild species. Toxins can also be produced by fungal activity before harvesting or during storage. Ironically, these mycotoxins, including dangerous carcinogens such as aflotoxin, are particularly prevalent in organic food, which has not been treated with fungicides.

It is clear that the public requires a higher level of assessment of the safety of GM food than conventional or organic foods and this is only possible because genetic modification is such a precise process. The products of the introduced genes are readily identified and their expression levels determined. The products may also be isolated in a pure form, either from the species of origin, from the transformed plant or after expression in a micro-organism. The pure protein can then be tested in detail and its presence in processed foods monitored. In contrast, it is virtually impossible to identify and characterize the changes in food composition that may result from conventional plant breeding. Consequently, we would argue that GM foods may be safer than food derived from non-GM varieties as the risks are readily quantified and monitored and GM foods are examined under a rigorous assessment system that goes beyond that applied to other foods.

Concluding remarks

Despite the safeguards applied to GM crops and foods, and the clear benefits that they are bringing, public acceptance in the UK is currently low. There are several reasons for this, including unease about food safety in general, caused by factors (BSE, *E. coli*, Salmonella, *etc*) that have nothing to do with GM, lack of information on the benefits, a well-organized anti-GM campaign lead by professional, multinational pressure groups (who have no responsibility for food production), and a succession of wild scare-stories. Much of the debate revolves around products that are not, and may never be, commercially available, the infamous 'terminator' crops and tomatoes containing fish genes being good examples. The industry itself must also accept much of the blame for public hostility, since the lack of labelling of GM products between late 1996 and 1999 led to the perception amongst the public that the technology was being imposed on them.

Governments continue to support research and development in plant biotechnology in the face of this hostility, and there are strong arguments to support this position. The most obvious is that GM crops are now well-established and very successful in large areas of the world, particularly the Americas and China, and other European countries are spending heavily in order to catch up with the UK and US in the science. GM crops are already playing a part in increased yields, improving nutritional quality, increasing the profitability of agriculture and reducing its dependence on high chemical inputs. It is almost inconceivable that this revolution in agriculture could be reversed at this late stage. Sooner or later, we will have to allow UK farmers to grow GM varieties if they are to compete.

References

1   Bevan M. Binary *Agrobacterium* vectors for plant transformations. *Nucl Acids Res* 1984; **12**: 8711–21
2   Barcelo P, Hagel C, Becker D, Martin A, Lorz H. Transgenic cereal (*Tritordeum*) plants obtained at high efficiency by microprojectile bombardment of inflorescence tissue. *Plant J* 1994; **5**: 583–92

3   Jefferson RA, Kavanagh TA, Bevan MW. Gus fusions: β-glucuronidase as a sensitive and versatile gene fusion marker in higher plants. *EMBO J* 1987; **6**: 3559–64

4   Tsien RY. The green fluorescent protein. *Annu Rev Biochem* 1998; **67**: 509–44

5   Dewar AM, Haylock LA, Bean KM, May MJ. Delayed control of weeds in glyphosphate-tolerant sugar beet and the consequences on aphid infestation and yield. Pest Manag Sci 2000; 56: 345–50.

6   de Maagd RA, Bosch D, Stiekema W. *Bacillus thuringiensis* toxin-mediated insect resistance in plants. *Trends Plant Sci* 1999; **4**: 9–13

7   Losey JE, Rayor LS, Carter ME. Transgenic pollen harms monarch larvae. *Nature* 1999; **399**; 214

8   Sangare A, Deng D, Fauquet CM, Beachy RN. Resistance to African cassava mosaic virus conferred by a mutant of the putative NTP-binding domain of the Rep gene (AC1) in *Nicotiana benthamania*. *Mol Breeding* 1999; **5**: 95–102

9   Napier JA, Michaelson LV, Stobart AK. Plant desaturases: harvesting the fat of the land. *Curr Opin Plant Biol* 1999; **2**: 123–7

10 Sayanova O, Smith MA, Lapinskas P *et al*. Expression of a borage desaturase cDNA containing an N-terminal cytochrome b(5) domain results in the accumulation of high levels of delta(6)-desaturated fatty acids in transgenic tobacco. *Proc Natl Acad Sci USA* 1997; **94**: 4211–6

11 Barro F, Rooke L, Bekes F *et al*. Transformation of wheat with high molecular weight subunit genes results in improved functional properties. *Biotechnology* 1997; **15**: 1295–9

12 Mor TS, Gomez Lim MA, Palmer KE. Perspective: edible vaccines - a concept coming of age. *Trends Microbiol* 1998; **6**: 449–53

13 Health and Safety Commission. *Genetically Modified Organisms (Contained Use) Regulations 1992 (SI 1992 No. 3217)*. London: HSE Books, 1992

14 Health and Safety Commission. *Genetically Modified Organisms (Contained Use) (Amendment) Regulations 1996 (SI 1996 No. 967)*. London: HSE Books, 1996

15 Department of Environment. *Genetically Modified Organisms (Deliberate Release) Regulations 1992 (SI 1992 No. 3280)*. London: DoE, 1992

16 Department of Environment. *Genetically Modified Organisms (Deliberate Release) (Amendment) Regulations 1996 (SI 1996 No. 304)*. London: DoE, 1996

17 Jonas D, Kaferstein FK. Genetic modification and food safety. *Biotech Dev Monit* 1995; **25**: 11–2

18 World Health Organization. *Application of the principles of substantial equivalence to the safety evaluation of foods or food components from plants derived by modern biotechnology*. Report of a WHO Workshop. WHO/FNU/FOS/95.1. Geneva: WHO, 1995

19 Raybould AF. Transgenes and agriculture – going with the flow? *Trends Plant Sci* 1999; **4**: 247–8

20 British Medical Association. *The Impact of Genetic Modification on Agriculture, Food and Health*. London: BMA, 1999

21 Advisory Committee on Novel Foods and Processes. *Report on the use of antibiotic resistance markers in genetically modified food organisms*. London: ACNFP, 1994

22 Bushby HVA. Quantitative estimation of rhizobia in non-sterile soil using antibiotics and fungicides. *Soil Biol Biochem* 1981; **13**: 237–9

23 Nordlee JA, Taylor SL, Townsend JA, Thomas LA, Bush RK. Identification of a Brazil nut allergen in transgenic soybeans. *N Engl J Med* 1996; **334**: 688–92

24 Astwood JD, Fuchs RL, Lavrik PB. Food biotechnology and genetic engineering. In: Metcalfe DD, Sampson HA, Simon RA (Eds) *Food Allergy*, 2nd edn. New York: Blackwell, 1996

Microbiological safety of water

D J Dawson* and **D P Sartory†**

Campden & Chorleywood Food Research Association, Chipping Campden, Gloucestershire, UK and †Quality and Environmental Services, Severn Trent Water Ltd, Shrewsbury, UK

Significant advances in water treatment over the last century have resulted in massive improvements in the microbiological safety of public drinking water supplies in the UK and the developed countries. Incidences of illness due to poor treatment or post-treatment contamination are rare, but when they occur tend to attract considerable media attention. A well managed water treatment works and supply system can provide high quality drinking water wherever in the world it is located. As a rule, throughout the world, private supplies tend to be of a poorer quality than public supplies, but poorly managed public supplies have the potential to make a large number of people ill and continued effort is needed to maintain and improve drinking water quality world-wide.

The history of water safety

The development of public water supplies, first seen in ancient times, assumed greater importance with the progressive increase in urbanisation. A public water supply has potentially great advantages, not only due to the convenience it brings but also in terms of health benefits deriving from its use in washing and cleaning. Potentially, however, a public water supply can be a risk to the health of large numbers of people due to the size of population exposed should contamination occur. This has been borne out by recorded outbreaks of disease, classically the outbreaks of cholera in European cities in the 19th century.

The first clear documented proof that public water supplies could be a source of infection for humans came from epidemiological studies of cholera carried out by Dr John Snow in the 1850s. Snow's study of an outbreak of cholera associated with a public water pump in Broad Street, London and his removal of the handle is the most famous, but his epidemiological study of the water supply areas of two London water companies is perhaps a more definitive piece of work. At that time, water was supplied to London by a number of small companies, many taking their water directly from the Thames. The Southwark and Vauxhall company obtained its water from the Thames at Battersea, whilst the Lambeth company obtained its water again from the Thames, but a

Correspondence to:
DJ Dawson, Campden & Chorleywood Food Research Association, Chipping Campden, Gloucestershire GL55 6LD, UK

© The British Council 2000

considerable distance upstream, above the major sources of pollution from human sewage. In one particular area of about 300,000 residents, the pipes of both companies were laid in the streets with houses connected to one or other source of supply. Snow's analysis of cholera deaths showed striking results: houses served by the Lambeth company had a lower incidence of cholera than the city of London in general, whereas those served by the Southwark and Vauxhall company had a very high incidence. As the other factors, including socio-economic conditions, were identical for each of the populations served by the two companies, Snow concluded that the water supply was the route by which the cholera agent was transmitted.

It is noteworthy that this work was carried out before the germ theory of disease had been fully developed, principally through the work of Robert Koch and Louis Pasteur. The causative agent of cholera, *Vibrio cholerae*, was finally isolated by Robert Koch some 30 years later in 1883. By the end of the 19th century the presence of the causative agents of the classical waterborne diseases of cholera, typhoid and dysentery had been identified in the faeces of patients, re-inforcing the link between faecally contaminated water and these diseases. Since that time, it has been recognised that the key to microbiologically safe drinking water is the exclusion of faecal contamination from the supply.

Outbreaks of cholera and typhoid in the 19th and the early 20th centuries led to the wide-spread use of filtration to treat water supplies followed by the gradual introduction of the use of chlorine, usually on an intermittent basis, from 1910 onwards. The Croydon typhoid outbreak in 1937 led to continuous chlorination of water being used almost universally on public supplies, the exception being those well or borehole sources with excellent microbiological quality. Today, all public water supplies in the UK contain disinfectant, normally chlorine, at a low level at the customer's tap. This helps to protect against contamination, which may occur if the integrity of the distribution system is breached (*e.g.* through burst mains or cross contamination).

The principles of water treatment were established in the 19th and early 20th centuries with surface water sources being subject to coagulation and filtration processes (or just filtration) to remove particles including bacteria, and a disinfection stage or stages to make the water microbiologically safe. Underground sources subject to natural filtration are typically of very high quality and normally a simple disinfection stage is sufficient. The introduction of variations to the treatment processes and alternative disinfectants, such as ozone and UV irradiation, resulted in a variety of options being available to treatment engineers. Traditional processes still form the core of advanced treatment today and it is their legacy that has made public supplies largely compliant with modern water quality standards in many countries.

Bacteriological indicators of contamination

Towards the end of the 19th century, it was increasingly realised that some bacteria were specifically associated with faecal matter, most notably *Bacterium coli* described by Theodore Escherich in 1885. As this organism appeared to occur in great numbers in all faeces, particularly compared to the enteric pathogens, it was suggested that detection of this *B. coli* in water would be indicative of the presence of faecal matter and, hence, the possible presence of enteric pathogens. Testing was based on the detection of fermentation of lactose at 37°C, characteristic of the organism. Over the years, however, it became apparent that *B. coli* was actually a group of closely related bacteria, the principal species of which is now named *Escherichia coli*, and the others are collectively known as the 'coliforms'. These bacteria are facultative anaerobes and tolerant of bile salts. *E. coli* is differentiated from the other coliforms by being able to ferment lactose and produce indole from tryptophan at 44°C. Although methods of isolation have changed over recent years, *E. coli* has remained the principal indicator of faecal pollution.

E. coli has, at least in temperate climates, the characteristics desirable of an indicator organism (*i.e.* it should be abundant in faeces, capable of easy isolation and examination and should not grow in the aquatic environment). In recent years, the enterococci, faecal bacteria of the genera *Enterococcus* and *Streptococcus*, have also been given a significant status as faecal indicators.

The use of bacterial indicators for drinking water quality assessment is well established and national and international standards have been established based upon them. Typically standards require that in supplied water *E. coli*, coliforms and enterococci are not detected in 100 ml samples taken on a regular basis. If these organisms are present in raw (untreated) water and can be shown to be absent in treated water from a particular treatment works, it is assumed that they have been removed successfully. The indicator principle assumes that any pathogenic organisms will also have been removed through the treatment works. It has been generally acknowledged that it is not normally practical to look for pathogens themselves in water due to the nature of the methods and the low levels that might be found.

This maxim generally holds and has helped to protect public health over many years. Outbreaks of bacterial enteritis linked to public supplies are very rare nowadays, only occurring when there has been gross post-treatment contamination of a supply. In some situations, however, it has been recognised that it is worth looking directly for pathogens, particularly in the case of the protozoan *Cryptosporidium*[1]. This organism has only been considered a significant pathogen of humans since 1976 and particularly following the advent of AIDS in the late

1970s. Waterborne outbreaks have been documented from the early 1980s onwards. As regards water treatment, it is removed in coagulation and filtration processes, but is very resistant to chlorine and, therefore, an absence of faecal indicators does not necessarily indicate an absence of *Cryptosporidium*.

Drinking water standards

Quantitative standards for water quality first emerged during the early part of this century. In the US, a bacteriological standard of less than 1 coliform per 100 ml was first expressed in 1914. In 1934, the first edition of the *Bacteriological Examination of Water Supplies* was published in the UK. This has become the primary reference for water microbiologists in this and many other countries and the sixth edition, under the title *The Microbiology of Water 1994: Part 1 – Drinking Water* was published in 1994[2]. (It is currently undergoing revision with regard to the forthcoming implementation of the new EU Directive on drinking water quality.) This document is referenced alongside the current regulatory standards and is useful for understanding the principles of drinking water microbiology in both regulatory and non-regulatory situations. Another key source of information is the World Health Organization's *Guidelines for Drinking Water Quality*, first published in 1984. An updated version of this 3 volume work was completed in 1996[3]. These volumes include detailed information on microbiological and chemical parameters and their pathogenic and toxic effects.

From these WHO guidelines (and their predecessors), standards have been derived in different parts of the world. These guidelines are not standards in themselves and must be dealt with in the context of the country in which they are employed. The EU Directive on drinking water quality, which was strongly influenced by WHO guidelines, was published in 1980[4] and led to a revision of the *Microbiology of Drinking Water* and ultimately in the UK, to the Water Supply (Water Quality) Regulations in 1989[5]. A new directive was adopted in 1998 which is expected to be implemented into national law in member states by the year 2000[6].

Obviously, it is not enough to have standards to work to in order to have safe drinking water; there must be an appropriate level of monitoring and reporting. The UK regulations contain comprehensive information on monitoring frequencies at treatment works, service reservoirs and consumer taps. The frequency of monitoring at treatment works depends upon the volume of water produced by that works and, in the case of customer taps, the volume of water or the population supplied within defined water supply zones. These are geographical areas with populations of less than 50,000 and containing reasonably uniform quality issues.

In England and Wales, the Drinking Water Inspectorate (DWI) is responsible for monitoring compliance with the regulations and a report on compliance is issued annually by the Chief Inspector. Compliance with UK legislation is very high, with 99.9% of samples being free from *E. coli*. In addition to the role of the DWI, health authorities are kept informed of abnormal water quality, which may affect public health, through the Consultants in Communicable Disease Control (CsCDC). Whereas chemical standards are set on a basis of life-time exposure and an occasional exceedence is not necessarily serious, microbiological standards are set on their potential immediate impact and the presence of *E. coli* in treated water is viewed very seriously. Depending on the situation, the finding of *E. coli* by water companies may lead to an advisory boil water notice being issued. Boil water notices have no legal status and the issuing of them is under the control of the water company, although the health authorities are often closely involved with the decision. Serious pollution incidents of drinking water may lead to the setting up of an Incident Management Team or Outbreak Control Team depending on the nature of the contamination. Representatives of water companies, health authorities and environmental health departments would all sit on such a group.

The Secretary of State (in reality the DWI) may take enforcement action if compliance with regulatory standards is breached. In practice, this does not occur if breaches are minor and trivial or if the water company makes immediate attempts to rectify problems. Enforcement action, if it does occur, involves the water company preparing a timetable of improvements to ensure that non-compliance with regulatory standards is halted. Under section 70 of the Water Industry Act 1991[7], the criminal charge of supplying water unfit for human consumption was introduced. Due diligence is allowable as a defence. Successful prosecutions have been brought against several water companies for supplying highly turbid water, alkaline water and water with a discernible chemical taste . In these cases, there is no evidence that the water was unsafe, but the water was deemed unfit for consumption in that customers felt that they could not use the water for drinking and domestic purposes. Prosecutions due to failure of bacteriological standards are extremely uncommon. In February 1999, a major water utility pleaded guilty of supplying raw river water to two properties in November and December 1997[8]. This was due to contractors connecting the water supply of the properties to a raw water pipe from the river to a reservoir by error. In this case, the water contained high levels of faecal bacteria.

Mechanical damage to a water main may cause depressurisation and could allow ingress of environmental material, although in the vast majority of cases the damaged main will still retain enough pressure to exclude extraneous material. It can be isolated and repaired without contaminated water reaching the consumer. During planned depressurisations for repair, relining or replacement, the risk of water contamination is minimised by specific hygiene procedures being followed by the water companies. These are developed in line with advice and key guideline documents, which require disinfection, flushing and sampling before the water mains are brought back into service. Water in the distribution network is also vulnerable to contamination if mismanaged on a customer's premises (*e.g.* an industrial site beyond the responsibility of the supplier). Mains water may be particularly vulnerable to contamination if the supply is in contact with contaminated water in a factory without the appropriate safety devices being fitted to prevent back-flow or back siphonage. Regulations are implemented by water companies to prevent wastage or contamination of water. Where water companies believe that regulations may be being broken, they may carry out inspections and insist on corrective work being carried out. Prosecution of industrial users is also an option.

World-wide, the situation exists whereby WHO guidelines on water quality are used to generate national regulations. In many cases, countries work directly to WHO guidelines. However, even if standards exist it does not mean they are being met. In many cases, the monitoring may be limited and this fact, combined with lack of data on compliance, makes it unclear how good drinking water quality is.

Private supplies in the UK are defined in the Water Industry Act 1991 as any supplies of water provided otherwise than by a statutorily approved water undertaker. The Private Supplies Regulations 1991[9] made under the Act require local authorities to take samples at certain frequencies dependent upon the size of supply. They also have powers to require improvements to be applied to unwholesome supplies. Although the standards set for private supplies are equivalent to those for public supplies, in practice the overall quality of private supplies is not nearly as good. Although some private supplies are well managed and produce excellent quality water, many will show intermittent faecal pollution. Since the monitoring of smaller private supplies is very infrequent, this may not be registered in analytical results and, even if it is, householders may not fit appropriate treatment to these water systems. This underlines the situation that the presence of standards does not necessarily guarantee good quality water.

The risk from contaminated water systems

Public health surveillance requires the monitoring of waterborne disease, but in practice the detection of many incidents is difficult. In England and

LIVERPOOL JOHN MOORES UNIVERSITY
LEARNING SERVICES

Wales, possible waterborne outbreaks are identified by health officials at a local level, *e.g.* through the CsCDC or Directors of Public Health. The Communicable Disease Surveillance Centre (CDSC) receives information from various sources about clusters of cases in England and Wales and the Drinking Water Inspectorate also has an interest in possible waterborne outbreaks.

Although after outbreaks have been identified there may be a hypothesis that water is associated with the illness, it is very difficult to prove beyond reasonable doubt that such a hypothesis is correct. Several factors contribute to this. Firstly, water samples are often taken retrospectively and samples taken from the time of the exposure are rarely available. Secondly, some organisms may be difficult to detect and, thirdly, case control studies on water supplies are hampered by the fact that most people have some exposure to water, even if only through washing vegetables or brushing teeth. This means that in a case control study when a population within an area has been ill, it will often be found that most of the population has been exposed to the risk factor under investigation. This is a very different scenario from a classic case control study where the cases have all visited for example a particular food outlet. It is thought that in the case of *Cryptosporidium*, that populations drinking certain water supplies may be exposed repeatedly to oocyst antigens and, therefore, develop some protective immunity. Outbreaks within the population may then reflect not only the possibility of higher levels of oocysts in the supply but variability in the immunity and exposure of the population, which may be hard to quantify[10]. Nevertheless, epidemiological studies can be used in certain cases to implicate the water supply; for example, when an outbreak can be traced to a particular treatment works where a population as a whole received various water sources.

Case control studies on an outbreak of cryptosporidiosis in Bradford in 1992 using both laboratory and neighbourhood controls showed an association between development of cryptosporidiosis and the consumption of unboiled tap water from the suspected treatment works[11]. In the instance of the North London 1997 outbreak, a case control study similarly indicated a link between the outbreak and tap water from a particular treatment works[12]. Various blends of this borehole water were supplied to different areas. Dose response data in both outbreaks and elsewhere, were used to indicate that water was the likely source of the pathogen, with increasing likelihood of illness being associated with higher consumption of the contaminated water. In the Bradford outbreak, there was a significant association between the amount of water usually drunk and the likelihood of illness. In the North London outbreak, a chi-squared test for trend with tap water consumed at home showed that the proportion of cases in the case control study increased significantly with consumption. The main problem with this sort of data is that there is a potential for significant recall bias by consumers. This is much less of a problem in the case of an outbreak being linked to a particular food outlet.

Problems with the recognition of water-borne disease has led to assignment of categories to disease outbreaks by the CDSC and the terms strongly, probably and possibly are used to describe association with water[13]. The criteria for classification of outbreaks under these descriptions are:

Strong association with water

Three scenarios exist for this category. In the first two, the pathogen in clinical cases must be found in the water, either in combination with analytical epidemiological evidence, or with descriptive epidemiology and the absence of an obvious alternative cause. In the third scenario, an analytical epidemiological study implicates the water supply and there have been water quality and/or water treatment problems but the pathogen has not been detected in water.

Probable association with water

This category includes the combination where descriptive epidemiology is good, there is no obvious alternative explanation and there is also evidence of water treatment and/or water quality problems. It also covers scenarios where analytical epidemiology has been carried out or the particular pathogen is found in the water in the absence of other evidence.

Possible association with water

Possible outbreaks are ones which occur in association with water quality and/or treatment problems but where there is no pathogen found in the water and no supporting epidemiology, or where descriptive epidemiology stands on its own without other evidence.

Outbreaks of water-borne disease

Although drinking water generally meets regulatory standards in developed countries and diseases such as typhoid and cholera are no longer spread by this route, there have still been outbreaks of water-borne gastrointestinal infection in countries with the most advanced water treatment systems. Outbreaks caused by protozoan pathogens such as *Giardia* and *Cryptosporidium*, bacteria such as *E. coli* O157 and

Campylobacter spp. and various viruses have been documented in recent years. Incidents involving water supplies typically attract considerable high profile media and public attention, giving the impression that water-borne outbreaks are common. In reality illness rates from contaminated water are a very small part of the disease burden in the UK.

In the last 10–15 years, *Cryptosporidium* has been the prime cause of water-borne disease associated with mains water supplies. This organism is very resistant to conventional disinfectants and can occur in mains supplies if water treatment is not fully effective. It is also a major problem in private water supplies. A study of 19 outbreaks due to drinking water in England and Wales between 1992 and 1995 comprised 10 outbreaks due to public supplies and 9 outbreaks due to private supplies[14]. The 10 outbreaks in public supplies were all caused by *Cryptosporidium*. Under the definitions ascribed by the CDSC, 7 were 'probably' associated with water and 3 'strongly' associated with water, including the Bradford outbreak previously mentioned.

Of the 9 outbreaks in private supplies, 5 were described as 'strongly', 2 'probably' and 2 'possibly' associated with water. In one outbreak, no pathogen was identified whilst the others involved *Campylobacter* spp. alone (5 outbreaks) *Cryptosporidium* alone (1 outbreak) or a combination of the two (1 outbreak). *Giardia* was identified as a cause of one outbreak in a Worcestershire village where the likely cause was direct faecal contamination of a shallow spring supply by grazing animals[15].

Water-borne disease from pathogenic *E. coli* strains is more likely in private rather than public supplies. Recent work has shown that this organism is as susceptible to chlorine as other *E. coli*[16]. In one recorded incident, isolation of *E. coli* O157:H7 from a well water in Canada was linked to a case of bloody diarrhoea in a 16-month-old child where water was the most likely route of infection[17]. In 1995, contaminated stream water was accidentally pumped by a local business into the mains supply of a village in Scotland resulting in 6 confirmed cases of *E. coli* O157 infection, 8 confirmed cases of *Campylobacter* spp. infection and 633 other people reporting gastrointestinal upset[18].

Outbreaks caused by small round structured or Norwalk type viruses have been described. In a 1994 incident, evidence suggested transfer of viruses from contaminated water into custard slices in a South Wales factory[19]. The mains water may have been contaminated due to an illegal connection between a pipe carrying river water and the mains water on the same industrial estate. Difficulties in the isolation of enteric viruses from environmental samples reduce the chances of demonstrating a link between water and viral illness; however, there is no suggestion from surveillance data that water-borne viral illness is nearly as prevalent as water-borne cryptosporidiosis.

References

1   Anon. *Cryptosporidium in Water Supplies*. Third Report of the Group of Experts to: Department of the Environment, Transport and the Regions & Department of Health. ISBN 1 85112 131 5, 1998

2   Anon. *The Microbiology of Water 1994, Part 1-Drinking Water*. Report on Public Health and Medical subjects. No. 71 Methods for the examination of waters and associated materials. London: Stationery Office, 1994

3   Anon. *Guidelines for Drinking Water Quality*. World Health Organisation International Programme on Chemical Safety. Geneva: WHO, 1996

4   Council Directive 80/778/EEC of 15 July 1980 relating to the quality of water intended for human consumption. *Official J EC* 1996; **L229**: 11–9

5   *The Water Supply (Water Quality) Regulations 1989*. Statutory Instrument No. 1147. London: HMSO, 1989

6   Council Directive of 98/83/EC of 3 November 1998 on the quality of water intended for human consumption. *Official J EC* 1998; **L330**: 32–54

7   *The Water Industry Act 1991*. London: HMSO, 1991

8   Anon. Anglian Water pleads guilty to charges of supplying water unfit for human consumption. Press Notice 110, 8 February 1999. Department of the Environment, Transport and the Regions, http://www.nds.coi.gov.uk/coi/coipress.nsf, 1999

9   *The Private Water Supplies Regulations 1991*. Statutory Instrument No. 2790. London: HMSO, 1991

10 Hunter PR, Quigley C. Investigation of an outbreak of cryptosporidiosis associated with treated surface water finds limits to the value of case control studies. *Communicable Dis Public Health* 1998; **1**: 234–8

11 Atherton F, Newman CPS, Casemore DP. An outbreak of waterborne cryptosporidiosis associated with a public water supply in the UK. *Epidemiol Infect* 1995; **115**: 123–31

12 Gray MJ. *Assessment of water supply and associated matters in relation to the incidence of cryptosporidiosis in West Herts and North London in February and March 1997*. Drinking Water Inspectorate, Department of the Environment, Transport and the Regions, Welsh Office, 1995

13 Tillett HE, de Louvois J, Wall PG. Surveillance of outbreaks of waterborne infectious disease: categorising levels of evidence. *Epidemiol Infect* 1998; **120**: 37–42

14 Furtado C, Adak GK, Stuart JM, Wall PG, Evans HS, Casemore DP. Outbreaks of waterborne infectious intestinal disease in England and Wales, 1992–5. *Epidemiol Infect* 1998; **121**: 109–19

15 Constantine CL, Hales D, Dawson DJ. Outbreak of giardiasis caused by a contaminated private supply in the Worcester area. In: Betts WB, Casemore D, Fricker C, Smith H, Watkins J (Eds) *Protozoan Parasites and Water*. London: Royal Society of Chemistry, 1994; 50-2

16 Kaneko M. Chlorination of pathogenic *E. coli* O157. *Water Sci Technol* 1998; **38**: 141–4

17 Jackson SG, Goodbrand RB, Johnson RP *et al*. *Escherichia coli* O157:H7 diarrhoea associated with well water and infected cattle on an Ontario farm. *Epidemiol Infect* 1998; **120**: 17–20

18 Jones IG, Roworth M. An outbreak of *Escherichia coli* O157 and campylobacteriosis associated with contamination of a drinking water supply. *Public Health* 1996; **110**: 277–82

19 Brugha A, Vipond IB, Evans MR *et al*. A community outbreak of food borne small round–structured virus gastroenteritis caused by a contaminated water supply. *Epidemiol Infect* 1999; **122**: 145–54

Preservation: past, present and future

Grahame W Gould

Formerly Unilever Research Laboratory, Colworth House, Bedford, UK

Foods deteriorate in quality due to a wide range of reactions including some that are physical, some that are chemical, some enzymic and some microbiological. The various forms of spoilage and food poisoning caused by micro-organisms are preventable to a large degree by a number of preservation techniques, most of which act by preventing or slowing microbial growth. These include freezing, chilling, drying, curing, conserving, vacuum packing, modified atmosphere packing, acidifying, fermenting, and adding preservatives. In contrast, a smaller number of techniques act by inactivating micro-organisms, predominantly heating (pasteurization and sterilization). Complementary techniques restrict access of micro-organisms to food products, e.g. aseptic processing and packaging. New and 'emerging' preservation techniques include more that act by inactivation. They include the application of ionizing radiation, high hydrostatic pressure, high voltage electric discharges, high intensity light, ultrasonication in combination with heat and slightly raised pressure ('manothermosonication'), and the addition to foods of bacteriolytic enzymes, bacteriocins, and other naturally-occurring antimicrobials. Major trends, reacting to consumers' needs, are towards the use of procedures that deliver food products that are less 'heavily' preserved, higher quality, more convenient, more 'natural', freer from additives, nutritionally healthier, and still with high assurance of microbiological safety.

With few exceptions, all foods deteriorate in quality following harvest, slaughter or manufacture, in a manner that is dependent on food type and composition, formulation (of manufactured foods) and storage conditions. The principal quality deterioration reactions, which are, therefore, the principal targets for preservation, are well known and relatively few (Table 1). They include some that are essentially microbiological, others that are chemical, enzymic or physical[1]. When preservation fails, the consequences range from extreme hazard, *e.g.* if any toxinogenic micro-organisms are not controlled, to relatively trivial loss of quality such as loss of colour or flavour. The most serious forms of quality deterioration include those due to micro-organisms, following the survival and/or growth of infectious pathogenic bacteria or the growth of toxinogenic ones[2]. The major food poisoning bacteria are listed in Table 2,

Correspondence to:
Prof. Grahame W Gould,
17 Dove Road, Bedford
MK41 7AA, UK

© The British Council 2000

Table 1 Principal quality deterioration reactions of foods

Microbiological	Enzymic	Chemical	Physical
Growth or presence of toxinogenic micro-organisms	Hydrolytic reactions catalysed by lipases, proteases, *etc.*	Oxidative rancidity	Mass transfer, movement of low MW compounds
Growth or presence of infective micro-organisms	Rancidity catalysed by lipoxygenases	Oxidative and reductive discolouration	Loss of crisp textures
Growth of spoilage micro-organisms	Enzymic browning	Non-enzymic browning	Loss of flavours
		Destruction of nutrients	Freeze-induced structural damage

Adapted from Gould[1].

along with their abilities to grow at low, chill cabinet/refrigerator temperatures, and their resistance to heating, *e.g.* during cooking in the home or food service establishment, or during processing in the factory[3].

Table 2 Major food poisoning bacteria and their temperature relationships

Minimum growth temperature	Heat resistance	
	Low[a]	High[b]
Low (0–5°C or so)		
Listeria monocytogenes (INF)[c]	*Clostridium botulinum* E and non-proteolytic B and F(TOX)[d]	
Yersinia enterocolitica (INF)		*Bacillus cereus* (INF and TOX)
		Bacillus subtilis (TOX)
Aeromonas hydrophila (INF)		*Bacillus licheniformis* (TOX)
Medium (5–10°C or so)		
Salmonella species (INF)		
Vibrio parahaemolyticus (INF)		
Escherichia coli enteropathogenic and verocytotoxigenic strains (INF)		
Staphylococcus aureus (TOX)		
Medium (10–15°C or so)		
		Clostridium botulinum A and proteolytic B (TOX)
		Clostridium perfringens (INF)
High (over 30°C)		
Campylobacter jejuni and *coli* (INF)		

[a]In excess of a 10⁶-fold inactivation of vegetative micro-organisms by pasteurization, e.g. at a temperature of about 70°C for 2 min.
[b]In excess of a 10⁶-fold inactivation of spores at temperatures ranging from about 90°C for most heat-sensitive types to about 120°C for 10 min for the most heat-tolerant types.
[c]INF – organisms that may contaminate foods, and may multiply in them, and which cause food poisoning by infection.
[d]TOX – organisms that may contaminate foods and multiply in them to form toxins that then cause food poisoning by intoxication.
Adapted from Russell and Gould[15].

Table 3 Changing consumer requirements and food industry reactions

Trends in consumer requirements

Improved convenience

Higher quality	– in preparation; storage; shelf-life
Fresher	– in flavour; texture; appearance
More natural	– with fewer additives
Nutritionally healthier	
Minimally packaged	
Safer	

Food industry reactions

Milder processing	– minimal over-heating
	– less intensive heating
	– non-thermal alternatives to heat
Fewer additives	– less 'chemical' preservatives

Use of 'hurdle' technologies or 'combination preservation' systems

Development and use of predictive models

- growth models, as a function of pH, a_w, temperature, preservatives
- survival models, as above
- thermal death models

Evaluation of natural antimicrobial systems as food preservatives

Less use of salt, saturated fats, sugar; more low calorie foods

Reduced, environmentally-friendly packaging

Elimination of food poisoning micro-organisms

Adapted from Gould[4].

Changes in the requirements of consumers in recent years have included a desire for foods which are more convenient, higher quality, fresher, more natural and nutritionally healthier than hitherto (Table 3). Food industry reactions to these changes have been to develop less severe or 'minimal' preservation and processing technologies (Table 3). However, minimal technologies tend to result in a reduction in the intrinsic preservation of foods, and may, therefore, also lead to a potential reduction in their microbiological stability and safety. Thus, an important challenge has been to ensure that new and improved technologies retain, or preferably improve on, the effectiveness of preservation and ensurance of safety that may otherwise be lost.

Major current preservation technologies

There is a limited range of techniques currently employed to preserve foods. These are commented on below, and listed in Table 4 in such a way as to emphasize the fact that most of them act by slowing down, or in some cases by completely inhibiting, microbial growth. Few act by

Table 4 Major existing technologies for food preservation

Techniques that slow or prevent the growth of micro-organisms	
Reduction in temperature	– chill storage; frozen storage
Reduction in water activity	– drying; curing with added salt; conserving with added sugar
Reduction in pH	– acidification (*e.g.* use of acetic, citric acids, *etc.*); fermentation
Removal of oxygen	– vacuum or modified atmosphere packaging
Modified atmosphere packaging	– replacement of air with CO_2; O_2; N_2 mixtures
Addition of preservatives	– inorganic (*e.g.* sulphite; nitrite)
	– organic (*e.g.* propionate; sorbate; benzoate; parabens)
	– bacteriocin (*e.g.* nisin)
	– antimycotic (*e.g.* natamycin)
Control of microstructure	– in water-in-oil emulsion foods
Techniques that inactivate micro-organisms	
Heating	– pasteurization
	– sterilization
Techniques that restrict access of micro-organisms to products	
Packaging	
Aseptic processing	

Adapted from Gould[1].

direct inactivation. A major trend is to apply these techniques in new combinations, in ways that minimize the extreme use of any one of them, and so improve food product quality. This has formed the basis of the successful 'hurdle technologies' of Leistner[5] that have fostered the development of new routes to food preservation around the world. While traditional hurdle technologies were developed empirically, new logical developments are being made supported by the use of mathematical models[6]. These are generated using data derived from large multifactorial experiments, and allow confident computer-aided predictions to be made, *e.g.* of the effects of parameters such as pH, a_w, temperature, preservatives, gas phase, *etc.* on the growth, survival, and thermal death of specific micro-organisms in foods[7].

Low temperature

As the temperature of a chilled food is reduced, the types of micro-organisms and their rates of growth are reduced also. Two particularly important temperatures are around 12°C, which represents the lower limit for growth of the strict anaerobes, *Clostridium perfringens* and the proteolytic strains of *Clostridium botulinum* (types A and some types of B), and 3°C, which is the lower limit for non-proteolytic strains of *C. botulinum* (types E and some types of B and F). A few years ago, this would have been the chill storage temperature below which no food poisoning micro-organisms would have been expected to multiply.

However, both *Listeria monocytogenes* and *Yersinia enterocolitica* can grow at temperatures below 1°C, so that indicated shelf-lives and sell-by dates can play an important role in ensuring safety, particularly when temperature control can not be assured, *e.g.* in the home[8]. Many types of spoilage micro-organisms may continue to grow at sub-zero temperatures, multiplying slowly at temperatures down to about –7°C. Badly stored frozen foods may, therefore, slowly spoil through the activities of micro-organisms, but not become dangerous if thawing has not occurred. At the temperature of properly stored frozen foods, nominally –18°C in many countries, microbial growth is completely prevented, although slow loss of quality may still occur through the activities of enzymes and through chemical reactions and physical changes (see Table 1).

Reduction in water activity

Water activity values (a_w) are widely used to predict the stability of foods with respect to the growth of micro-organisms and the chemical, enzymic and physical changes that lead to quality deterioration[9]. Values range from 1 (pure water) to zero (no water), equivalent to equilibrium relative humidities (ERH) on a scale from 100% to 0%. The water activity of foods is reduced by drying or by adding solutes such as salt, as in cured products, or sugars, as in conserves, or by combinations of these treatments. Small reductions, *e.g.* to about 0.97, are sufficient to prevent the growth of some important spoilage micro-organisms, *e.g.* *Pseudomonas* species that grow at high a_ws, and rapidly spoil foods such as fresh meat stored in air. Cured meats generally have a_ws sufficiently reduced to ensure longer *Pseudomonas*-free shelf-lives. Slow souring, caused by lactic acid bacteria occurs instead. If the a_w is lower still, below about 0.95, as in some salamis and dry-cured meat products, even these are inhibited, and slow spoilage by low a_w-tolerant micrococci takes over. These and similar relationships are widely used to explain and predict the storage stability and safety of foods. Of the food poisoning micro-organisms, *Staphylococcus aureus* is the most tolerant, with a low a_w limit for growth of about 0.86 in air, but only 0.91 anaerobically, so that it may grow and produce enterotoxin in relatively low a_w foods if other conditions are conducive, *e.g.* temperature and time of storage. At a_w values below 0.86, few bacteria, and no bacteria of public health concern, can grow, and food is spoiled by yeasts or moulds, some of which can multiply slowly at a_ws as low as 0.6. Below this a_w, no micro-organisms are able to grow. Shelf-stable dried foods are generally formulated around a_w 0.3, where lipid oxidation and other chemical changes are minimal.

An interesting extrapolation of a_w-control of microbial growth into the clinical area was made by Herszage and his colleagues in Buenos Aires[10]. He built on the ancient uses of honey and other highly soluble solutes by promoting the treatment of infected wounds with cane sugar. The sucrose was not highly absorbed into underlying tissues, but served to reduce the a_w within a wound, and apparently without interfering with macrophage activity, sufficiently to prevent the growth of pathogens, including *Staph. aureus*. Efficacy was demonstrated in a number of clinical studies[11], and the procedure was said to have potential value, *e.g.* where particularly antibiotic-resistant micro-organisms were involved, or in third world countries where sugar is much cheaper than antibiotics.

Vacuum and modified atmosphere packaging (MAP)

The effectiveness of vacuum and MAP derive firstly from the removal of oxygen, with the consequent inhibition of strictly oxidative micro-organisms. Fermentative organisms continue to multiply but they do so more slowly and, for some types of foods, they have less unpleasant consequences for food quality. Special attention is always given to the possibility of encouraging the growth of strictly anaerobic food poisoning micro-organisms, such as *C. botulinum*, so that for foods such as 'sous vide' products, which are vacuum packed and pasteurized rather than sterilized, minimal heat treatments and tight temperature control in distribution are recommended[12]. Carbon dioxide is widely used in MAP foods because it has a specific antimicrobial activity, acting as a preservative that uniquely dissipates when the food pack is opened[13]. For example, much supermarket meat is packed in gas mixtures containing about 70% O_2 and 30% CO_2. The O_2 maintains the meat in the bright red oxymyoglobin colour that consumers prefer, while the CO_2 slows down the growth of Gram-negative spoilage bacteria so as to about double the useful shelf-life.

Acidification

Many yeasts and moulds are able to multiply at very low pH values, *i.e.* well below pH 2, so that they predominate in the flora of spoiling acidified foods. Few bacteria grow below about pH 3.5 or so. Those that do are adapted to acid environments, *e.g.* the lactic acid bacteria, and indeed are employed in numerous acid-generating food fermentations such as those for yoghurts, cheeses and salamis. A particularly important pH for food safety is pH 4.5, because it is the pH below which *C. botulinum* is unable to multiply. Consequently, in thermal processing,

Table 5 Most-used food preservatives

Preservatives	Examples of foods in which they are used
Weak lipophilic organic acids and esters	
Sorbate	Cheeses, syrups, cakes, dressings
Benzoate	Pickles, soft drinks, dressings
Benzoate esters (*e.g.* methyl, propyl)	Marinaded fish products
Propionate	Bread, cakes, cheese, grain
Organic acid acidulants	
Acetic, lactic, citric, malic, *etc.*	Acidulants for low pH sauces, mayonnaises, dressings, salads, drinks, fruit juices and concentrates
Mineral acid acidulants	
Phosphoric, hydrochloric	Acidulants, as above
Inorganic anions	
Sulphite (SO_2, metabisulphite)	Fruit pieces, dried fruits, wine, meat (British fresh sausages)
Nitrite	Cured meats
Antibiotics	
Nisin	Cheese, canned foods
Natamycin (pimaricin)	Soft fruit, dry-cured meats
Smoke	Meats and fish

Adapted from Russell and Gould[15].

it is not necessary to heat foods that are more acid than this to the same extent as higher pH 'low acid' foods. Below about pH 4.2, other food poisoning and spoilage bacteria are mostly controlled. However, recently the spore-forming bacterium *Alicyclobacillus acidoterrestris*, capable of growth at pH values as low as 2, has caused spoilage problems ('disinfectant taints') in some low pH foods.

Survival of micro-organisms at low pH may be important, even if they are unable to multiply. For example, *Escherichia coli* O157 has an acid tolerance that may have contributed to some food poisoning outbreaks in which the vehicle was a low pH food, *e.g.* American (non-alcoholic) apple cider. Furthermore, acid tolerance may aid passage of such organisms through the stomach. Food processors are aware that acid tolerance may be increased by prior exposure to mild acidification, or even by seemingly unrelated stresses, such as mild heating[14].

Preservatives

Most of the preservatives that are used in foods are acids (Table 5), such as the weak lipophilic organic acids (sorbate, benzoate, propionate) or the inorganic ones (sulphite, nitrite). All are more effective at low rather than at high pH[15]. Indeed, with the possible exceptions of the alkyl esters of *p*-hydroxybenzoate ('parabens'), there are no wide-spectrum antimicrobial food preservatives that are effective at near-neutral pH. There is a well-established rationale for the effectiveness of the weak acids and for their synergy with hydrogen ions, *i.e.* with low pH. This derives from the fact that in their unionized forms, which are favoured at low pH, they are able to readily equilibrate across the microbial cell membrane and access the cytoplasm of the cell. The pK value of the common weak acid preservatives range from 4.2 (benzoic) to 4.87 (propionic), so that at pH values much above these activity is greatly reduced. At the pH of most foods, micro-organisms maintain an internal pH higher than that of their surroundings. Consequently, on entering the cytoplasm, the undissociated acids tend to dissociate, delivering hydrogen ions along with the particular anion. The additional hydrogen ions may be exported by the micro-organisms, but this is energy-demanding, so cell growth is restricted. If the energy supply is overcome, then the pH of the cytoplasm eventually falls to a level that is too low for growth to continue. In addition, the accumulated anion may have specific antimicrobial effects[16].

From the point of view of practical food preservation, it is, therefore, sensible to include a weak organic acid whenever possible, then to acidify the food product as much as is organoleptically acceptable to capitalize on the weak acid-low pH synergy, then to vacuum pack it if possible because this will restrict the amount of energy that is available for the extrusion of hydrogen ions, then to reduce the a_w as much as possible, because this will place additional energy requirements on the cell, and so on. In this way, many empirical preservation 'combination technologies' can be rationalized, and new, logically-based ones sought.

Heat

Pasteurization at times and temperatures sufficient to inactivate vegetative micro-organisms, and sterilization at times and temperatures sufficient to inactivate bacterial spores, remain the bases of large industries around the world[17]. With the slow acceptance of irradiation for food preservation in most countries, heat remains the only substantial means for inactivating micro-organisms in foods. However, most of the new and 'emerging' technologies that have been investigated and promoted in recent years act by inactivation, but without the need for substantial heating.

New and emerging food preservation technologies

Natural additives

A few natural additives are widely used (Table 6)[18,19]. For instance, egg white lysozyme is employed at levels in excess of 100 tonnes per annum to prevent 'blowing', by lysing vegetative cells of *Clostridium tyrobutyricum* outgrowing from spores in some cheeses. Activation of the lactoperoxidase system has been shown to be useful to extend the shelf-life of bulk milk in those countries in which pasteurization soon after milking is not possible and refrigerated transport systems are poorly developed. The small post-transcriptionally modified peptide bacteriocin, nisin, is increasingly used to prevent spoilage of some cheeses and to prevent spoilage of some canned foods by thermophilic spore-forming bacteria such as *Bacillus stearothermophilus* and *Clostridium thermosaccharolyticum*. More than 40 other bacteriocins have been discovered and some are being evaluated for food use. Hundreds of herb, spice and other plant-derived compounds have been described and shown to have antimicrobial properties in laboratory studies[20]. While some of them are effective in foods, their efficacy is often reduced because of binding of the compounds to food proteins, partition into fats, *etc.*

New physical procedures

It is likely that new physical procedures will provide the most effective alternatives to heat. Some of them are already in commercial use, while other are attracting substantial research and development support (Table 6)[4].

High hydrostatic pressure

The application of high hydrostatic pressure is now well-established for the non-thermal inactivation of vegetative bacteria, yeasts and moulds in foods, by 'pressure pasteurization'[21]. Vegetative forms of micro-organisms are generally sensitive to pressures in the region of 400–600 MPa (Megapascals) or so (equivalent to 4000–6000 atmospheres), though with large differences in the sensitivities of different species and sometimes large strain-to-strain variations too. Foods so treated include jams, fruit juices, dressings, and avocado dip (guacamole). The advantage of the treatments is that, whereas pressure may greatly alter the state of macromolecules in foods, such as proteins and poly-saccharides, it has little effect on small molecules, so that flavours and odours remain relatively unaltered and 'fresh-like'.

Table 6 New and emerging technologies for food preservation

Natural additives

Animal-derived antimicrobials	– lysozyme
	– lactoperoxidase system
	– lactoferrin; lactoferricin
Plant-derived antimicrobials	– herb and spice extracts
Microbial products	– nisin
	– pediocin
	– other bacteriocins and culture products

Physical processes

Gamma and electron beam irradiation
High voltage electric gradient pulses ('electroporation')
High hydrostatic pressure
Combined ultrasonics, heat and pressure ('manothermosonication')
Laser and non-coherent light pulses
High magnetic field pulses

High pressure has so far been exploited mainly for the preservation of foods in which spores are not a problem, *e.g.* foods in which the pH is too low for spores to outgrow, or which are stored for limited times at chill temperatures. These limitations result from the fact that bacterial spores are far more tolerant to pressure than are vegetative cells. However, it has been found that pressure can be highly synergistic with mild heating for the inactivation of spores. This seems to occur because pressure, in some as yet unknown manner, actually triggers spores to germinate. Having germinated, they lose their resistance to pressure, and to heat, so that the two physical processes applied together inactivate many more spores than either alone. Further development along these lines, and the possibility of other synergies (*e.g.* pressure has been shown to be synergistic with nisin) may eventually allow it to be used as an alternative to heat-sterilization of foods, and possibly of some pharmaceuticals too. Pressure was first evaluated for vaccine production.

Ultrasonication

Ultrasonication at high enough intensities has long been known to inactivate vegetative bacteria and to reduce the heat resistance of spores; the effect is amplified by increasing the temperature. However, as the temperature is increased, the relative magnitude of the amplification becomes reduced. It is thought that this occurs because, as the vapour pressure rises, it has the effect of reducing the effectiveness of cavitation (the rapid formation and collapse of tiny bubbles), which is the main vehicle of killing. However, application of a slight overpressure (*i.e.* a few atmospheres) has been reported to overcome this fall in effectiveness, so that the amplification is maintained at higher temperatures. The combination procedure ('manothermosonication'), therefore, has been claimed to have potential for reducing pasteurization and sterilization temperatures for pumpable liquid and semisolid foods[22].

High voltage electric discharges

High voltage electric discharges ('electroporation') are most effective for the inactivation of vegetative bacteria, yeasts, and moulds, while spores are much more tolerant. The cell membrane is one of the most important structures controlling many of the vegetative cell's homeostatic mechanisms. It is not surprising, therefore, that electroporation, which breaches this structure, has such a lethal, and essentially non-thermal, effect on vegetative cells. Voltage gradients in the region of 20–60 kV/cm are used, delivered in a series of microsecond pulses, at pulse repetition rates sufficiently low to avoid too much heating. Foods such as milk and fruit juices can be pasteurized using this technique in flow-through continuous treatment cells[23]. The reason for the resistance of spores is not known for certain, but probably results from the fact that the central cytoplasm of spores is thought to be relatively dehydrated. This would reduce its conductivity, and make difficult the development of a sufficiently high voltage gradient to breach the surrounding membrane.

High intensity light

High intensity laser and non-coherent light pulse generators have been developed for the decontamination of surfaces of foods and packaging materials, and possibly transparent foods also[24], as well as in dentistry[25]. The killing effect results partially from the UV content for some applications and partially from intense but local heating for others. Additional non-UV and non-thermal effects have been claimed by some researchers.

High intensity magnetic field pulses

Exposure to high intensity oscillating magnetic fields has been reported to have a variety of effects on biological systems ranging from selective inactivation of malignant cells[26] to the inactivation of bacteria on packaging materials and in foods[27]. Treatment times are very short, typically from 25 ms to a few milliseconds, and field strengths are very high, typically from 2 Tessla to about 100 Tessla at frequencies between about 5–500 kHz. Efficacies of treatments did not exceed about 100-fold reductions in numbers of vegetative micro-organisms inoculated into milk (*Streptococcus thermophilus*), orange juice (*Saccharomyces* spp.), bread rolls (mould spores) and no inactivation of bacterial spores has been reported[27], so the practical potential for the technique, as it has been developed so far, appears to be limited[28].

Irradiation

The use of ionizing radiation, including gamma radiation from isotopes such as ^{60}Co, and electrons and X-rays from machine sources, is legal for disinfestation, to prevent sprouting of bulbs and tubers, and for antimicrobial pasteurization of foods in nearly 40 countries. Doses allowed have generally been up to 10 kGy (kilogray). Recently, the World Health Organization recommended that there are no toxicological or other hazards associated with higher doses, so that there should be no upper dose limit imposed for the irradiation of foods[29]. The technology is relatively simple to apply, with straightforward inactivation kinetics and geometry that makes dose control and processing requirements much easier than for many heat processes. The potential value to consumers, in the area of prevention of food poisoning through the elimination of pathogens such as *Salmonella* and *Campylobacter* from some foods of animal origin and some sea foods, is substantial. However, this is not widely recognized by consumers, so that slow acceptance by the public continues to restrict its introduction in most parts of the world.

Conclusions

While the most-employed preservation technologies have a long history of use, there is currently a real need for improved techniques, to meet the developing needs of consumers. Some improvements are being derived from the use of established techniques in new combinations or under improved control, and other improvements are being derived essentially from the development of new techniques. These are finding, at first, new and attractive, but niche, markets. It is expected that these will expand as experience in the new techniques is gained. If the resistance of bacterial spores to some of the new techniques could be overcome, and in a manner that was widely proven and accepted to be safe, then the potential markets could be immeasurably larger. A particular attraction of the newer techniques is that they act by inactivation rather than by inhibition. With regard to reducing the incidence of food poisoning disease, the introduction of effective inactivation techniques that lead to the elimination of the pathogens must be the ultimate target of primary food producers, processors, distributors, and retailers. Occasional lapses of hygiene will continue to occur in the food service establishment and in the home, but would be of no public health consequence if the organisms of concern did not enter these premises in the first place.

References

1 Gould GW. (Ed) Mechanisms of Action of Food Preservation Procedures. Barking: Elsevier, 1989
2 Lund BM, Baird-Parker AC, Gould GW. (Eds) The Microbiological Safety and Quality of Foods. Gaithersburg, MD: Aspen, 2000

3 Gould GW, Abee T, Granum PE, Jones MV. Physiology of food poisoning microorganisms and the major problems in food poisoning control. Int J Food Microbiol 1995; **28**: 121–28

4 Gould GW. (Ed) New Methods of Food Preservation. Glasgow: Blackie, 1995

5 Leistner L, Gorris LGM. Food preservation by hurdle technology. Trends Food Sci Technol 1995; **6**: 41–6

6 Baranyi J, Roberts TA. Mathematics of predictive microbiology. Int J Food Microbiol 1995; **26**: 199–218

7 Baranyi J, Roberts TA. Principles and application of predictive modeling of the effects of preservative factors of microorganisms. In: Lund BM, Baird-Parker AC, Gould GW. (Eds) The Microbiological Safety and Quality of Foods. Gaithersburg, MD: Aspen, 2000; 342–58

8 Herbert RA, Sutherland JP. Chill storage. In: Lund BM, Baird-Parker AC, Gould GW. (Eds) The Microbiological Safety and Quality of Foods. Gaithersburg, MD: Aspen, 2000; 101–21

9 Christian JHB. Drying and reduction in water activity. In: Lund BM, Baird-Parker AC, Gould GW. (Eds) The Microbiological Safety and Quality of Foods. Gaithersburg, MD: Aspen, 2000; 146–74

10 Chirife J, Scarmato G, Herszage L. Scientific basis for use of granulated sugar in treatment of infected wounds. Lancet 1982; i: 560–1

11 Selwyn S, Durodie J. The antimicrobial activity of sugar against pathogens of wounds and other infections of man. In: Simatos D, Multon JL. (Eds) Properties of Water in Foods. Dordrecht: Martinus Nijhoff, 1985; 293–308

12 Notermans S, Dufrenne J, Lund BM. Botulism risk of refrigerated processed foods of extended durability. J Food Protect 1990; **53**: 1020–24

13 Molin G. Modified atmospheres. In: Lund BM, Baird-Parker AC, Gould GW. (Eds) The Microbiological Safety and Quality of Foods. Gaithersburg, MD: Aspen, 2000; 214–34

14 Wang G, Doyle MP. Heat shock response enhances acid tolerance of Escherichia coli O157:H7. Lett Appl Microbiol 1998; **26**: 31–4

15 Russell NJ, Gould GW. (Eds) Food Preservatives. Glasgow: Blackie, 1991

16 Eklund T. The antimicrobial effect of dissociated and undissociated sorbic acid at different pH levels. J Appl Bacteriol 1983; **54**: 383–9

17 Pflug IJ, Gould GW. Heat treatment. In: Lund BM, Baird-Parker AC, Gould GW. (Eds) The Microbiological Safety and Quality of Foods. Gaithersburg, MD: Aspen, 2000; 36–64

18 Davidson PM, Brannen AL. (Eds) Antimicrobials in Foods. New York: Marcel Dekker, 1993

19 Dillon VM, Board RG. (Eds) Natural Antimicrobial Systems and Food Preservation. Wallingford, Oxon: CAB International, 1994

20 Hoover DG. Microorganisms and their products in the preservation of foods. In: Lund BM, Baird-Parker AC, Gould GW. (Eds) The Microbiological Safety and Quality of Foods. Gaithersburg, MD: Aspen, 2000; 251–76

21 Ledward DA, Johnston DE, Earnshaw RG Hasting APM. (Eds) High Pressure Processing of Foods. Nottingham: Nottingham University Press, 1995

22 Sala FJ, Burgos J, Condon S, Lopez P, Raso J. Effect of heat and ultrasound on microorganisms and enzymes. In: Gould GW. (Ed) New Methods of Food Preservation. Glasgow: Blackie, 1995: 176–204

23 Zhang Q, Qin BL, Barbosa-Canovas GV, Swanson BG. Inactivation of E. coli for food pasteurization by high strength pulsed electric fields. J Food Proc Pres 1995; **19**: 103–18

24 Dunn JE, Clark RW, Asmus JF, Pearlman JS, Boyer K, Parrichaud F. Method and apparatus for preservation of foodstuffs. Int Patent 1998: WO88/03369

25 Rooney J, Midda M, Leeming J. A laboratory investigation of the bactericidal effect of a Nd:YAG laser. Br Dental J 1994; **176**: 61–4

26 Costa JL, Hoffman GA. Malignancy treatment. US Patent 1987: 4,665,898

27 Hoffman GA. Inactivation of microorganisms by an oscillating magnetic field. US Patent 1985: 4,524,079 and Int Patent 1985: WO85/02094

28 Barbosa-Canovas GV, Pothakamury UR, Swanson BG. State of the art technologies for the sterilization of foods by non-thermal processes: physical methods. In: Barbosa-Canovas GV, Welti-Chanes J. (Eds) Food Preservation by Moisture Control: Fundamentals and Applications. Lancaster, PA: Technomic, 1995: 493–532

29 Patterson M, Loaharanu P. Food irradiation. In: Lund BM, Baird-Parker AC, Gould GW. (Eds) The Microbiological Safety and Quality of Foods. Gaithersburg, MD: Aspen, 2000; 65–1002

Consumer perception and understanding of risk from food

Barbara Knox

Northern Ireland Centre for Diet and Health, The University of Ulster, Coleraine, County Londonderry, UK

The study of risk perception has been punctuated with controversy, conflict and paradigm shifts. Despite more than three decades of research, understanding of risk assessment remains fragmented and incoherent. Until recently, food and eating has been viewed as a low-risk activity and perceived risk surrounded matters of hygiene or lack of food. Consequently, theories of risk have been constructed with reference to environmental and technological hazards, such as nuclear power, whilst neglecting food issues. However, following a decade of 'food scares', attention has moved towards the study of food risk. Within this, food risk research has focused almost exclusively upon attempting to explain the divergence of opinion that exists between experts and the lay public whilst neglecting to address it. The following discussion provides a brief historical overview of theories and approaches that have been applied to the study of risk perception, continues with a summary of findings derived from food risk research and concludes with a discussion of methodological issues and some projections for future research.

Correspondence to:
Dr Barbara Knox,
Northern Ireland Centre
for Diet and Health, The
University of Ulster,
Coleraine,
County Londonderry
BT52 1SA, UK

Risk is an important determinant of food choice and correspondingly, estimates of risk are strongly related to estimates of consumption[1]. Food risk has become particularly salient in the wake of a decade of 'food scares' (such as: alar residue in apples, 1988; salmonella in eggs, 1988; and bovine spongiform encephalopathy (BSE) in beef, 1996), which have served to seriously undermine public confidence in the food industry and government regulatory bodies. Consumer concern over food safety has steadily increased since the 1970s[2,3], yet only recently have risk perceptions been explored in relation to food. This recent attention may well reflect the vested interests of government and funding bodies who are eager to introduce new technology, such as food irradiation and genetically modified foods, into food production in the knowledge that the success of these new technologies will largely depend upon public acceptance.

Risk: a historical perspective

Theories of rational choice/quantitative risk

Historically, theories of risk have assumed that public perception of risk is constructed rationally and have focused upon associated probabilities, costs and benefits, the best example of which is Kahneman and Taversky's expected utility theory[4]. Also known as prospect theory, expected utility theory was derived from Von Neuman and Morgenstern's (1944), mixed-motive game theory which arose out of the experimental study of strategic thinking and decision-making within the context of conflict[5]. Gaming studies were undertaken within laboratory constraints and results were expressed and interpreted in terms of mathematical models. This approach, therefore, failed to embody the social and cultural context of decision-making with the result that the approach has proved to be of little utility for the prediction of behaviour. It is now generally acknowledged that perceived risk is influenced by a wide range of qualitative factors rather than statistical rationale and probabilities, yet attempts to model risk assessment mathematically persist[6–8].

Individual differences approach

The individual-differences approach, which has focused upon the effect of cognitive style upon risk perception through psychometric measures, has also failed to find any evidence that risk is quantitatively or rationally assessed.

Starr (1969) was first to point out the importance of dispositional and cognitive factors, such as volition and perceived control in the perception of technological risk[9]. Following on from Starr, the idea that risk perceptions are biased by heuristics (rules of thumb or operating principles) was suggested by Kahneman and Taversky[4], who then set out to test this idea. Although as far back as 1974, Kahneman and Taversky found no relationship between objectively calculated risk judgements and public risk perceptions, research has persisted in the search for rules through which to predict and influence public response.

Expanding further upon Starr's model of technological risk, Slovic and colleagues treated risk as a psychological construct and set out to define and quantify the nature of heuristic bias in risk perception through psychometric means[10]. Risk was defined in terms of benefit to society, magnitude of risk and acceptability of risk, and assessed in relation to dimensions of risk including voluntariness, dread, perceived control, severity, personal and social consequences and familiarity. However, risk assessments appeared to be related to only two of these dimensions, 'dread' and 'severity', and these factors have yet to be fully defined in relation to food risk concepts.

The work of Frewer and colleagues over the last decade has concentrated almost exclusively upon food risk, much of it devoted to testing Slovic's psychometric model of risk perception and expanding it to include the phenomenon of optimistic bias. The underlying premise in this research is that through better understanding of the rules and biases of perception, communication between food regulatory authorities and the public might be enhanced.

One such optimistic bias is the tendency to overestimate certain risks and underestimate others. Within certain contexts, such as that of health risk behaviour, there is a tendency to view others as more at risk of danger than oneself. This may partly explain why health messages have so little impact. Moreover, there is some evidence to suggest that optimistic bias or 'unrealistic optimism' cannot be countered through information and that it can actually be exacerbated through health promotion messages[11].

Frewer and colleagues have, therefore, attempted to explain optimistic bias in relation to perceived control over risk. Whereas environmental and technical risks, such as potential risk from food biotechnology, are characterised by low perceptions of control, life-style and dietary health risks are associated with greater perceptions of control[12,13]. Man-made hazards, such as BSE and potential hazards from biotechnology are perceived as unlikely to be properly regulated and, therefore, difficult to control. Consequently, it was hypothesised that optimistic bias or 'unrealistic optimism' would be greater in situations perceived as under personal control, such as health or food risk. To test this idea, Frewer and colleagues analysed risk assessments for a range of potential hazards of a technical, bacteriological, chemical and life-style nature that varied in terms of perceived control[14]. However, contrary to what the model would have predicted, the high fat diet, over which perceived control would be high, was rated overall the riskiest hazard. The relationship between perceived risk and perceived control is clearly complex. Later work has suggested that the perception of risk in relation to perceived control may be offset by perception of need and benefit[15]. Another possible explanation is that optimistic bias is related to perceived control, but it is mediated by 'reactance'[16]. In the face of a threatening communication, reactance may occur such that an individual may change his or her attitude in a direction contrary to that advocated in order to restore the perception of control.

Although research into optimistic bias appears equivocal, the evaluation of food risk perceptions has provided some support for Slovic's model. However, questionnaire structure has tended to be biased toward the theory[13,15], allowing only limited scope for unanticipated factors to arise during the process of inquiry. Furthermore, studies of this type have been criticized for the almost exclusive use of factor analysis and other perceptual mapping techniques, allowing researcher bias to intrude into the analysis through the category labels that are attributed to factors[17]. For example, it has been argued that the 'dread' dimension, defined by Slovic in relation to the psychological construction of risk, is analogous to the discrepancy between 'lay' and 'expert' risk perception, a discrepancy that causes the public to experience anxiety expressed as dread[18]. Furthermore, optimistic bias may represent a proxy for perceived control[14] rather than a separate entity, and may provide an adaptive way of reducing anxiety and coping with a situation that is not perceived as controllable. The model has since been expanded to include 'trust' within the context of risk communication. There is still no theory behind the psychometric approach[19].

The individual differences approach has been favoured politically, because of its potential to explain the apparent irrationality of lay risk perceptions, and the implication that the public can be educated to overcome perceptual bias and to accept more rational assessments of risk. However, psychometric approaches which measure cognitive and dispositional variables have demonstrated only limited explanatory power in the case of food risk[20,21], so that qualitative approaches are gaining increasing favour.

Sociological theory of risk

The sociological view holds that the rich array of social meanings surrounding risk perceptions render the quantitative assessment of risk impossible. Risk, particularly technological risk, which includes food biotechnological risk, is often imposed upon the public by an elite authority such as government, science and industry, hence, power can become the over-riding issue leading to conflict[22,23]. This conflict finds expression not only in the polarization of lay and expert risk assessments, but also in the different schools of academic thought that guide research.

Risk research has concentrated almost exclusively upon the so-called 'irrational' views of the general public, whilst the private beliefs and perceptions of scientists and civil-servants have largely been ignored. This focus upon the lay perception of risk reflects the interests of risk managers and research funding bodies seeking to influence public opinion[24]. In addition, the topic of risk perception has been neglected in favour of risk quantification, and risk assessment based exclusively upon probability and rationality has provided little opportunity for active lay input into research data that have been collected[25]. Sociologists have attempted to overcome these biases by studying risk within the wider social and ideological context. Recent work looking at the effect of experience upon risk perception suggests that social factors may be more important than physical and psychological factors in determining risk perceptions[26]. The sociological approach takes into account the role and perceptions of regulating and policy bodies, the scientific community and the media.

Cultural theory of risk

Risk assessment is a social phenomenon based upon culturally determined ideas. Social and cultural factors determine what risks are salient. Communication regarding risk probabilities is seldom successful in reducing lay risk concerns because the quantitative construction of risk represents only one aspect of public risk assessment. It has been argued that the quantitative approach has led to a focus upon the failings rather than the richness of human perception[27]. Within this is the implication that the lay view is somehow inferior.

According to cultural theory, risk perception is ideologically driven whether it be the lay public, the media, the government or the scientific elite[28]. Risk perceptions are an expression of four different socially determined 'thought worlds' or ideologies: (i) the 'atomised' perspective, which is expressed through a fatalistic attitude; (ii) the hierarchical view, characterised by trust in authority; (iii) the individualistic or rational view; and (iv) the egalitarian or critical view[29]. These views are dynamic, such that people shift from one perspective to another depending upon the issue.

Food is embedded in our social and cultural practices within which it holds symbolic significance. In particular, meat holds a varying degree of significance across cultures[30]. Food choices and food risk perceptions are, therefore, motivated by culturally relevant ethical concerns. Food-related risk is, therefore, likely to be construed in a way that is unique 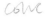 and may vary by food type. Exploration of food risk perceptions across societies would establish the degree to which risk perceptions are culturally determined. Both social and cultural theories have yet to be fully explored in relation to food risk.

The marketing viewpoint

Having only recently entered the research arena, market researchers have attempted to put risk in context and observe it in relation to different decisions of product choice, including food.

Product involvement, the degree to which a product purchase reflects personal goals, values and needs, is reflected in risk perceptions and this may be particularly true of food. In one study, different product classes including consumable and electrical goods were correlated for both perceived risk and product involvement[31]. The only food item that was included in the study, tinned soup, received highest ratings in terms of both risk and product involvement. Although only one food was evaluated in this study, this high level of product involvement is a reflection of the importance ascribed to food. Food is deeply embedded in our social and cultural fabric and frequently acts as a vehicle through which to express personal, social and cultural identity. Given the high degree of involvement associated with food, it is perhaps not surprising that ethical concerns direct public food risk perceptions.

Schutz and Weidmann (1998)[32] compared perceptions of personal versus environmental risk for a range of 30 different products including electrical goods, clothing items, medicines and food items such as organic vegetables, butter, and genetically modified strawberries[32]. Food tended to be perceived largely in terms of personal risk, except for genetically modified foods, which were considered risky both on a personal and environmental level. However, there was a correlation between personal and environmental risk assessments, suggesting that both personal and environmental issues are considered when making risk judgements.

In one of very few studies to consider emotion in relation to risk, Chaudhuri (1998)[33] attempted to bring together the information processing approach, which is objective and rational, and the experiential approach, which is subjective[33]. It was found that the degree of emotion associated with products varied by product class. Luxuries tended to receive higher risk ratings than essential items, however, essential items, such as food, became viewed as risky if associated with negative emotion. This suggests that objective and subjective factors are considered together and interact in the perception of food risk. Further research is required in order to gain deeper insight into the nature of such interactions.

The perception of risk from food

The bovine spongiform encephalitis (BSE) scare

Recently, consumer confidence in government food regulation has been seriously undermined. Food regulatory bodies had been aware of the potential risk of BSE for some time, an awareness based upon strong epidemiological evidence, however, until 1996, any suggestion of risk to the public was discounted by government, the scientific community and policy makers through media sources. Denial, indecision and lack of preparation characterised the management of the BSE crisis. In effect, the British government misled the public from 1988 until 1996, while exposing them to serious health risk from beef. Was this a case of ignorance or of putting industrial interests over public health concerns? In hindsight, given the uncertainties associated with the risk from BSE infected meat, the lay public appeared as well placed as the scientific elite to assess and manage the risk[25]. Given the cultural emphasis upon the quantitative rational approach to the assessment of risk, it is of note that no quantitative analysis of the effectiveness of the culling exercise and subsequent risk of BSE transmission, has yet been published[25]. The incident has changed the face of public food risk perception for the future.

The only study that appears to have made direct qualitative inquiry into public perceptions of BSE at the time of the crisis, Keane and Willets (1996) has indicated polarised views[34]. While many viewed BSE as the result of society going against nature, others saw BSE as purely a media creation. Whereas the former attitude may constitute a moral stance against technological interference in natural processes, the latter may reflect an 'atomised' perceptual set, characterised by a fatalistic view of risk.

Attitudes toward meat appear intrinsically linked to ideological beliefs with regard to the natural world[30]. In this sense, the feeding of meat to ruminants represented a flagrant breach of cultural taboo, hence, the strong public reaction. 'Mad cow' disease arose out of unnatural animal husbandry practices, hence, the 'unnaturalness' of genetic modification has proved a major barrier to public acceptance. Consumer rejection of genetically modified (GM) foods may reflect this generally accepted taboo against unnatural food production practices.

Genetic modification and food

Uncertainty typifies lay perceptions of risk from both BSE and GM foods. In the absence of quantitative information, the public must rely almost exclusively on qualitative concerns when deciding whether or not to eat beef or GM foods. Fears of the consequences of science 'meddling with nature' have been brought about through the BSE food scare. The BSE crisis demonstrated the power of 'nature' to 'strike back' and genetic modification seems to have tapped into the same type of fear[35].

Investigation by the Consumers' Association, combining the approaches of survey by interview and focus group discussion, revealed that during 1994 only 21% of people had heard of gene technology and only 17% understood the term[36], but that by 1996, 41% understood the meaning of the term. Since then, a classic risk conflict scenario has evolved, evidenced by the polarized views of experts and the lay public.

As in the case of BSE, public risk perceptions of food biotechnology appear directed towards ecological and ethical issues. Concerns have been raised regarding antibiotic-resistant genes[37] and other environmental issues such as herbicide-resistant plants[38]. On ethical grounds, the public appears more willing to accept genetically modified products in which the genetic material has been derived from a plant source as opposed to taken from an animal source[15,39]. Qualitative studies have clearly demonstrated the nature of consumer ethical concerns. Consumers view genetic modification as 'unnatural', that it is 'meddling with nature' and that science is 'playing God' by altering the genetics of nature[35–37]. This may reflect the apparent cultural taboo against unnatural production processes.

The public believes that the only people to benefit from genetic engineering will be food producers and manufacturers. In contrast, the scientific community and the food industry present genetic modification as a 'saviour' technology capable of solving world food shortage and production problems[40,41]. Genetic modification could also be used to enhance the nutrient content of foods[37] and help to eliminate known food-borne allergens[42]. In attempting to present a philosophical rationale for GM foods, Robert Shapiro, chief executive of the Monsanto Company, drew an analogy between information technology and gene technology arguing that both are merely concerned with the transfer of information[40]. The innovative idea of linking genetic modification conceptually with 'consumer-friendly' information technology assumes a rational approach and appears unfounded given that food attitudes are culturally embedded and construed differently to other types of risk. Consumers are suspicious of the motives of the food industry and biotechnologists because the two groups appear to be working from 'unsound value systems'. Whereas science and industry view the consumer as lacking understanding, a problem which could be overcome through public education, the consumer views science and industry as commercially driven and the technology as being imposed upon them without consultation.

During 1996, two genetically modified products, tomato puree and soya produced by the Monsanto Company for use as an ingredient in other food products, went on sale for the first time in Europe[36]. Although there was no legal requirement to label such products, the companies concerned took the decision to do so voluntarily. Nevertheless, conflict between consumers and industry surrounds the issue of the labelling of GM foods and ingredients. A recent survey found that 62% of scientists oppose mandatory labelling of foods containing GM ingredients[43]. The Food Advisory Committee and the Advisory Committee on Novel Foods and Processes saw no requirement for labelling herbicide-resistant soya produced by the Monsanto Company. They argued that labelling was unnecessary as the ingredient was safe and that is was impossible to determine the approximate amount of GM soya contained, as it was unsegregated from normal soya.

The Novel Food and Novel Ingredients Regulation came into force during 1997 allowing food manufacturers, if they wished, to label products as 'may contain GM ingredients'. However, consumers do not want ambiguous statements but clear and precise labelling to indicate which foods have been genetically modified[36,44,45]. Food labelling increases consumer perceived control. Information enables the public to choose or to reject GM foods if desired, otherwise the risk becomes involuntary, beyond personal control and thus may be perceived as more threatening[46]. The current debate surrounding GM foods provides a unique opportunity through which to study food risk perceptual processes prospectively both in context and in relation to existing theory.

The communication of food risk perception

Consumer concern over food risk has increased while at the same time trust in government and industry to control and monitor technological development has been seriously eroded, further amplifying risk perceptions. This has driven research into the communication of risk perception.

Communication appears to enhance trust only under certain conditions[6]. Frewer and colleagues have applied the elaboration likelihood model[47] to the study of risk communication and the effect of trust in the information source upon attitudes to GM foods. According to the theory, persuasion can occur on one or both of two interacting levels or channels – deep and peripheral. Information itself is processed at a deep level, while contextual factors surrounding the information, such as perceived credibility of the source, are processed at a peripheral level, influencing how the information is interpreted. An initial study that considered perceived risk from food poisoning and from excessive alcohol consumption found that the perceived credibility of the source had no effect upon persuasiveness of the risk message[48]. More recently, comparison was made between information sourced either from a consumer organization (trusted) or government (less trusted). The persuasiveness of the information was also varied. However, contrary to what the model would predict, it was information which was 'high in persuasiveness' from the consumer organisation, and 'low in persuasiveness' from government sources, which was most trusted[49]. Perhaps government authorities come across to the public as 'trying too hard' when attempting to communicate risk messages, and in doing so, appear dishonest.

Consistent with the idea of 'trying too hard', qualitative exploration has suggested that the least trusted sources are those perceived to exaggerate or distort information, those with an apparent vested interest, and those motivated to self-protection. The most trusted sources were those which are moderately accountable to others, those which have little vested interest in promoting the viewpoint and those which are only somewhat self-protective[12].

Understanding of public perception of risk is crucial to the success of food safety communication and the uptake of new technology. Toward this end, we need to know more about how people define and interpret risk and the ideological framework within which risk decisions are expressed.

Conclusions

Whereas quantitative and psychometric models of risk perception provide some insight into how risk perceptions are constructed at the cognitive and dispositional level, social and cultural theories provide a framework through which to understand such perceptions. However, people do not think and behave in mechanistic ways, consequently, appreciation of public response to food safety issues requires some understanding of the subjective perceptions and meanings ascribed to such issues, as well as the wider cultural and social forces operating to determine public response to food safety issues. Taken together, the evidence implies that risk cannot be studied in isolation as a discrete entity, but that risk concepts run like a common thread, linking a diverse range of decision-making factors.

Despite the importance of risk perception in determining food choice, very few studies of risk have been applied to food specifically. Theories and models have been adapted from research into financial, nuclear or environmental risk. Given that health risk, and particularly food risk, is likely to be uniquely construed, even food product specific, it would seem appropriate to first go back and explore food risk qualitatively within the context of food purchase and choice, and to develop specific theoretical models accordingly. Theories of food choice provide a framework through which to understand and predict human dietary behaviour. Models of food choice clearly must incorporate the perception of risk as a decisional factor.

The private views of scientists, civil servants and industrialists have been largely ignored[2]; however, what little research there is, suggests that scientists hold ethical arguments against genetic engineering and share many consumer reservations[43]. Given the suggestion that the public perception of risk is subject to optimistic bias, is it not conceivable that government and scientific personnel representing official groups are expressing the same optimistic bias through their emphasis upon the probabilities of risk, whilst apparently disregarding the intuitive ethical views of consumers, when communicating risk messages? This apparent neglect of consumer concerns has served to undermine consumer confidence in the safety of the food supply. Risk perceptions require exploration within the social and cultural context in which they are embedded. This means that the views and interactions of all parties involved in the risk assessment and management forum need to be fully considered. Only then can it be determined if the discrepancy between lay and expert assessments of risks is perceived or actual.

Risk is a 'fuzzy' concept[19], which has yet to be described or explored in all its facets. Co-ordinated interdisciplinary collaboration is required in the endeavour to encompass the scope and complexity of risk perception and the nature of any interactions therein. Furthermore, risk assessment is dynamic, the processes of which require definition by means of prospective, longitudinal research[51], surrounding food-related 'live issues'. Meanwhile, there is a growing market for food products with enhanced safety attributes.

Acknowledgement

The author wishes to acknowledge the assistance of Corrina Donnelly in gathering some of the cited literature. A full bibliography can be obtained from the author.

References

1 Raats M, Sparks P. Unrealistic optimism about diet-related risks: implications for interventions. *Proc Nutr Soc* 1995; **54**: 737–45
2 Tait J. Public perception of biotechnology hazards. *J Chem Tech Biotechnol* 1988; **43**, 368–72
3 Payson S. Using historical information to identify consumer concerns about food safety. *Technological Bulletin US Department of Agriculture* 1994; **1835**: 1–19
4 Khaneman D, Taversky A. Prospect theory: an analysis of decision under risk. *Econometrica* 1979; **47**: 263–91
5 Hamburger H. *Games as Models of Social Phenomena*. San Francisco: WH Freeman, 1979
6 Sato Y. Special issue on social action and structure. *Sociol Theory Methods* 1999; **13**: 155–68
7 Govindasamy R, Italia J. Predicting consumer risk perceptions towards pesticide residue: alogistic analysis. *Appl Econom Lett* 1998; **5**: 793–6
8 Rai S, Krewski D. Uncertainty and variability analysis in multiplicative risk models. *Risk Analysis* 1998; **18**: 37–45
9 Starr C. Social benefit versus technological risk. What is our society willing to pay for safety? *Science* 1969; **165**: 1232–8
10 Slovic P, Fischhoff B, Lichenstein S. Rating the risks. *Environment* 1979; **21**: 14–39
11 Weinstein N, Klein W. Resistance of personal risk perceptions to debiasing interventions. *Health Psychol* 1995; **14**: 132–40

12 Frewer L, Howard C, Hedderley D, Shepherd R. What determines trust in information about food related risks? Underlying psychological constructs. *Risk Analysis* 1996; **16**: 473–86

13 Sparks P, Shepherd R. Public perceptions of the potential hazards associated with food production and food consumption: an empirical study. *Risk Analysis* 1994; **14**: 799–805

14 Frewer L, Shepherd R, Sparks P. The interrelationship between perceived knowledge, control and risk associated with a range of food-related hazards targeted at the individual, other people and society. *J Food Safety* 1994; **14**: 19–40

15 Frewer L, Howard C, Hedderly D, Shepherd R. Methodological approaches to assessing risk perceptions associated with food-related hazards. *Risk Analysis* 1998; **18**: 95–102

16 Brehm J. *A Theory of Psychological Reaction*. New York: Academic Press, 1966

17 Brown J. Introduction: approaches, tools and perceptions. In: Brown J. (Ed) *Environmental Threats: Perception, Analysis and Management*. London: Belhaven Press, 1989

18 Wynne B. Frameworks of rationality in risk management: towards the testing of naïve sociology. In: Brown J. (Ed) *Environmental Threats: Perception, Analysis and Management*. London: Belhaven Press, 1989

19 Sjoberg L. A discussion of the limitations of the psychometric and cultural theory approaches to risk perception. *Radiat Protect Dosimetry* 1996; **68**: 219–225

20 Sjoberg L. Worry and risk perception. *Risk Analysis* 1998; **18**: 85–93

21 Urban D, Hoban T. Cognitive determinants of risk perceptions associated with biotechnology. *Scientometrics* 1997; **40**: 299–331

22 Freudenburg W, Pastor S. Public responses to technological risk: toward a sociological perspective. *Sociol Q* 1992; **33**: 389–412

23 Kasperson R, Renn O, Brown HS *et al*. The social amplification of risk: a conceptual framework. *Risk Analysis* 1988; **8**: 177–87

24 Freudenburg W. Risk and recreancy: Weber, the division of labour, and the rationality of risk decisions. *Social Forces* 1993; **71**: 909–32

25 Jasanoff S. Civilization and madness: the great BSE scare of 1996. *Public Understand Sci* 1997; **6**: 221–32

26 Rogers G. The dynamics of risk perception: how does perceived risk respond to risk events? *Risk Analysis* 1997; **17**: 745–57

27 Douglas M. *Risk Acceptability According to the Social Sciences*. London: Routledge, Kegan Paul, 1985

28 Plutzer E, Maney A, O'Connor R. Ideology and elites' perceptions of the safety of new technologies. *Am J Politic Sci* 1998; **42**: 190–209

29 Douglas M. *Essays in the Sociology of Perception*. London: Routledge, Kegan Paul, 1982

30 Fiddes M. *Meat: A Natural Symbol*. London: Routledge, 1991

31 Dholakia U. An investigation of the relationship between perceived risk and product involvement. *Adv Consumer Res* 1997; **24**: 159–67

32 Schutz H, Weidmann P. Judgments of personal and environmental risks of consumer products – do they differ? *Risk Analysis* 1998; **18**: 119–29

33 Chaudhuri A. Product class effects on perceived risk: the role of emotion. *Int J Res Marketing* 1998; **15**: 157–68

34 Keane A, Willets A. *Concepts of Healthy Eating: An Anthropological Investigation in South East London*. Goldsmiths: University of London, 1996

35 Grove-White R, MacNaughton P, Mayer S, Wynne B. Uncertain world: genetically modified organisms. In: University of Lancaster. *Food, Public Attitudes in Britain*. Lancaster: Centre for the Study of Environmental Change (CSEC), 1997

36 Davies S. *Gene Cuisine – a consumer agenda for genetically modified foods*. Consumers' Association Policy Report. London: Consumers' Association, 1997

37 Burke D. What biotechnology can do for the food industry. *Food Sci Technol Today* 1997; **11**: 202–9

38 Sheppard J. Spilling the genes – what we should know about genetically engineered foods. *Splice of Life Publication*. London: The Genetic Forum, 1996

39 Kusnesof S, Ritson C. Consumer acceptability of genetically modified foods with special reference to farmed salmon. *Br Food J* 1996; **98**: 39–47

40 Shapiro R. How genetic engineering will save our planet. *Futurist* 1999; **33/34**: 28–9

41 Clarke A. The impact of biotechnology in a changing world. *Aust Biotechnol* 1996; **7**: 96–100

42 Jones L. Food biotechnology: current developments and the need for awareness. *Nutr Food Sci* 1996; **6**: 5–11

43 Rabino I. Ethical debates in genetic engineering: US scientists attitudes on patenting, germ-line research, food labelling, and agri-biotech issues. *Politics Life Sci* 1998; **17**: 147–63

44 International Food Information Council (IFIC) Consumer confidence in biotechnology. Current FDA Labelling Policy. *Aust Biotechnol* 1997; **7**: 101

45 Saint V. Objectives and purpose of consumer information in Community legislation. *Eur Food Law Rev* 1997; **4**: 377–87

46 Frewer L. Trust and risk communication. Health, AIR-CAT 4th Plenary Meeting: *Ecological, Safety Aspects in Food Choice* 1988; **4**: 10–5

47 Petty R, Cacioppo J. *Attitudes, Persuasion: Classic, Contemporary Approaches*. USA: William Brown, 1981

48 Frewer L, Howard C, Hedderley D, Shepherd R. The elaboration likelihood model and communication about food risks. *Risk Analysis* 1997; **17**: 759–70

49 Frewer L, Howard C, Hedderley D, Shepherd R. Reactions to information about genetic engineering: impact of source characteristics, perceived personal relevance, and persuasiveness. *Public Understanding Sci* 1999; **8**: 35–50

50 Lin J. Demographic and socio-economic influences on the importance of food safety. *Agr Resource Econom Rev* 1995; **24**: 190–8

51 Raats M, Sparks P. Unrealistic optimism about diet related risks: implications for interventions. *Proc Nutr Soc* 1995; **54**: 737–45

Risk communication: factors affecting impact

Glynis M Breakwell

Social Psychology European Research Institute, School of Human Sciences, University of Surrey, Guildford, UK

The impact of risk communication depends upon a complex interaction between the characteristics of the audience, the source of the message, and its content. Audience perception of risk is influenced by demographic factors (e.g. age, gender), personality profile, past experience, and ideological orientation. It is also affected by cognitive biases (e.g. unrealistic optimism) and lay 'mental models' of the hazard. For food hazards, the important dimensions of risk are controllability, novelty and naturalness. The source must be trusted for a risk message to be effective. Trust is associated with believing the source is expert, unbiased, disinterested, and not sensationalising. To maximise impact, risk communications must have a content which triggers attention, achieves comprehension and can influence decision-making. It must be unambiguous, definitive and easily interpretable – rarely achievable particularly when risk is shrouded in scientific uncertainty. Risk messages initiate social processes of amplification and attenuation, consequently their ramifications are rarely controllable.

Public concerns about the safety of food have grown enormously in recent years. The average consumer is now faced with a plethora of messages that suggest that food is dangerous. In some cases, it is the natural constituents of the food that are said to be hazardous: fat, sugar, alcohol. In others, it is the unnatural constitution of food that generates anxiety: genetically modified organisms – so-called, Frankenstein foods. Some types of food processing arouse suspicion, for instance, irradiation. Additives (for example, colourings) are claimed to have unanticipated health consequences. Above all, contaminants (like BSE, salmonella, listeria) are feared. Food is now widely recognised to be risky.

Achieving effective risk communication concerning food is consequently becoming increasingly important. 'Risk communication' is the label used to refer both to the content of any message concerning a hazard and the means of delivering that message. Typically, risk communication may provide an estimate of the likelihood that a hazard will result in something undesirable happening and/or an estimate of the extent of the damage that may be caused. Risk communication can be considered effective if it alerts the target audience (whether the public in

Correspondence to:
Prof. G M Breakwell,
SPERI, School of Human
Sciences, University of
Surrey, Guildford,
Surrey GU2 7XH, UK

© The British Council 2000

general or particular at risk populations) as to what is hazardous, the extent of the danger and what should be done to protect oneself. It should do this without arousing unnecessary anxiety. Some of the factors which determine the efficacy of risk communication efforts have been systematically examined by social scientists and this paper summarises some of their findings.

Risk perception

In order to understand the impact of risk communication, it is useful to know something about the basis for risk perception. In general, judgements about perceived risk and its acceptability are a function of: (i) a variety of qualitative aspects of the hazards, such as levels of perceived control and voluntariness, or catastrophic potential; and (ii) demographic characteristics, individual attitudes, or cultural and institutional affiliations[1,2].

There is some evidence that these general principles apply to perception of food hazards[3,4]. Hazards are typically conceptualised on two key dimensions[5]. The first reflects the level of dread they arouse and is associated with assessments of whether the hazard: (i) is controllable; (ii) involves involuntary exposure; (iii) has impact which is globally catastrophic; (iv) impacts upon future generations; (v) is inequitable in consequences; or (vi) has an increasing probability of occurrence.

The second reflects level of knowledge of those exposed and is associated with whether the hazard: (i) is new; (ii) observable; (iii) known to science; or (iv) has delayed effects.

Fife-Schaw and Rowe[4] showed that many food hazards were conceptualised by the public in terms of these two dimensions (which they characterised as control and awareness). However, they also found a third dimension was important in the conceptualisation of food hazards: the extent to which the hazard was considered naturally occurring or a product of human interference. Figure 1 illustrates how different food hazards might sit within this three dimensional matrix. Of course, their position in the matrix reflects how they are perceived by the public and not necessarily how they would be located by a technical risk assessment. Since in thinking about food hazards, people focus upon these three dimensions, in constructing risk communication messages it is also necessary to take them into account.

Gender, ethnicity, age, socio-economic status and geographical region are potential sources of demographic variation in risk perception. To date, however, the only established differences in food risk perception are associated with gender. Women perceive most food hazards to entail greater risk than do men. The difference is greatest with regard to

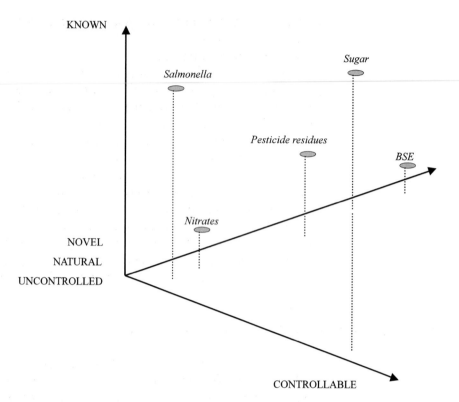

Fig. 1 Three dimensions of risk perception of food hazards.

technological hazards (for example, genetic modification)[6]. There is also some evidence that older people are more concerned about the risks of food poisoning (perhaps because they are targeted for information about such hazards given their susceptibility)[7].

Other types of individual differences have been found to be tied to risk perception. For instance, there is a relationship between the personality trait of venturesomeness, past experience of specific hazards and perceived characteristics of certain voluntary and involuntary hazardous activities[8]. Involuntary risks are more likely to be perceived as more unfamiliar and uncontrollable by those who have greater personal experience of hazardous activity. Greater venturesomeness is associated with perceiving involuntary risk activities as having delayed effects and being unfamiliar. Adherence to particular belief systems also affects risk perception. Not surprisingly perhaps, individuals who have 'green' environmentalist beliefs are more likely to perceive environmental hazards to be more serious and uncontrollable. Anthropological work[9] has suggested a series of five 'world views' or social orientations characteristic of different cultures that will predispose individuals to have differing perceptions of risks: hierarchical, egalitarian, individualist, fatalist and hermit. Differences in personality type, past experience, general attitudes and world view may need to be taken into account in designing risk communications which have optimal impact.

However, the relationship between risk perception and personal involvement with a hazard is not simple. For instance, if the object which is jeopardized is of great personal importance and the risk cannot be controlled by the individual, under-estimation of the degree of risk will often result[10]. This suggests that denial (or motivated reconstrual) may play a part in risk perception. A well-documented bias in risk perception supports this suggestion. Weinstein[11] summarises evidence that people display unrealistic optimism (labelled optimistic bias) about their personal risk levels. Essentially, most people consider themselves less likely to suffer from any particular hazard than other similar people. Optimistic biases are prevalent in life-style food hazards (such as high fat diets and domestic food poisoning)[12]. This and other cognitive biases in personal risk perception are important since they may seriously hinder efforts to communicate about risks and to promote risk-reducing behaviours.

The structure of risk communication

There is an extensive body of social psychological research which examines the factors that affect the persuasiveness of any communication. The effectiveness of a message is a function of the interaction of: (i) characteristics of the audience; (ii) characteristics of the source of the message (most importantly its perceived competence and trustworthiness); and (iii) content of the message. This interaction is complex. With regard to risk communication, some aspects of the interaction have been analysed.

Mental models of hazards

Some characteristics of the audience that are likely to be important in risk communication have been summarised above. In addition, considerable work has been done to develop methods which allow examination of the 'mental models' which individuals use in their appreciation of hazards[13]. The 'mental models' approach seeks to identify for a particular hazard both accurate and inaccurate beliefs that are held by a target population. These are then used as the basis for developing risk communication material that will correct misunderstandings. In this approach, the object is to bridge the gap between lay and expert models of the risk by adding missing concepts, correcting mistakes, strengthening correct beliefs and minimising peripheral ones. The approach is claimed to adhere to three tenets: (ii) the audience needs to be offered a basic understanding of the exposure, effects, and mitigation processes relevant to making decisions about the hazard; (ii) the existing beliefs of the audience are assumed to affect and interpret any new information; and (iii) new information must be presented in a such a way as to be consistent with the levels of under-standing (textual or other) that is manifest in the audience.

Essentially, the mental models approach argues that people have an intuitive understanding of risks and that they can be helped to a better appreciation, and consequently be placed in a position to make more informed decisions, if they are given new information in a format that is consistent with their initial belief system. The mapping of the initial belief system about the hazard that is the target for risk communication is thus crucial[14,15]. There are now several publications which describe in detail how mental models may be corrected[16,17].

The particular value of the mental models approach for risk communication is that it requires one to think in terms of a complex interacting system of beliefs which underpins risk appreciation. In order to have its desired impact, any information provided by a risk communication must be designed so as to take account of the way in which the entire system of beliefs will respond. Successfully shifting one belief in the system may not ultimately bring about the desired outcome because other elements in the system dampen any impact of movement in one. Figure 2 depicts a very basic lay mental model of the perceived risk of food poisoning associated with eating chicken. It should be noted that this is not a simple causal model that links the food source to exposure to illness. It recognises that exposure can be controlled by certain hygienic and preparative precautions. It also recognises that failure in hygiene precautions can result in exposure without direct consumption of the food source (e.g. through transmission via cutting boards, unwashed hands, or

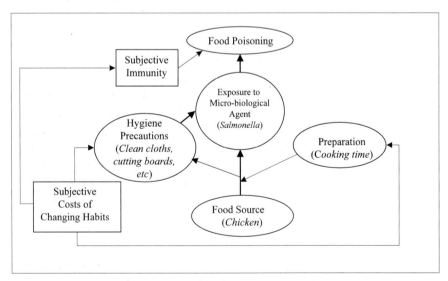

Fig. 2 Simplified mental model of a food hazard.

dish-cloths). Most importantly, it has as an integral part of the model subjective assessments of the costs of taking precautions and assumptions about personal immunity from illness caused in this fashion. Assessments of subjective immunity may even result in re-interpretation of apparent symptoms of food poisoning. If the person harbours expectations of immunity, symptoms can be re-interpreted as the product of over-eating or drinking too much. Any effort at risk communication directed at the person who held a mental model of high subjective immunity would need to take account of the motivational as well as the informational elements it entails.

The source of the risk communication

Impact of the characteristics of the source of risk communication have also been examined. The source of a risk message must be trusted if the communication is to have its desired impact. Trust is associated with believing that the source is expert, knowledgeable, unbiased, has no vested interest in the hazard and is not seeking to sensationalise the hazard. The public have been shown to hold quite strong opinions about the level of trust they attribute to different sources of information about food hazards[7]. Some hazards aroused greater distrust than others irrespective of the source, notably natural toxins, genetic engineering and pesticide residues (it should be noted that the data quoted here were collected prior to recent upsurges in concern about organophosphates and GM crops). Nevertheless, across the overall range of hazards, university scientists proved the most trusted source, with medical doctors a close second and consumer organisations third. The least trusted source was tabloid newspapers, followed by MPs and government ministers and then government ministries. However, trust in sources did vary across hazard types. Distrust increased when, for particular hazards, sources were expected to have vested interests or less knowledge. Medical sources were more trusted in medically-related areas, less so in technological risk assessment. This suggests that the choice of source for risk communication should be carefully matched to the nature of the hazard. Such information suggests that the public clearly has a sophisticated understanding of the motives that may predispose sources to bias their risk communication.

Content of the message

The impact of the content of the risk communication message has been studied. Much empirical research has focused upon the design of hazard warnings, and particularly upon product warning labels. There is now a large literature upon the manner in which information should be presented in order to have maximum intelligibility[18]. This work has in the main used an information processing paradigm. Information processing conceptualisations make the assumption that, when new information is given to an individual, it must trigger attention, then achieve comprehension and can only then influence decision making (though the nature of this influence will depend upon a subjective evaluation of the costs and benefits of any change). Given these assumptions, the information processing paradigm has resulted in much research which has catalogued the design features of messages which may increase the likelihood that they gain the audience's attention. This work has highlighted the significance of novelty, font size, icons, signal words, colour, contrast and location in designing hazards warnings. However, the attention grabbing power of any single characteristic has been found to be dependent upon both physical and social context. There appear to be no foolproof design features that will inevitably work to galvanise attention. Turning to issues of comprehensibility, in many respects, the conclusions drawn are unremarkable: information needs to be unambiguous, definitive and easily interpreted by those who need to attend to it. This tends to argue again for the need to pay attention to the mental models of the hazard held by the target audience. Evidence about what must be done in order to motivate individuals to change their behaviour once they have attended to and comprehended risk information is less conclusive. Changes in levels of knowledge about a hazard are not found to correlate simply with modifications in behaviour[19]. Familiarity with and habituation to a hazard are particularly likely to reduce the effectiveness of hazard warnings. This is particularly important in relation to food safety hazards since the source of danger is such a ordinary part of everyday life.

Recent research has focused specifically upon the effect that admissions of uncertainty have upon the reception of risk information. This is obviously of considerable importance since for many types of hazard the actual risks are uncertain. The health risks associated with various meat products following the identification of BSE have not been completely determined. There is still great scientific controversy about what is safe and what is not. In such a situation, the risk communicator has to decide how to express uncertainty. Decisions must be taken in the knowledge that the public in general wants certitude when dealing with hazards. Studies thus far suggest that the impact of admissions of uncertainty may result either in the information offered being taken more seriously and trusted or in the information being ignored or rejected[2]. The way that an admission of uncertainty is interpreted depends on who is making the admission. A trusted source that admits uncertainty may lose absolute authority but enhance credibility. An untrusted source that admits uncertainty may become more suspected since the expression of uncertainty may be interpreted as a desire to hide the full facts[20]. The impact of admissions of uncertainty also appears to depend upon how the admission emerges. If it is freely given, it is more likely to enhance trust. If given only after unexpected disclosures by other sources or under duress, it is likely to damage trust. The dilemmas facing risk communicators when they admit uncertainty cannot be eliminated. Yet neither can the need to acknowledge uncertainty. Much more research is needed that will examine how and when uncertainty should be explained.

Social amplification of risk

The major obstacles to anticipating and controlling the impact of any risk communication arise because it does not occur in a social vacuum. Once public, information about a hazard is subject to all of the normal social influence processes. The Social Amplification of Risk Framework (SARF) was devised in 1988[21-25] in order provide a more comprehensive and systematic approach to analysing how risk and risk events interact with psychological, social, institutional, and cultural processes in ways which intensify or attenuate risk perceptions and concerns and, thereby, shape risk behaviour, influence institutional processes and affect risk consequences. Examples of hazards which have been subject to social attenuation of risk might include naturally occurring radon gas, automobile accidents, and smoking. Social amplification of risk perceptions appears to have occurred in relation BSE/CJD and GM foods.

Figure 3 provides a simplified schematic representation of the elements considered to interact within the SARF. In the SARF, a hazard or risk event is said to become known either through direct experience or, more frequently, through communication via others (whether informal social networks or institutional information providers, such as the media or education systems). These sources of communication create the risk representation. In generating the representation of the risk they enhance, filter and reconfigure information. Once available, this initial risk representation will be subject to further processes of refinement, re-interpretation and elaboration both at the level of the individual (psychological filters) and of the cultural or social group (social filters). These processes of psychological and social filtration are not independent; they interact, sometimes re-inforcing, sometimes counteracting each other. The revised risk representations they produce may stimulate changes in behaviour at both the individual and societal levels. Individuals may cease some activities, organisations may change their structures or alter commercial plans, governments may introduce political or legislative

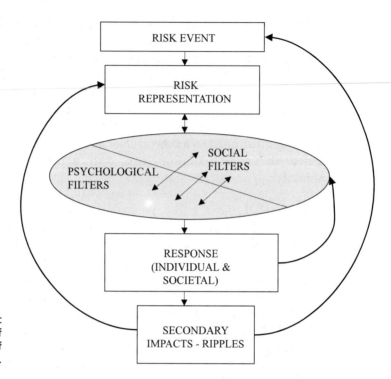

Fig. 3 Schematic representation of social amplification of risk framework.

change. Each type of behavioural response may have secondary impacts (ripple effects). Changes in individual patterns of consumption may cause major disruption of markets, legislative revision may encourage up-swing in litigation, new political policies may engender social disorder. These ripple effects mean that changes in risk representations can have substantial geographical and temporal extension impacts. The system is also reflexive. Secondary impacts may modify the nature of the original hazard or significantly modify the way it is represented subsequently. Individual and societal responses may serve to shift how psychological and social filters are operating to mediate risk representation.

The SARF is a useful analytical tool when considering how risk communication messages may need to work. At first sight, it suggests that risk communication is not a controllable process. The originators of a message may feel that they can rarely do much more than set it adrift on a sea of social amplification and attenuation. However, there is no reason for complete despair. In relation to specific hazards, it may be possible to identify how the risk representation will be modified as it is transmitted on by various social agents. For instance, the role of the media in risk amplification already has been reasonably well-documented for some hazards[26,27]. Interestingly, it has been shown that the extent of media coverage is not related, in any simple manner, to increases in public concern about a hazard. Trust in the media concerned may be mediating the tendency for public anxiety to grow. If this type of analysis can be done systematically for other parties in the process, it may be possible to use SARF to improve the design of risk communication. The SARF currently includes no predictive model of the relationships between different mediators of risk representations or how they influence each other. It does not incorporate any of the many theories that try to explain how social influence occurs. Development of SARF to explain the processes underlying amplification/attenuation so as to allow causal pathways to be tested is overdue.

The SARF is useful in emphasising that risk communication is not a one-way process. It is not even a just two-way process. It is a multi-dimensional process. In the so-called 'information society' the choice of sources for risk representations is virtually infinite. The opportunities for individuals or relatively powerless groups to respond to risk representations and to be heard by others is growing as the channels of communication become more diverse (particularly through the internet). This suggests that official sources of risk communication may expect even less control in the future than they have currently. It also suggests that instead of regarding amplification and attenuation processes as aberrations that need to be eliminated, official sources of risk communication will need to position their messages carefully within the system, capitalising upon processes they recognise to be inevitable.

References

1 Pidgeon N, Hood C, Jones D et al. Royal Society Report on Risk Analysis, Perception, and Management. London: Royal Society, 1992: (Chapter 5)
2 Pidgeon N, Beattie J. The psychology of risk and uncertainty. In: Calow P et al. (Eds) Handbook of Environmental Risk Assessment and Management. Oxford: Blackwell Science, 1997
3 Sparks P, Shepherd R. Public perceptions of food-related hazards: individual and social dimensions. Food Quality Pref 1994; 5: 1–10
4 Fife-Schaw C, Rowe G. Public perceptions of everyday food hazards: a psychometric study. Risk Analysis 1996; 16: 487–500
5 Slovic P. Perception of risk. Science 1987; 236: 280–5
6 Frewer L. Demographic differences in risk perceptions and public priorities for risk mitigation. Interim Report to the UK Ministry of Agriculture, Fisheries and Food. London: MAFF, 1998
7 Frewer L, Howard C, Hedderley D, Shepherd R. What determines trust in information about food-related risks? Underlying psychological constructs. Risk Analysis 1996; 16: 473–86
8 Twigger-Ross CL, Breakwell GM. Relating risk experience, venturesomeness and risk perception. J Risk Res 1999; 2: 73–83
9 Douglas M, Wildavsky A. Risk and Culture. Berkeley CA: University of California, 1982
10 Bonaiuto M, Breakwell GM, Cano I. Identity processes and environmental threat: the effects of nationalism and local identity upon perception of beach pollution. J Community Appl Social Psychol 1996; 6: 157–75
11 Weinstein N. Optimistic biases about personal risks. Science 1989; 246: 1232–3
12 Frewer L, Shepherd R, Sparks P. The interrelationship between perceived knowledge, control and risk associated with a range of food related hazards targeted at the self, other people and society. J Food Safety 1994; 14: 19–40

13 Fischhoff B, Bostrom A, Jacobs Quadrel M. Risk Perception and Communication. Oxford: Oxford University Press, 1997

14 Bostrom A, Fischhoff B, Morgan M. Characterizing mental models of hazardous processes: a methodology and an application to radon. J Social Issues 1992; **48**: 85–100

15 Jungermann H, Schutz H, Thuring M. Mental models in risk assessment: informing people about drugs. Risk Analysis 1988; **8**: 147–55

16 Atman C, Bostrom A, Fischhoff B, Morgan M. Designing risk communications and correcting mental models of hazardous processes, Part 1. Risk Analysis 1994; **14**: 779–87

17 Bostrom A, Atman C, Fischhoff B, Morgan M. Evaluating risk communications: completing and correcting mental models of hazardous processes, Part 2. Risk Analysis 1994; **14**: 789–98

18 Wolgater M, Laughery K. Warning! Sign and label effectiveness. Science 1996; **5**: 33–7

19 Breakwell GM. Risk estimation and sexual behaviour: a longitudinal study of 16–21 year olds. J Health Psychol 1996; **1**: 79–91

20 Miles S, Frewer L. Effective communication and food-related hazards. Report to the UK Ministry of Agriculture, Fisheries and Food. London: MAFF, 1998

21 Kasperson R, Renn O, Slovic P et al. The social amplification of risk: a conceptual framework. Risk Analysis 1988; **8**: 177–87

22 Renn O. Risk communication and the social amplification of risk. In: Kasperson R, Stallen P. (Eds) Communicating Risks to the Public. Dordrecht: Kluwer, 1991

23 Kasperson R. The social amplification of risk: progress in developing an integrative framework. In: Krimsky S, Golding D. (Eds) Social Theories of Risk. Westport, CT: Praeger, 1992

24 Burns W, Slovic P, Kasperson R et al. Incorporating structural models into research on the social amplification of risk: implications for theory construction and decision making. Risk Analysis 1993; **13**: 611–23

25 Kasperson R, Kasperson J. The social amplification and attenuation of risk. Ann Am Acad Political Social Sci 1996; **545**: 95–105

26 Macintyre S, Reilly J, Miller D, Eldridge J. Food choice, food scares and health: the role of the media. In: Murcott A. (Ed) The Nation's Diet. New York: Longman, 1998

27 Eldridge J, Reilly J. Risk and relativity: the case of BSE. Paper at Social Amplification of Risk Workshop, Windsor, UK, 1999

Understanding life-style and food use: contributions from the social sciences

Anne Murcott

Sociology, South Bank University, London, UK; Director, Economic & Social Research Council (UK) Programme, The Nation's Diet

The contribution of social sciences to the study of life-style and food use in Britain is illustrated by drawing on recent evidence of purchasing patterns, reports of the organisation of meals, snacks, eating out and images of the origins of food. Work discussed underlines a considerable degree of empirical complexity, demonstrates that the supply side as well as demand should be taken into account, and illustrates the manner in which even supposedly highly voluntaristic spheres of consumption activity may none the less be circumscribed. The article is prefaced by briefly contrasting the approach to 'life-style' adopted by market researchers, public health professionals and social theorists. It concludes with the proposal that in order to understand the complexity surrounding human food use, we may be advised to consider ensuring that the descriptive and conceptual tools being used can capture that complexity.

This article illustrates the contribution of selected social sciences to the study of life-style and food use in Britain. Its underlying purpose is to indicate that between them, the social sciences represent diverse types of research approach that may enhance understandings of the health of a nation, its food chain and its population's dietary selection. What follows is an overview of some recent, evidence-based insights which assume no prior acquaintance with any of the social sciences. In introducing recent contributions from human geography, economics, sociology and media studies, this article seeks to complement other, more tightly-focused examinations of social, psychological or economic topics in this volume. Though the substantive focus here is parochially British, it is anticipated that readers will be able to draw on material for regions with which they are familiar to apply the analytical outlooks made available here.

It will be useful to bear in mind that several considerations intended to illuminate the current 'state of the art' have been taken into account in selecting the material to follow. One is a concern to illustrate the wide diversity to be found amongst disciplines that fall under the generic heading social sciences[1]. In terms of their epistemology, approach to

Correspondence to:
Prof. Anne Murcott,
Sociology, HSS (Erlang),
South Bank University,
103 Borough Road,
London SE1 0AA, UK

British Medical Bulletin 2000; **56** (No. 1): 121–132

© The British Council 2000

research design, modes of procedure and technicalities of method, this group of disciplines lies between, but also spans, the gap between CP Snow's 'two cultures'. In these respects they run from those lying very close to some of the biomedical sciences – psychology is an example – to those that display much greater affinity with the humanities – for instance social anthropology or social history[2]. Second, is a concern to high-light topics that are less usually taken into account when contemplating the implications of life-style for diet and health, but which, none the less, are relevant – for instance those associated with the supply side, the structure of production and distribution of food, together with the regulatory climate within which they are to operate. A third consideration is not simply to illustrate the steady increase in the volume of contributions from the social sciences. It is also to emphasise the increased recognition that understanding human food use requires attention to substantial empirical complexity. Correspondingly, this demands an analytical complexity, of which reflection on the terminology being used is a necessary component. A corollary of this complexity is renewed confirmation that, realistically, there is no single set of ready answers for understanding human behaviour in respect of diet – or indeed anything else – any more than there are fool-proof blueprints for engineering change – dietary or otherwise.

Life-style

Although 'life-style' is widely accepted as relevant to health, food purchase and dietary choice, defining it presents some difficulty. The word is used in such a multiplicity of circumstances it may come as little surprise to find a prophecy made as long ago as 1981 that it 'will soon include everything and mean nothing, all at the same time'[3]. Yet getting to grips with the difficulty is integral to understanding life-style and food use. To begin so doing, this section sketches differences in the degree of precision with which (i) market research, (ii) public health, epidemiology and health promotion and (iii) a modern strand of social theory, have used the word in relation to health and food use.

Market research

Good access to the use to which market research puts the word life-style is not readily available to academics, and systematic scrutiny of the obtainable reports and journals to establish a well-substantiated analysis has, as far as is known, yet to be undertaken. At the same time, a usage illustrated by Lowe almost 20 years ago continues to be widely reported in and perpetuated by the mass media. More than anything else, this usage is allusive.

In an article, in whose title he chose to include the word life-styles[4], Lowe lists the following changes in Britain's eating habits: (i) new meal patterns; (ii) what is being prepared?; (iii) who is preparing the meal?; (iv) snacks; (v) take-away foods; (vi) eating out; (vii) foreign foods; and (viii) health foods.

He took the view that these were related to the preceding three decades of social changes in British society, including alterations in values and the growth of new social attitudes leading to 'new life-styles which in turn have produced new demands and expectations from meals and food'. Drawing on commercial research data collected by Taylor Nelson, the company he represented, Lowe's article illustrates the way that contrasts between social attitudes which he described as 'return to nature' and 'acceptance of disorder', can lead to both contrasts as well as 'convergence in the market place'. In other words, it is possible to buy the same items, *e.g.* 'health foods', in the name of dramatically different allegiances – respectively: a commitment to 'healthy' and 'natural' food; the pursuit of novelty or excitement. It is to be noted that the article happens to exclude all technical discussion, and correspondingly, offering neither discussion nor definition of life-style is able to treat its meaning as self-evident. It is likely that the phenomena to which Lowe refers may correspond to those with which public health experts are also concerned when discussing life-style. Where they differ is that the purposes of market research – purposes associated with work that is only ever conducted in so far as it addresses someone's life as a consumer of commercially supplied goods and services by those providing a commercial service for an industrial client's requirements for information about markets – reduces the need to stop and define terms.

Epidemiology/public health/health promotion

Academics in this field have, however, addressed the definition of life-style. Hetzel and McMichael were sufficiently convinced of its significance for the cover of the 1988 edition of their book *The LS Factor* to read: 'of all the health issues affecting our society today the life style factor is the most crucial'[5]. They admitted that the word presented difficulty, and arguably their efforts at defining it proved awkward. In practice, they enumerate several life-style factors (in the plural) noting that those which have been 'studied extensively include: diet, alcohol consumption, cigarette smoking, physical activity, sexuality and reproductive behaviour'. Associated with this well-established use of 'life-style' in epidemiology and public health[6], a distinction is made between two main elements of health promotion[7]. One has been described as structural, an approach covering fiscal policies, legislative or environmental measures – commentators give as examples of the latter two, measures governing the use of seat belts and regulating the positioning of out-fall waste pipes, respectively. The other is based on 'life-style approaches', which centre on the individual not the group, and are geared to 'the identification and subsequent reduction of behavioural risk factors associated with morbidity and/or premature death'.

Life-style approaches typically rest on an assumption that some behaviour under scrutiny carries more or less risk to health, is enacted voluntarily, and is a matter of option or choice – albeit, if correlated with adverse health consequences, choice that is held to be ill-educated or uninformed. Several commentators have argued that there has been an undue emphasis on life-style approaches at the expense of the structural, which in any case, they add, cannot adequately be confined to regulation or to the effect of the physical environment[8]. So doing, they note, is to neglect a great body of evidence that socio-economic factors, including income, employment status, occupation, and housing persistently affect health. Such structural factors contrast with life-style by acting as constraints, limiting the scope for voluntary action and, thereby, shaping the behaviour of the individual. For some, then, the public health agenda is to extend beyond what is regarded as the individualistic focus of life-style.

Social theory, identity, modernity

In the hands of social theorists[9], life-style is the focus of considerable debate, where definitions are more likely to be ostensive than precise, part of a much broader discussion about modernity, *i.e.* the distinctive state of society toward the end of the 20th century. Here, health and food use tend to be included by way of illustrating abstract discussion, and are presented alongside reference to contemporary aesthetic and ethical concerns about identity and nature, dress and décor, or how to conduct oneself at work.

By referring back to its origins in the early years of this century, Giddens, as one of the leading contemporary social theorists, suggests that the notion of life-style risks being corrupted by consumerisms and trivialised by marketing. Life-style, he argues, is much more than that. Moreover, it is not just a collection of routine practices that are incorporated into usual ways of dressing, eating, frequenting favoured haunts and so forth. Life-style implies choice within a plurality of possible options, and is 'adopted' rather than 'handed down'[10].

For Giddens, life-style is more than about how to act, it is also about who to be. In other words, life-style is about identity. There is an active, creative even inventive element to life-style. Rather than being obedient, passive followers of fashion, people are well aware, *i.e.* self-conscious, of the artificiality of life-styles and can choose to don or discard them. This active element is reflected in the adoption of the expression 'food use' in place of 'food habits'.

Like the contrast drawn by those in public health, *etc.*, social theorists also distinguish between life-style as involving the realm of choices – albeit of considerable complexity – and the limits placed on those choices by economic constraints of, at the extreme, social disadvantage. But Giddens, in particular, views that distinction from a strikingly different angle. He implies that in modern society, such constraints are no longer liable to be accepted fatalistically. Possibilities for the pursuit of a type of life-style which are denied by economic deprivation are regarded as just that, possibilities. As a result, life-style routines may themselves be created as part of resistances to exclusion and deprivation; and, in less dramatic form, a resolute decision to by-pass research findings on the wisdom of a low-fat-low-sugar-low-salt, high fibre diet is, Giddens claims, conduct which none the less forms part of a distinctive life-style – precisely because the world now consists of a plurality of choices within which people may choose whether to opt for alternatives.

Life-style and food use in Britain: some recent evidence

The brief sketch just presented exposes different degrees of precision in the use of the notion of life-style. In the process, it suggests that attempts to understand food use and life-style are liable to be inadequate if the relation, the tension even, between voluntary active choice and constraints limiting that choice is ignored. It is with a consideration of constraints that this selected overview of recent evidence from the social sciences begins. Except where indicated by the provision of a full reference, the evidence derives from 18 research projects funded under the Economic and Social Research Council (UK) Research Programme *The Nation's Diet* 1992–98. For the sake of brevity, the separate publications are not referenced, although the principal researchers concerned are named[11].

Systems of supply, images of origins

Economic constraints limiting active expression of food use is not solely a matter of the level of an individual's resources on the demand, or consumption, side of the economic equation. It is also a matter of the supply side, where changes may alter how far those resources can stretch. One of the notable features of food retailing in late 1980s and early 1990s Britain was the growth of superstores on edge-of-city sites. Critics became concerned that not only was this contributing to a decline in town centres but with it, reduced access to food shops for sectors of the population unable to afford appropriate transport. Regulations introducing tightened land-use planning (1993, 1994, 1996) which prioritised the viability of town centres would, it was believed, among other things reduce the severity of economic constraint. But in his analysis of the underlying economic geography of the broader competitive trends, Wrigley shows that by the end of 1997 at least, the effect remained muted, and somewhat mixed. Certainly retailers had, to some extent, 'returned to the high street'. But higher operating costs – despite the inclusion on the shelves of a larger proportion of 'value added' items – depressed the achievement of satisfactory returns on investment. At the same time, the workings of the regulatory framework in practice, still meant that new, out-of-town development was set to continue.

A more complicated example of the intertwining of supply and demand is demonstrated by Fine who records, for instance, the irony that though purchases of low-fat foods are increasing, levels of purchase of cream and high fat dairy products have remained steady. Part of his work can shed some light on the conundrum that, despite improved public awareness of advice to eat less fat, actual levels of intake for the population overall have altered little. A well-established conclusion is drawn by psychologists that attitudes or knowledge do not neatly lead to corresponding behaviour. Fine's innovative economic analysis approaches the matter rather differently. He brings supply and demand together in taking the length of the whole food chain into account, to include examining both its production and consumption constituent parts. First he is able to confirm that familiar variables, notably income, are indeed correlated with whether or not households purchase different foods. But he also showed that socio-economic variables are related to patterns of purchase which differ from one type of food to another, echoing the structures of supply. Instead of a single food chain for all foods, Fine argues that it is necessary to develop analyses in terms of a separate production chain for each group of foodstuffs, meat, sugar, dairy products, etc., reflecting back again in separate consumption parts of each chain. Behind each are major differences in the complex pattern of incentives associated with relations between primary producers, processors/manufacturers and retailers, combined with the workings of agriculture policies, and the presence, absence or changes in marketing boards.

Pursuing the question of new products, Fine takes the case of the dairy system of provision. Trends over the last two decades in this chain of production involve restructuring which can be credited with making 'healthier' products available. Skimmed milk production has increased, and vegetable oils have been substituted for butter. The resulting surplus butterfat has, however, remained in the food system, ending up in more extensive production of cheese or diverted to new products, such as desserts or 'up-market' ready prepared meals. In a separate part of his analysis, Fine shows that there are also systematic variations in purchasing patterns for new products. Those households which spend more on food are those most likely to buy food items newly on the market. But, he finds, that it is these same households which are also most likely to continue buying 'older' products the novelties might have supplanted. The scene is now set for a plausible, though still speculative, interpretation in terms of the social theorists' creativity in life-style. Echoing a political and commercial allegiance to 'consumer choice' and reflecting the plurality of options and milieu in which people can adopt one life-style or another, a self-conscious pursuit of 'healthy' activities during the week can co-exist, in the name of balance, with an equally self-conscious pursuit of stylish or more self-indulgent relaxation at weekends. This switching between styles of eating, is found in Warde's work on eating out which is most commonly thought of as some type of special occasion, as well as in Caplan's study where tourists to West Wales regarded their time off as a short holiday, not simply away from work and home, but also away from the attentiveness to dietary advice. As a result, **both** skimmed milk and thick cream are added to the same shopping basket.

These two examples of studies demonstrate the manner in which the structure and nature of the food supply literally figures in patterns of food purchase. In contrast are studies of people's images of the food supply, particularly of the origins of food. It is assumed that in some, as yet imperfectly specified fashion, such images not only form an integral part of life-style and food use, they also affect purchasing patterns and, thereby, the patterns of what actually gets eaten. Investigating the former, Cook and colleagues[12] noted twin stereotypes of 'the consumer': on the one hand is the sovereign, super-informed consumer which the industry is urged to understand and be responsive to; on the other is that of a consumer ignorant of the origin or the nutritional composition of foods, who is kept less well informed, *e.g.* by limited product labelling. They uncovered images of geographical origins of foodstuffs to show that the reality may well include both these, but that there is a range of quite sophisticated images that cross-cut them. Far from being ignorant about the origins of foods, people have wide-ranging and socially differentiated images, deriving, mosaic-fashion, from childhood recollections, experience of travel, mass media coverage of food issues, even school geography lessons. It is no doubt the case that the actual complexity of the food-chain and its modern, global character, powerfully militate against any but the professional experts being able to approach complete actual knowledge. Instead, people develop images of foods' origins that serve as a shorthand, which, Cook suggests, can account for the well-recognised trust in brand names, reliance on the recommendations of popular TV chefs, or the recent growth of farmers' markets in British cities.

That the mass media represent one of the sources of people's images of the food supply, is familiar – not least in the common accusation that journalists are responsible for sensationalist reporting of threats to food safety that plays on the ignorance of a gullible public. It is an accusation, however, that is not well based on evidence. Research in the area repeatedly confirms that the mass media do not tell people what to think, though they may well tell people what to think about. When the mass media bring a topic to the attention of their audiences, evidence regularly indicates that people do not passively 'believe all they read in the newspapers'. Eldridge showed that the manner in which people interpret media coverage of *Salmonella enteritidis,* bovine spongiform encephalopathy, and associated images of the food supply, was mediated by several types of factor. One duly reflected the widely reported scepticism of official advice, but finds that such scepticism is likely to be re-inforced by quite other sources of information, for example first-hand acquaintance with the catering or other sector of the industry. Less frequently noticed, however, is his finding that a positive image of the food-chain prevailed. In practice, safety problems were regarded as temporary, with people treating the reduction in mass media attention as signalling that the difficulties had been successfully resolved and a secure or safe supply had been restored. In turn, this allowed people relief from restrictions on buying or eating.

Meal patterns, snacks and eating out

It is highly likely that when Lowe[13] presented his paper 20 years ago, his London audience immediately recognised his reference to 'new meal patterns'. Meals – especially family meals – were then, and are now, held to be disappearing, replaced, in the market researcher's evocative phrase, by 'grazing'[14]. The prospect repeatedly evokes dismay in public commentary lest it presage not only a nutritional decline but also some type of social disintegration, a decline in the quality of family bonds. Before evaluation of either type of decline can be initiated, however, the changes alluded to need to be substantiated.

For a topic so widely covered, it is striking that adequate quality trend data are not obviously available. What is becoming apparent, however, is that the very concern about a supposed decline in family meals itself may not be new: evidence of its expression is vividly reported in a study of a small American town in the 1920s. Recent British work is starting, piece by piece, to build up a picture which suggests people are making a self-conscious distinction between what is practicable – grazing – and what is important for family life – a continued allegiance to the idea of family meals, which then become slightly special occasions. Whether it is couples who have just set up house together, women who go out of their way to accommodate one household member's dietary changes (whether for medical or non-medical reasons) African Caribbean Londoners for whom it is an important aspect of black identity, the importance of family meals may turn out to be more robust than has been feared. If further work supports this suggestion, then the social theorists' meaning of life-style which emphasises a plurality of choices, a creative response to a multiplicity of options, might be the most suitable definition to adopt when characterising emerging trends.

Evidence that family meals at home in the evening continue to be valued is found in a pioneering study of both primary and secondary school-based eating by Burgess. Conducted in the wake of policy changes that have sought to replace universal welfare/state provision with family responsibility and 'consumer choice', his work offers a view on food use and life-style among the young. Legislation in Britain now permits schools to cease standard provision, although, as in the case of one of the primary schools in Burgess' study, space and supervision for children to eat at midday is made available. This would seem to maximise the opportunity for choices from home to be manifest in what each child ate, leading, in principle, to the anticipation of considerable variety in the food pupils daily carried into school. In practice, institutional arrangements limited the types of food that could be included, for it has to be conveniently carried by a child below 11-years-old, be storable unrefrigerated for some 3 h, and easily eaten without either cutlery or plates.

Small wonder that the study's best description for school dinner time was a 'large indoor picnic' comprising a selection of snacks, which, far from reflecting any anticipated wide variety, conformed to a standardised format. What parents actually sent to school entailed compromises between their notions of nutritional adequacy, the practicalities of lunch box storage, and familiarity with their own child's preferences. Compromises took into account two further dimensions which re-introduces the question of constraint to the closing stages of this short article: what could be afforded and acute sensitivity to their children's anxieties about being different from their friends. These two dimensions also introduce a distinction between financial and non-financial constraints. Both are found to be at issue in final case to be mentioned here. This case is the first known academic study out in the UK of eating out – another item in Lowe's list of new life-styles and changes in British eating habits.

There is a view that the activities involved in consumption allow the majority a considerable degree of discretion, greater even than in most other aspects of modern life. It may be that this view has served as a spur to what public health critics argue is an overemphasis on life-style as a realm of voluntary action. For many, such discretion is a norm both for shopping for specific items and also for engaging in specific leisure pursuits of which eating specific foods may be a particular instance. If that is held to be the case, then as all these coincide, they support an idea that eating out allows more freedom from restriction that any other sphere of modern life. There are several associated features of eating out. For example, as part of the commercial rather than domestic sphere, it means that the relation between the diner and the cook is contractual, shorn of mutual family obligations and household practicalities where a shared meal also tends to entail a shared menu. Again, the conventions of eating in a commercial outlet provide for diners selecting different dishes from one another at the self-same meal.

All this helps underscore eating out as an occasion for maximum individual discretion, optimal circumstances for active, creative life-style choice. So it is the more surprising that Warde finds any evidence of constraint among those able to afford to eat out. Yet he reports that there are those who commonly claim that they were often constrained as to what they ate, in the sense that they had little or no voice in decisions about whether or where to eat out. It then become clear that the non-financial constraints of day-to-day cultural conventions and norms of appropriate behaviour come into play. It is the social complexities of decision-making – negotiations between couples, the 'give-and-take among friends – that turn out differentially to affect the 'say' people have in what they actually get to eat. In this fashion, the 'freedom' to choose is limited in one of the very sectors of modern life which at times is considered to constitute the epitome of aesthetic stylishness, creativity and plurality of choices that the word 'life-style' is held to connote.

Concluding observations

This article has indicated that the three separate spheres of market research, public health/health promotion and modern social theory, approach and use the word life-style in rather different ways. In the world of market research, there may be little need to analyse its meaning. Work can proceed by allusion, apparently anticipating shared assumptions. By contrast, experts in public health and health promotion propose that structural as well as individualistic concerns should explicitly be addressed. Thus, they seek to ensure that an emphasis on option or choice, does not lead to neglecting the constraints that limit the scope for voluntary action. Different again, certain modern social theorists are approaching the matter the other way on. They propose that life-style is also about identity, in that it entails a self-conscious, creative act of choice.

Briefly identifying these differing usages here, is emphatically not to be confused with adjudicating between them. Any such evaluation is not intended, and in any case would represent an untenable intellectual exercise. The present purpose of making comparisons is to expose two matters for careful consideration. First, it is to underline the absence of, and difficulty in achieving, an adequate and agreed definition of the word 'life-style' when seeking scientifically to describe modern dietary habits or food purchasing patterns. Second, as the main part of the article aims to illustrate albeit in compressed and selected form, the realm to which 'life-style' has been used to refer is characterised by considerable empirical social, economic and political complexity. Thus, if we are trying to understand that self-same complexity, we may be very well advised to start by matching our descriptive and conceptual tools to its multi-dimensional nature – and in the process avail ourselves of this component, among the others, of the contribution to be made by the social sciences in efforts to improve understandings of the health of a nation, its food-chain and its population's food use.

Acknowledgements

Grateful acknowledgement is made to Gill Ereaut for comments on key sections of this article, and to Roger Dickinson for ruminative conversation.

Notes and References

1 Murcott A. Food choice, the social sciences and The Nation's Diet Research Programme. In: Murcott A. (Ed) *The Nation's Diet: the social science of food choice*. Harlow: Addison Wesley Longman, 1998; 1–22
2 A fine fictional illustration of just this span is represented by Djerassi C. *Cantor's Dilemma* New York: Penguin, 1989
3 Sobel ME. *Lifestyle and Social Structure* quoted in Chaney D. *Lifestyles* London: Routledge, 1996
4 Lowe M. Influence of changing lifestyles on food choice. In: Turner M. (Ed) *Nutrition and Lifestyles*. London: Applied Science, 1980; 141–8
5 Hetzel B, McMichael T. *The LS Factor* Ringwood, Vic: Penguin, 1988
6 See also Jacobson B, Smith A, Whitehead M. *The Nation's Health: a strategy for the 1990s*. London: The King's Fund Centre, 1988

7 Bunton R, Macdonald G. *Health Promotion: disciplines and diversity* London: Routledge, 1992
8 Blaxter M. *Health & Lifestyles* London: Tavistock/Routledge, 1990; Nettleton S. *The Sociology of Health & Illness* Cambridge: Polity, 1995 and see also Jacobson, Smith, Whitehead *op cit*
9 For an introduction see Chaney *op cit*
10 Giddens A. *Modernity and Self-Identity* Cambridge: Polity, 1991
11 Readers are directed to Murcott A. (Ed) *The Nation's Diet: the social science of food choice* Harlow: Addison Wesley Longman, 1998, an edited volume introducing the work of the Programme and which, together with the website www.sbu.ac.uk/~natdi provides an extensive bibliography
12 Cook I, Crang P, Thorpe M. Biographies and geographies: consumer understandings of the origins of foods. *Br Food J* 1998: **100**: 162–7
13 See note 4
14 Murcott A. Family meals: a thing of the past? In: Caplan P. (Ed) *Food, Health and Identity* London: Routledge 1997; 32–49

Economic aspects of food-borne outbreaks and their control

Jennifer A Roberts

Collaborative Centre for Economics of Infectious Disease, Health Services Research Unit, Department of Public Health and Policy, London School of Hygiene and Tropical Medicine, London, UK

This paper begins with a discussion of the definition of an outbreak. It considers the portion of outbreaks in the general pattern of food-borne infectious disease. The methods used to identify outbreaks are described and the importance of the potential benefits and the economic impact of outbreak recognition and control and are discussed. The paper concludes by illustrating the economic impact of intervention using three infectious diseases botulism, *Salmonella* and *Escherichia coli* O157 as case studies of outbreaks.

What is an outbreak? An outbreak is said to occur when two or more cases of an infectious illness are linked by epidemiological, clinical or microbiological evidence. A food-borne outbreak is one caused or thought to be caused by food or water. Food-borne infections have been rising steeply over the past decades and, although better identification of organisms and possibly better reporting has contributed to this trend, there does appear to be a growing problem. Concern about food-borne infection was heightened in the UK in the late 1980s following the identification of *Salmonella enteritidis* in eggs. This led to the setting up of the Committee on Microbiological Safety of Food (Richmond Committee)[1] and to the Study of Infectious Intestinal Disease in England,[2] a microbiological, epidemiological and economic assessment of disease. Reports of infectious intestinal disease have continued to rise. *Campylobacter* spp. and *Salmonella* spp. account for a large portion of cases but more virulent forms of infections such as *Escherichia coli* O157:H7 have emerged as important risks. However, in 1997 and 1998, there was a fall in reports of *S. enteritidis* and *Salmonella typhimurium* outbreaks. Much of this disease burden is likely to be food or water borne.

It has been estimated that the cost of intestinal infections for England is £750 million[2]. The burden of infection is felt by those infected, those whom they might infect and those who care for them either informally at home or as part of the formal health services. Preventive policies for

Correspondence to:
Dr Jennifer A Roberts,
Collaborative Centre for
Economics of Infectious
Disease, London School
of Hygiene and Tropical
Medicine, Keppel Street,
London WC1 7HT, UK

© The British Council 2000

food-borne infectious intestinal disease need to address all points along the food-chain, particularly critical points that have been found to be risky and have hazardous consequences. This may be part of a formal hazard analysis and critical control point (HACCP) system. HACCP identifies steps in the process that are critical and assesses the consequences to health that may arise if mistakes occur[3]. If possible, strategies to reduce hazards should be in place. This endeavour involves commercial producers, farmers and market gardeners and private individuals who garden or who collect food-stuffs for consumption, manufacturers and purveyors of food and those who prepare food for consumption. If at any point in the system prevention fails an outbreak may occur.

Notification of disease

There are three systems of notification of infectious disease in the England and Wales. The first is based on clinical reports. Every doctor in clinical practice has a statutory duty to report certain infectious diseases and food poisoning to the consultant in communicable disease control (CCDC). The second is the national surveillance scheme of laboratory-confirmed infections reported by public health and NHS laboratories to the Centre for Communicable Disease Surveillance (CDSC) at the Public Health Laboratory Service (PHLS). The third is a national surveillance system for general outbreaks that relies upon reports of outbreaks by the CsCDC to the CDSC at the PHLS. Food poisoning is also reported to CDSC at the PHLS by environmental health departments of local authorities. Reported cases reflect only a small portion of illnesses experienced in the community.

The proportion of diseases identified using community surveys and those identified using notification systems of infectious intestinal disease vary by infectious group. The study of Infectious Intestinal Disease in England[2] found that cases in the community were identified by notification systems more frequently for salmonellas than for viruses, particularly small round structured viruses (SRSV). One in 3 cases of salmonellosis and 1 in 7 campylobacteriosis cases were reported compared to 1 in 1567 for SRSV, possibly because of the relatively short duration of illness associated with SRSV. For each case visiting the GP, there were approximately 6 cases in the community.

These findings support the view that food-borne infections are under-reported. Unfortunately, because there was no easy way of collecting suspect food products for testing from the cases or controls recruited to the Infectious Intestinal Disease Study, it was not possible to estimate the proportion of cases that were food-borne from that study.

In the US, it has been estimated that between 6.5 million and 33 million illnesses and up to 900 deaths occur each year from food-borne microbes (namely, bacteria, parasites, viruses and fungi)[4]. The risk of fatality from a food-borne event for the population has been estimated in the US to be 1/29,000[5].

Identification of outbreaks

Identification of an outbreak might occur in a number of ways. Possibly most outbreaks are discovered by cases reported to CsCDC by alert individuals – general practitioners, hospital doctors and microbiologists. A good example of a rapid response was the one that led to the identification of an outbreak of *E. coli* O157 in Lothian in 1994[6]. In this outbreak, a hospital doctor, a GP and a microbiologist contacted the CCDC within hours of each other to report that they had seen suspicious cases or, in the case of the microbiologist, had identified the organism. National surveillance is frequently the only way of detecting an outbreak where cases are spread widely across the country. An example of this type of identification was a *Salmonella agona* outbreak identified in North London, and traced to other areas in Europe, Canada and the US and tracked back to a manufacturer in Israel[7]. Increasingly, given the growth of electronic data bases and linked reporting, scanning for higher than expected reports may prove useful in the identification of outbreaks. A surveillance system, linked to a public health network that can investigate and implement control strategies, can contribute directly to the interruption of an epidemic and to the reduction in the risk of future epidemics[8].

Outbreaks make up only a small proportion of cases of infections notified to the public health laboratory service. The number of outbreaks identified varies by organism for a number of reasons: length of illness, the likelihood of tests being taken and the microbiological sensitivity and specificity of the testing. The identification of outbreaks often depends upon the ability to link cases microbiologically. The ability to do this varies by organism. Sub-types of salmonella can be accurately identified. Such identification facilitates investigations. Identified outbreaks of salmonella make up about 10% of reported cases. A similar percentage of *E. coli* O157 cases are identified as outbreaks possibly because of the seriousness of the illness and the availability of highly specific tests that make it easy to match cases and associated food or environmental samples. Only 0.2% of *Campylobacter* cases are linked with outbreaks[9]. This is largely because it has proved impossible to sub-type campylobacters isolated in clinical practice, from foods and from the environment. A number of campylobacter infections may well be part of undetected outbreaks.

Benefits to identification of outbreaks

Outbreaks are costly, attract media attention and cause alarm. The costs of not identifying an outbreak, however, may be even more substantial. The main benefit from outbreak recognition is to prevent further spread. The economic benefits that result from an intervention will vary by outbreak. The net benefits depend on the costs of the investigation compared to the benefits accruing from interrupting the outbreak.

Identifying and controlling an outbreak may reduce the number of cases infected, improve clinical care and provide opportunities for prevention of other outbreaks thus reducing the long-term and short-term morbidity and costs. If the outbreak arose from a single source and was self-limiting, no primary cases may be avoided but the number of secondary cases may be reduced and lessons may be learnt that may affect future practice and prevent recurrences. An example of this type of outbreak often recounted is that of the wedding breakfast at which chickens, cooked the previous day and packed in the boxes in which they were delivered when raw, infected all the wedding guests with salmonella. No doubt the caterer and the wedding party learnt from this. Single source outbreaks may contribute more to prevention of disease if the contaminated product can be removed rapidly from the shelves. This happens quite frequently. Good examples of interventions of this kind include an outbreak of botulism traced to contaminated hazelnut conserve used to flavour yoghurt. This was removed from the food chain[10]. Another was an identification of an outbreak of *Salmonella napoli* in chocolate bars[11]. This resulted in 80% of a consignment being withdrawn from sale. These examples are discussed as case studies below.

Often the outbreak is caused by a continuing source that would cause infection indefinitely. The outbreak of *S. agona* caused by a fault in the production process is an example of this[7,12]. Outbreaks can also arise from a recurring source perhaps in a private water supply. These can be modified by interventions and advice, *e.g.* advice about boiling water during outbreaks due to *Cryptosporidium*[13].

The lessons learnt from an outbreak may lead to improvements in practice or regulation that can prevent further epidemics or outbreaks occurring. The improvements might modify or remove the source of infection, *e.g.* facilities for hand-washing at farm centres or children's zoos may reduce the likelihood of infections due to *Campylobacter* and *E. coli* O157:H7[14] or recommendations or advice about preparation and storage procedures – pasteurisation processes with relation to *Listeria*[15] or to changes in production procedures – *S. agona*[7] and botulism outbreaks[10].

Identification of the infective agent can modify treatment and so reduce morbidity and mortality. The identification of the infective agent could reduce the likelihood of misdiagnosis and unnecessary surgical interventions in cases with acute abdominal pain, such as that associated with campylobacter and *E. coli* O157. Rapid identification of infections such as *Cryptosporidium* may provide important clinical information for the management of those with reduced immunity.

Advice to infected individuals, those who look after them and to institutions who employ them or look after them is very important in containing an outbreak and avoiding secondary spread. This can result in: (i) isolation of patients to reduce the spread of infection, *e.g.* isolation in cases of listeriosis in mother and baby units; (ii) limiting person-to-person spread, *e.g.* exclusion from work or school, advice to formal and informal carers; and (iii) suggesting institutional interventions, *e.g.* ward closures, cleaning to reduce contamination of air or water.

Information, and advice to the public and industry that is accurate and timely can reduce public and professional concern associated with scare stories and outbreaks, *e.g.* handling of the panic about the perceived threat of 'super bug' and the 'flesh-eating bacteria'. Credible management of the potential threat can allow adjustments and changes to be made to behaviour or manufacturing practice, *e.g.* an outbreak of salmonella in kebanos sausages was handled promptly by taking products off the shelves. Subsequently, the product was manufactured using a pasteurisation process so limiting further outbreaks from that source[16].

High profile outbreaks can provide a catalyst for change. Arguably the Lanarkshire outbreak of *E. coli* O157 provided a catalyst for changes that led not only to changes in regulations relating to retail practices but added to the political pressure for a food standards agency[17].

An outbreak that goes unrecognised will not recoup the benefits outlined above.

Economic aspects

Evaluating infectious disease control consists of evaluating an absence – the avoidance of any infection potentially frees up resources that can then be used for other purposes. A full economic appraisal of an outbreak would seek to cost and analyse the intricate web of activities and value their contribution. Evaluations, typically in the form of cost of illness studies, provide minimum estimates of the value to society of the avoidance of disease. Some infections have a significance in the popular imagination, cultural and value systems that imply that society would be willing to pay more than the mere resource costs of the illness in order to avoid them. Policy making takes place in the context of such culturally determined fears and beliefs. Estimations of the costs of illness, together with descriptions of the disease characteristics, could provide information that could form a basis for using a willingness to pay approach to estimating benefits. Such estimates of the value society places on avoiding infection would allow an economic evaluation to take the form of a full cost-benefit study that would indicate the rate of return to intervening in an outbreak.

As willingness to pay studies are difficult to undertake, the most useful approach at present appears to involve assessing the opportunity costs of the resources forgone because of the infection. A bed used by someone suffering unnecessarily from an infection, given the pressure on resources in the health sector, deprives someone else of treatment. Intervention may reduce illness and so save resources of the public health laboratory services, the resources of the health care sector, including hospital, GP and community services, and the time and resources of people infected and those who care for them[18].

Few studies have offered a comprehensive account of the implications of an outbreak. Attempts were made to cost the intervention including costs to the patient and the family, the NHS, and public health departments were made in the costs of S. *napoli* outbreak[11], the national study of salmonellosis[19] and the E. *coli* O157 study[6]. Few estimate the costs of the intervention, few trace out the costs beyond the health sector and few project the costs to encompass the long-term sequelea of the illness[20].

Studies of outbreaks usually allow a more comprehensive range of costs to be included. Each outbreak, however, is different and the estimates may not be generalisable. On the other hand, estimates using epidemiological surveys will usually exclude the costs of investigating cases and the costs to third parties resulting from the illness[2]. Estimates

Table 1 Estimates of the costs of intestinal infectious disease in England

Cost category	Costs per case (£) All intestinal infectious disease	Costs per case (£) Salmonella
Those visiting a GP		
National Health Service		
GP costs	44.8	47.8
Hospital costs	17.6	84.0
Costs to cases and carers		
Direct costs	15.5	34.3
Indirect costs (including time off work)	174.9	440.3
Total	253.8	606.5
Costs of community cases who did not see a GP		
Costs to cases and carers		
Direct costs	3.9	3.8
Indirect costs (including time off work)	30.6	40.0
Total*	34.5	43.8

Adapted from the *Report of Infectious Intestinal Disease in England*[2].
*Subject to rounding errors.

based on reported cases will represent a different cost profile from those based on a community survey[2]. Some studies have concentrated only on hospital costs of illness[21]. These cases represent the most severe and most expensive cases. Those who see a GP will cost more than those who do not and those who do not have been found to be less severely ill[2]. Table 1 indicates the distribution of costs of infectious intestinal disease in England[2]. It is clear that the costs of all intestinal infectious disease, that includes many short-term virus infections, is much lower than the costs of cases with salmonella.

It is possible to estimate the contribution of early detection and control both from self-limiting and potentially continuous sources.

Case studies

Case studies will be used to illustrate the impact of interventions that have taken place.

Botulism

Rapid and successful intervention prevented illness and the high costs associated with an outbreak of botulism in hazelnut flavoured yoghurt. The intervention to remove the source of infection reduced the outbreak by at least one half, probably more, as, in addition to the removal of yoghurt from the shelves, a can of infected hazelnut conserve that would have been used to produce more yoghurt was taken out of the food-chain. The process of producing hazel nut conserve was also changed limiting the likelihood of recurrence from this source. The rapid identification of the source of infection was of paramount importance in this outbreak. Successful identification can save in the order of £22,000 per case to the health sector alone. The high mortality and high health care costs make this the second most expensive infectious disease in the acute phase of illness. The intervention was likely to have saved over £606,000 to the health sector and £4–10 million in total, using the lowest value of lives lost[8]. The cost of the intervention was largely the cost of the time of the consultant investigating the outbreak and the costs of testing the cases and food samples. The cost of the investigation was unlikely to have been more than £6000 including the removed products from the shelves.

Salmonellosis

A national outbreak of salmonellosis due to chocolate contaminated with *S. napoli* occurred. As a result of the detection and control of this outbreak 80% of a consignment of chocolate from Italy was withdrawn from sale and the outbreak with its attendant cost limited[11]. At 1995 prices, the value of this intervention would have been £8.7 million in health care cost, £4.8 million in public health costs, and £13.5 million in costs to patients and families. The cost of the intervention yielded a 3.5-fold rate of return. The measured benefit related to the UK but the intervention no doubt prevented many cases in continental Europe.

A more recent intervention to prevent salmonellosis, *S. agona*, similarly interrupted an outbreak. The savings were primarily in Israel where some 2000 cases were avoided – cost savings in UK prices of some £600,000 to the health care sector alone and some £10–16 million in total. The intervention also may have led to changes in production methods and so reduced the likelihood of imports from this source causing problems in the future[7,12].

E. coli O157

An outbreak of *E. coli* O157:H7 in Lothian in 1994[6] was brought under control in 36 hours by the timely intervention of those involved and the rapid identification of the source. The cost of the outbreak was very large. The hospital costs associated with treating 71 cases during the acute phase and the subsequent 12 months was £600,000. Some cases were in hospital for over 6 months. Two cases left hospital on dialysis and one has since had a kidney transplant. Had the intervention not occurred to remove the milk supplies ready for distribution from the food-chain, it is likely that more cases would have been infected adding to the costs and suffering of those affected. The pay off to the intervention was thus likely to have been high. However, this outbreak also points to the importance of primary prevention in organisms of such high pathogenicity[17].

Conclusions

It is unlikely that we can reduce food-borne infections entirely. We could, however, reduce them by using adequate control procedures. The adoption of well designed sensitive system of hazard and critical control points (HACCP)[3] to stages of food production could limit hazards and risks of infection along the food-chain[17]. When primary prevention fails, then rapid detection of outbreaks, intelligent investigation to locate the source and controls to limit the spread are vitally important and investment in this activity is likely to have a high pay off both in the short and long-term.

The food-borne outbreak studies described indicate the potential benefits that arise from early recognition and control of outbreaks. Good surveillance systems to identify outbreaks are essential. Surveillance costs have not been estimated as they are complex and embedded in clinical and public health medicine. They are, however, likely to be small compared to the enormous costs of infection. The pay off to investment in outbreak detection, investigation and control is many fold.

References

1   Committee on the Microbiological Safety of Food. *Report of the Committee on the Microbiological Safety of Food* (Richmond Committee). London: HMSO, 1990
2   Infectious Intestinal Disease Study Executive. *Report on the Intestinal Infectious Disease in England*. London: Department of Health, 2000
3   Baird-Parker AC. Development of industrial procedures to ensure the microbiological safety of food. *Food Control* 1995; **6**: 29–36
4   Roberts T, Unnevehr L. New approaches to regulating food safety *Foodreview* 1994; **17** Issue 2: 2–8
5   Alchrich L. Food-safety policies balancing risk and costs *Foodreview* 1994; **17** Issue 2: 9–13
6   Roberts JA, Upton PA. *E. coli O157 – The Socio-economic Impact*. Lothian Health Edinburgh, 2000
7   Killalea D. *An Outbreak of Salmonella agona Infection due to a Contaminated Kosher Snack Food*. London: Communicable Disease Surveillance Centre, Public Health Laboratory Service, 1995
8   Roberts JA. *The Economics of Surveillance*. A Report to the Public Health Laboratory Service. London: PHLS, 1996
9   Wheeler JG, Sethi D, Cowden JM *et al*. on behalf of the Infectious Disease Study Executive Study of Infectious Intestinal Disease in England. Rates in the community, presenting to general practice and reported to national surveillance. *BMJ* 1999; **318**: 1046–50
10 O'Mahony M, Mitchell E, Gilbert RJ *et al*. An outbreak of foodborne botulism associated with contaminated hazelnut yoghurt *Epidemiol Infect* 1990; **104**: 389–95
11 Roberts JA, Sockett PN, Gill N. Economic impact of a nation-wide outbreak of salmonellosis: cost-benefit of an early intervention. *BMJ* 1989; **341**: 1227–30
12 Stoat T, Green MS, Meron D, Salter PE. *An International Outbreak of Salmonella caused by Salmonella agona Traced to a peanut-flavoured Snack*. Israel: Centre for Disease Control 1995
13 PHLS. Outbreaks of water borne infectious intestinal disease in England and Wales. *CDR Wkly* 1996; 27th June: 223
14 Dawson A, Griffin R, Fleetwood A, Barrett NJ. Farm visits and zoonoses. *CDR Wkly* 1995; 26th May: R81–R86
15 Newton L, Hall SM, McLauchlin J. Listeriosis surveillance: 1992. *CDR Wkly* 1993; **3**: 10th September: R144–R146
16 Mahony M. Personal communication, 1996
17 Pennington Group. *Report on the Circumstances Leading to the 1996 Outbreak of Infection with E. coli O157 in Central Scotland: The implications for Food Safety and the Lessons to be Learnt*. Edinburgh: The Stationery Office, 1997
18 Donaldson C. *Theory and Practice of Willingness to Pay for Health Care*. Health Economics Research Unit discussion paper 01/93. Aberdeen: University of Aberdeen, 1993
19 Sockett PN, Roberts JA. The social and economic impact of salmonellosis. A Report of a National Survey in England and Wales of laboratory confirmed infections. *Epidemiol Infect* 1991; 107: 335–47
20 Buzby JC, Roberts T, Mishu Allos B. *Estimated Annual Costs of Campylobacter-associated Guillain-Barré Syndrome*. United States Department of Agriculture, Report No 756, 1997
21 Djuretic T, Ryan MJ, Wall PG. The costs of in-patient care for acute infectious intestinal diseases in England from 1991–1994 *CDR Wkly* 1996; 6: R78–R80

Control of vegetative micro-organisms in foods

James S G Dooley* and **Terry A Roberts†**

*School of Applied Biological and Chemical Sciences, University of Ulster, Coleraine, County Londonderry, UK and †Reading UK

Microbes share our food whether we want them to or not. We need to control microbial proliferation in foods in order to avoid spoilage, to enhance flavour and, most importantly, to reduce the risk of food-borne illness. A broad spectrum of interventions are available to control microbial growth, but the most widely used is temperature. The use of temperature to control metabolically active bacteria is discussed briefly in the context of current practices. The marketing and legislative climate has provided an impetus to develop an ever-widening range of systems for microbiological control. This short review highlights some of the problems associated with such novel control systems, including selection of new spoilage agents or food-borne pathogens, and the difficulties of monitoring the efficiency of microbial control in the light of a better understanding of bacterial physiology.

Micro-organisms are inextricably linked with the food we eat. We may sometimes employ rigorous processing procedures to eliminate them but in the main we tend to accept their presence and have decided to adopt a strategy of containment rather than elimination. We, therefore, allow for the presence of undesirable micro-organisms in raw materials but attempt to control the microbial population of foodstuffs that are offered for sale or consumption. Control of vegetative (*i.e.* metabolically active) micro-organisms in food-stuffs is exercised for a number of reasons including prolonging shelf-life by minimising spoilage, or encouraging the growth of organisms that have a desirable trait, such as imparting a particular flavour to the food. However, the primary reason for control is to enhance safety by preventing the growth or activity of disease causing organisms.

Food-borne bacterial pathogens and disease

*Correspondence to:
Dr Terry A Roberts,
59 Edenham Crescent,
Reading RG1 6HU, UK*

Periodic reviews indicate that diseases caused by food-borne bacterial pathogens are a world-wide, and increasing, public health problem[1-4], varying with demographics, industrialisation and centralisation of food production and supply, travel and trade, and microbial evolution and adaptation. Symptoms vary greatly from mild to severe or occasionally fatal gastro-enteritis. Food-borne disease is usually acute, but can also become chronic with long-term sequelae.

In spite of the ubiquitous nature of food-borne illness, relatively few bacteria are recognised as significant food hazards. Until the mid-1990s, in many countries the combined annual total number of outbreaks of illness attributed to salmonellae, *Staphylococcus aureus* and *Clostridium perfringens* often represented 70–80% of the reported bacterial disease outbreaks. With improved refrigerated storage during food distribution and use, *Staph. aureus* and *C. perfringens* now cause illness only when the food has been temperature abused. Improved refrigeration has also lengthened the shelf-life of foods leading to concerns that psychrotrophic pathogens may increase to dangerous levels without spoilage being evident to the consumer. Micro-organisms of most concern are non-proteolytic strains of *C. botulinum* types B, E and F, *Listeria monocytogenes* and *Yersinia enterocolitica*, all of which cause little or no deterioration of the food supporting their growth.

Botulism is the result of ingesting pre-formed toxin, usually the result of spores of *C. botulinum* surviving a process, germinating and growing under conditions in the food that do not prevent multiplication of vegetative cells. While botulism is relatively infrequent, it remains a serious concern because of its life-threatening nature and the impact on trade in the incriminated product type. Over many years, home-canned or home-prepared foods have mainly been responsible for the disease. In recent years, commercially prepared products have been implicated due to faulty processing and/or inappropriate storage temperatures and examples include: inadequately heat-processed hazelnut yoghurt[5], unheated chopped garlic-in-oil, containing no acidulants or preservatives[6], commercially roasted eggplant (aubergine)[7], and a commercial cheese sauce[8].

Disease caused by *L. monocytogenes*, although not common, can be severe with a high mortality rate. Listeriosis is most common in at-risk populations such as pregnant women, infants and the immunocompromised. The organism is ubiquitous in agricultural and food processing environments. Foods implicated in outbreaks have included raw milk products, ready-to-eat meat products, frankfurters, sausages, smoked fish and vegetables. Disease caused by *Y. enterocolitica* occurs world-wide and is often associated with the consumption of raw or undercooked pork.

Salmonellae have long been considered the most important food-borne pathogen in many countries. Foods commonly implicated in outbreaks of salmonellosis include meat and poultry, eggs and egg products, milk and milk products, seafood, fresh produce and spices. In recent years, the incidence of disease caused by *Campylobacter jejuni/coli* has exceeded that due to salmonellae in several countries[9]. Outbreaks of campylobacteriosis are most commonly associated with undercooked poultry as well as cross-contamination of various foods from raw poultry. Other foods and untreated water have also been implicated.

Escherichia coli strains are a common part of normal microbial flora of animals, including man. Most strains are harmless, but some strains cause diarrhoea, while strains bearing particular virulence properties have emerged as a serious hazard, consumption of low numbers causing life-threatening illness. During the last two decades enterohaemorrhagic *E. coli* (EHEC), especially *E. coli* O157:H7, has emerged as a serious food-borne hazard. EHEC infection can be severe causing bloody diarrhoea, haemolytic uraemic syndrome (HUS), and even death. The disease typically affects children, and the infective dose is low. The reservoir of *E. coli* O157:H7 is the intestinal tract of ruminants and a common source of infection is undercooked ground (minced) beef. However, other foods have been implicated, including fresh vegetables, unpasteurised milk and recreational waters. Outbreaks have also been traced to unpasteurised apple juice, vegetable sprouts, yoghurt, fermented sausage, and contact with farm animals[10].

Bacillus cereus and other *Bacillus* spp. have been responsible for food-borne disease, but normally cause problems only after poor handling and/or temperature abuse. Some strains are able to multiply and produce enterotoxin at domestic refrigeration temperatures.

Where raw fish is a major part of the diet, disease caused by *Vibrio parahaemolyticus* is frequent. However, disease caused by *V. parahaemolyticus* and other *Vibrio* spp. has been reported in western countries, but the vehicle of transmission is usually processed rather than raw sea-foods. *Vibrio cholerae* is endemic in many tropical countries and water plays a major role in the epidemiology of cholera.

Shigella spp. Also represent an important public health problem in many third-world countries. Cases of shigellosis reported in developed countries are often associated with travelling. As the reservoir of *Shigella* spp. is restricted to humans, the source of infection is food or water contaminated by human carriers.

Microbial contamination of food and food processing

Most food preservation processes developed empirically, *e.g.* converting milk into cheese, curing pork, salting and drying fish. Micro-organisms were first observed and described by Leeuwenhoek in 1683, and only in 1837 did Pasteur first associate bacteria with food spoilage. The demonstration that diseases are transmitted via foods also came in the

19th century. Hence, for most of man's history, food spoilage and disease transmission have been dealt with in ignorance of the responsible agents.

Raw agricultural products carry a wide range of microbes making up the 'primary contamination', varying with commodity, geographic region, and production and harvesting methods. Crop and animal diseases are controlled stringently because losses affect producers, but the two major concerns for the food industry attributable directly to microbes are: (i) losses of products before consumption due to spoilage; and (ii) costs associated with food-borne disease.

From the point of view of the food processor, the primary microbial contamination of animals and plants is rarely under such control that complete freedom from particular hazardous microbes can be guaranteed. Nor does mechanization necessarily improve hygiene or the microbiological conditions of foods. Modern mechanized slaughter-houses have not provided raw meat that is less heavily contaminated with bacteria, partly because the emphasis remains on high through-put rather than high standards of hygiene.

Efforts continue to minimize the occurrence of microbes able to cause illness, but attempting to control this initial flora is often less cost-effective than applying well-established preservative measures later in the food-chain. With available technology there seems little prospect that complete freedom of particular microbes from new foods will ever become possible; indeed, intensive animal production has in some cases worsened the situation considerably, *e.g.* with respect to salmonellae.

Hence food processors identify the microbes of concern that could be present and consciously take measures to either kill them, or to ensure that they are unable to multiply in their products. Further processing (*e.g.* slicing and repacking) often recontaminate meat products with bacteria of human origin, commonly *Staph. aureus* and occasionally salmonellae and *L. monocytogenes*.

Animals have long been recognised as a major source of several pathogens, faeces being the origin of salmonellae, campylobacters, entero-toxigenic *E. coli*, *C. perfringens*, *C. botulinum* and *L. monocytogenes*. Although it has long been recognised that fruit and vegetables can be contaminated with soil, only in recent years has the association of produce with food-borne illness become obvious and frequent[11].

Control strategies: inactivation of vegetative cells

Brown (this issue) deals with control of bacterial spores. It should be emphasised that, if spores survive a heat process, control of that micro-organism during food storage is by preventing multiplication of its vegetative cells.

The most certain means of controlling bacteria in foods is to inactivate them by heating. Their resistance to heat varies with the species and with the environment in which they are heated. Products of low pH can be rendered stable and safe by lower heat processes than those of neutral pH, because bacterial spores are more sensitive to heat in acid conditions. Some bacteria of concern are unable to grow at acid pH values (*e.g. C. botulinum* will not grow below pH approximately 4.5 except under

Table 1 Growth-limiting conditions for common food-borne bacterial pathogens

	Growth temp min. (°C)	Growth temp opt. (°C)	Growth temp max. (°C)	°C	Heat D-value minimum	pH min.	pH opt.	pH max.	Inhibited by % NaCl	a_w	Ref.
Aeromonas spp.	>0<4	26–35	>42<45	55	0.2	<4.5	7.2	?	>5<6	0.96	[53]
*B. cereus	10[†]	30–40	55	Spores		5	6–7	8.8	ca 10.5	0.93	[53]
*B. cereus	10[†]	28–35	50	Spores		4.35			ca 10	0.912	[54]
Campylobacter spp.	32	42–43	45	60	0.2–0.4	4.9	6.5–7.5	ca 9.0	–	?	[53]
Campylobacter spp.	32	42–45	45	55	0.74–1.0	4.9	6.0–8.0	9.0–9.5	>1.5<2.0	0.99	[54]
C. botulinum (prot.)	ca 10	35	ca 47	Spores		4.6	6.5–7.0	–	ca 10	0.935	[53]
C. botulinum (prot.)	ca 12	30–40	48	Spores		4.6	7	9	ca 10	0.935	[54]
C. botulinum (non-pr.)	ca 3.0	27–30	ca 33	Spores		ca 5.0	6.5–7.0	?	ca 5.0	0.97	[53]
*C. perfringens	12	43–47	ca 52	Spores		5.5–5.8	7.2	8.0–9.0	ca 10	0.935	[53]
*C. perfringens	12	43–45	50	Spores		5	6.0–7.5	8.3	ca 6.0	0.964	[54]
E. coli	ca 7.0–8.0	35–40	44–46	60	0.75	4.4	6.0–7.0	9	ca 8.0	0.95	[53]
L. monocytogenes	ca 0	37	45	70	0.1–0.2	4.4	7	9.4	ca 11.5	0.92	[53]
L. monocytogenes	0	25.3	45	70	0.14–0.27	4.4–4.6	6.5–8.0	9.5	ca 10	0.935	[54]
Salmonellae	4.8–5.2[‡]	35–43	46	60	0.2 (a)	3.8	7.0–7.5	9.5	9.5	0.94	[53]
				90	40–80 (b)						[53]
Salmonellae	5.1	37	45–47	60	0.06–0.1	4	6.5–7.0	9	ca 8.0	0.95	[54]
Shigellae	ca 6.0	47	?	–	–	4.9	–	9.4	ca 5.0	0.97	[53]
Staph. aureus	ca 7	37	48	60	5.0–15.0	4	6.0–7.0	10	ca 14.0	0.83	[53]
Staph. aureus	11	37	48	61.7	20	4	6.0–7.0	9.8–10	ca 14.0	0.83	[54]
V. parahaemolyticus	5	37	43	55	2.5	4.8	7.8–8.6	11	ca 10.0	0.935	[53]
V. parahaemolyticus	12.8	37	42–43	60	ca 1.0	4.5–5.0	7.5–8.5	11	ca 8.5	0.948	[54]
Y. enterocolitica	–1	25–37	42	55	ca 2.0	4.2	7.2	>9.6<10.0	> 5<7	0.964	[53]
Y. enterocolitica	0 to –1	32–34	44	62.8	0.1–1.0	4.6	7.0–8.0	9	>5<7	–	[54]

Tabulated values are for single controlling factors when other factors are close to optimal. In reality control is achieved by combinations of sub-optimal growth conditions.

*Spores: if spores survive a process, control during food storage is by preventing multiplication of the vegetative cells.

[†]Most strains ca 10°C, some strains grow at 4–5°C.

[‡]Salmonellae: most serotypes fail to grow below 7°C.

(a) Salmonellae: when heated in 'wet' environments.

(b) Salmonellae: when heated in 'dry' environments such as chocolate.

prot. = proteolytic; non-pr. = non-proteolytic; max. = maximum; opt. = optimum; min. = minimum unusual circumstances not normally found in foods). Hence pH also plays an important role in food preservation.

Inactivation occurs more rapidly with increasing temperature. The death rate of vegetative bacteria increases 10-fold for every (approximately) 5°C increase in temperature within the lethal range. Most vegetative pathogens are inactivated almost instantly above about 70°C unless heating occurs at low water activities, *e.g.* as occurs in chocolate, when the heat resistance increases very substantially (Table 1).

Thermal treatment processes are designed around a limited number of parameters, *e.g.* time, temperature, pH, and a_w. They are calibrated with selected test organisms to achieve a particular reduction in numbers (*e.g.* 4-decimal [4-D] reductions of *L. monocytogenes*). For example, the process for milk pasteurisation in the US is 71.7°C for 15 s[12]. This combination of temperature and time will assure the destruction of *Coxiella burnetii*, as well as other non-sporeforming pathogens that are known to occur in raw milk. In other foods, specific heat treatments may be required. For example, in the US, minimum heat processes (any one of 16 time and temperature combinations equivalent to instant heating to 63°C) targeted at killing salmonellae must be used for the manufacture of pre-cooked roast beef joints for chilled or frozen distribution[13,14]. A similar requirement (equivalent to instant heating to 70°C) is mandatory for fully cooked meat patties[15], aimed at destruction of *E. coli* O157:H7.

Design of thermal treatment processes must also take into account subsequent storage conditions such as use of modified atmospheres and vacuum systems, *etc.* Whilst *L. monocytogenes* is the target organism for 'short shelf-life' chilled foods, psychrotrophic strains of *C. botulinum*, which are able to multiply and produce neurotoxin even at 4–5°C, are the main organisms of concern in perishable, 'extended shelf-life' chilled foods (shelf-life at chill longer than 10 days), including the so-called *'cuisine sous-vide'* products.

The UK Advisory Committee on the Microbiological Safety of Foods (ACMSF), in its report on vacuum packaging and associated processes[16], made a series of recommendations on the safety of 'extended shelf-life' vacuum-packed foods. These were the use of a heat treatment such that all components receive a minimum heat process of 10 min at 90°C (6-D reduction of group II [psychrotrophic] strains of *C. botulinum*); or to reduce the a_w of all components to 0.97 (equivalent to 3.5% w/w sodium chloride) or less; or to reduce the pH to 5.0 or less; or to use a combination of preservation treatments capable of giving equivalent security against group II strains of *C. botulinum*[17]. Similar requirements to these are incorporated in the guidelines recently published by the European Chilled Foods Federation[18]. National guidelines or regulations for vacuum-packed and other extended shelf-life meat products exist in many countries including the US[19], Canada[20], Australia[21] and Europe[22,23].

The cooking process given to industrially produced cooked meats will effectively destroy all vegetative bacterial pathogens, viruses, parasites and most vegetative spoilage micro-organisms. 'Faecal streptococci' (enterococci) and certain lactobacilli are relatively heat resistant and often survive commercial pasteurisation processes and multiply slowly, even under good refrigeration.

Recognising that such processes will not destroy all organisms, specific cooling requirements are also specified. For meat joints this requires them to be rapidly and continuously cooled such that the time between temperatures 48.9°C and 12.8°C does not exceed a total of 6 h, with cooling continuing until a temperature of 4.4°C is reached; this is intended to prevent the growth of spore-forming bacteria. In the UK, there are Department of Health guidelines for the manufacture of pre-cooked chilled and frozen foods for catering[24], and trade guidelines for pre-cooked chilled meals and meal components sold through retail outlets[25]. These guidelines specify both cooking and cooling requirements and also hygienic practices to prevent contamination of the cooked product. Similar guidelines have been developed by other countries and can be useful sources of information[26,27]. The cooking process required for products with a shelf-life of 10 days or less is a heat process equivalent to heating to a minimum of 70°C for 2 min. This will give at least a 6 decimal [6-D] kill of *L. monocytogenes*[28].

Control strategies: growth limitation

Vegetative bacteria multiply less rapidly as the temperature falls and maintaining the storage temperature at, or below, the minimum temperature for growth is the most common means of preventing their growth. Storing foods in vacuum packs or under modified atmospheres, commonly containing carbon dioxide, extends shelf-life.

Meat and meat products represent a group of foodstuffs associated with a wide variety of growth limitation strategies and a good understanding of the microbiological processes involved is being developed. Vacuum packing meat extends the shelf-life by preventing the aerobic Gram-negative portion of the flora (*e.g. Pseudomonas, Acinetobacter, Psychrobacter* spp.) multiplying and allowing the facultative anaerobes (*e.g. Lactobacillus, Carnobacterium, Leuconostoc* spp.) to dominate. The extent of microbial growth is determined by the food pH, film permeability to oxygen and carbon dioxide, temperature and the microbes' tolerance of carbon dioxide. On meat of pH 6.0 and above,

Brochothrix thermosphacta grows anaerobically to about $10^7/cm^2$, and *Shewanella putrefaciens* grows when the pH is 6.0 and above, but not when the pH is 5.8 or below. Different mixtures of oxygen, nitrogen and carbon dioxide are used for a wide range of foods.

Spoilage of meat by psychrophilic clostridia has only relatively recently been recognized and is characterised by the production of hydrogen and carbon dioxide causing pack distension, and of butanol, butanoic acid, ethanol, acetic acid and a range of sulphur containing compounds[29,30]. Thus new sets of growth limiting storage conditions are selecting for novel spoilage agents. The isolate/strain of Dainty *et al.* was shown by 16S rRNA sequencing to be a new species *C. estertheticum*[31]. Yet another new psychrotrophic species, *C. algidicarnis*, spoiled vacuum-packed cooked pork[32]. The use of microbiological population analysis based upon interrogation of 16S rRNA databases has proved to be exceedingly useful in identifying novel spoilage organisms and some pathogens. Such technology will be at the forefront of the future food microbiology research as it will allow for rapid recognition of emerging hazards based upon changing food products or processes.

Spoilage of meat stored in air is due to formation of a complex mixture of esters, branched-chain alcohols, sulphur-containing compounds, amines, unsaturated hydrocarbons and ketones[33]. Meat of normal pH, vacuum packed and stored refrigerated develops a relatively inoffensive sour acid odour, while high pH meat tends to develop sulphydryl, putrid and faecal odours[33]. 'Greening' of meat is caused by the formation of sulphmyoglobin from hydrogen sulphide, formed by *Shew. putrefaciens*, *Enterobacteriaceae* or *Lactobacillus sake*, reacting with oxymyoglobin.

Freezing prevents growth of vegetative bacteria, but should not be relied upon to eliminate pathogens. Most vegetative bacterial pathogens survive for many months in frozen foods. Thawing frozen foods is a crucial stage because bacteria at the surface of the frozen food multiply at the thawing temperature. Ideally thawing should be under refrigeration, but the time taken to thaw large items, *e.g.* a large Christmas turkey, often tempts consumers to try to accelerate thawing by holding the food under warm conditions. In the case of chicken and turkeys, thawing without refrigeration, followed by inadequate cooking, has led to outbreaks of salmonellosis. Another cause of illness has been cooking a large turkey that has not thawed in the centre.

Cured meats have an extended shelf-life because sodium chloride and curing salts, *e.g.* sodium nitrite, combine to prevent multiplication of spoilage bacteria and slow greatly the growth of pathogens. Many fermented meats have a low pH value due to production of lactic acid during the fermentation[34], although in those that are subsequently mould-ripened, the pH can rise again during ripening to near 7.0.

Control strategies: some future developments

At every stage of food processing, temperature plays a critical role. Increasingly, traditional products and processes are changed to accommodate the wish for improved textural properties after lower heat processes, curing with reduced levels of salt and nitrite, and foods from which established preservatives have been removed. Developments in other methods of food preservation are dealt with elsewhere in this issue. While many new techniques show promise as alternatives to heat, few are yet in widespread commercial use. Thus, greater and greater reliance is being placed on temperature control as the main factor controlling the growth of spoilage microbes and those able to cause food-borne illness.

In recent years, changing eating patterns and technological developments in food production, processing and preservation have increased enormously the variety of products available. Many are sold 'ready-to-eat' and are not, therefore, subjected to heating immediately before consumption which would kill the occasional vegetative pathogenic bacteria[35]. Some products spend weeks in distribution and storage before being offered for sale alongside the fresh product. The food industry has developed novel products, modified formulations and devised alternative means of packaging (vacuum, modified atmosphere). There are pressures to extend even further the shelf-life of foods held under chill and continuing demands for longer shelf-life products, coupled with minimal heating and reduced, or no preservatives/additives.

The development of microbes on foods has long been recognized to be a response to physical and chemical conditions such as pH, available water, gaseous atmosphere, temperature, preservatives and numerous other factors. Much effort has been directed to defining conditions that limit growth, since understanding those conditions appeared to proscribe conditions that would extend shelf-life and minimise the growth of microbes associated with food-borne illnesses. As a consequence tables of 'minimum' values are readily available for key spoilage and pathogenic bacteria (Table 1). In most instances, these data have been generated when other controlling factors are near optimal, *e.g.* the minimum water activity when the pH value is near 7 and incubation temperatures are optimal, which is unrealistic if the concern is safe food storage.

Stable and safe foods are the consequence of preservative factors acting in combination, often at levels which singly would not be inhibitory. Our understanding of the relative contributions of factors to give safe and shelf-stable food products remains surprisingly poor.

Biological control systems

There is no doubt that the development of rigorous physical and chemical methods of food preservation has been one of the most important contributions to food safety in the latter half of the 20th century. At this stage, one might reasonably conclude that, within a properly controlled environment, application of appropriate techniques would result in microbiologically safe foods. This may well be the case if the range of foods available were to remain static, but in a consumer-led industry considerable pressure is applied to replace traditional preservation methods particularly the use of chemical additives. There has been considerable interest in the use of a class of bacteria-specific toxins known as bacteriocins. These are usually low molecular weight proteins that are synthesised by a particular strain of bacteria to be active against related strains. The spectrum of activity can vary quite widely. Some strains of *E. coli* can produce bacteriocins (called colicins) that are only active against other *E. coli* strains[36]. On the other hand, many lactic acid bacteria produce bacteriocins with a much broader spectrum of activity, some even targeting food borne pathogens such as *L. monocytogenes*. In principle they would make ideal food additives as they are natural bacterial products released by organisms, such as lactic acid bacteria, that would be present in many foods. They also have not been demonstrated to have toxic effects on mammalian cells and would, therefore, behave as 'magic bullets' only attacking specific groups of undesirable bacteria[37,38].

There are few general characteristics shared by bacteriocins as a group. There is still continuing debate on nomenclature and it is common to have molecules with different names reclassified when nucleic acid or protein sequencing studies reveals them to be identical. As a working system, many researchers utilize a four group classification for these low molecular antimicrobial proteins.

Group I

This group is characterised by proteins with post-translationally modified serine and threonine amino acids which allow the formation of unusual thioether lanthionine rings. There are many examples of these bacteriocins but the best known is the 'lantibiotic' nisin.

Group II

These are very low molecular weight, heat stable proteins. They are characterised by the presence of a consensus leader sequence (Gly–Gly^{-1}–Xaa^{+1}) that is essential for the correct export and processing of the molecule. Pediocin AcH is probably the best known member of this group.

Groups III and IV

These are less well characterised than the previous sets but they generally contain higher molecular weight proteins (up to 30 kDa) and are normally heat labile. Group III molecules can be distinguished from Group IV by the absence of carbohydrate or lipid moieties.

In spite of an extensive scientific literature on the antimicrobial efficacy of many bacteriocins in laboratory systems, there have been few commercial applications to date. This is a reflection of the difficulty in obtaining large quantities of sufficiently well-characterised preparations that would be suitable for use as a food additive, and the absence of toxicological evaluation. Nisin has been added to a range of foods particularly dairy products[39]. It is active against vegetative bacteria such as *L. monocytogenes* and also has an effect against endospore formers such as clostridia. It has been demonstrated to permeabilize cell membranes in a time- and concentration-dependent manner suggesting an oligomerisation of inserted monomers to form hydrophilic diffusion channels[40]. The mechanism of action against spore-forming bacteria is less well understood and the process is less efficient.

Nisin and pediocin AcH have been demonstrated to have synergistic effects with both thermal[41] and non-thermal antimicrobial processes[42,43]. The immediate future for bacteriocins looks to be in combination with other processes. However, the genetics of these proteins are well known and recombinant organisms expressing heterologous bacteriocins (with a wider range of bacteria attacked) have been described. However, in the current climate of hostility towards the use of any genetic manipulation associated with food, it is unlikely that recombinant organisms will be a commercial strategy for some time to come.

Control – future challenges

Food microbiology developed via studies on the main commodities such as milk, meat, poultry, fish, fruit and vegetables, without appreciation of the main factors controlling microbial growth. Factors are sometimes claimed to be important without convincing evidence of their contribution, *e.g.* competition between pathogens and the spoilage flora is less widespread than believed. Most foods are nutrient rich, and it has been shown that microbial growth is largely determined by a relatively small number of factors, *e.g.* pH, a_w, temperature, atmosphere, particular organic acids. This realisation has led to efforts to model microbial death and growth responses as a function of those factors. The resulting models give a quick 'first estimate' of the microbial response and are being used in many aspects of product design and development, shelf-life assessment, HACCP and risk assessment. The greatest advantage of models is that they can be used to test the consequences of changing a number of factors at the same time and, with the power of modern computers, the answers are almost instantaneous. A disadvantage is that the predictions may not be precise and may only indicate a trend, but knowing that trend quickly is highly advantageous when reformulating or modifying or evaluating storage conditions. Care should be taken that the controlling factors included in the model are those relevant to the foods in question, and models should be validated by comparing predictions from the model with microbial responses in different foods before reliance is placed on them[44–47].

In order to improve control methods, it is necessary to have standard, reproducible assays to assess the impact of a treatment on microbial cell viability. As knowledge of microbial physiology has gradually increased, some of the most basic concepts, such as what actually constitutes a dead cell, have been revisited. The discipline of food microbiology has centred on the manipulation of various environmental parameters to influence microbial populations in foods. This has been measured by traditional culture techniques relying on organisms forming colonies on solid nutrient media. The assumption is that each viable bacterial cell will always give rise to a single colony. This central tenant of microbiology has been increasingly challenged with evidence pointing towards the generation of sub-populations of injured organisms following sublethal administration of physical or chemical control methods. Injury to cells will prevent their growth in simple enumeration assays and, as such, the efficacy of certain processes can be significantly overestimated. An injured cell retains the capacity for multiplication and there are numerous procedures for reviving such cells[48,49]. The current trend in food processing is towards the use of milder treatment conditions. This has meant that evaluation of sublethal injury is now more pertinent than ever to the critical analysis of all processes aimed at controlling vegetative micro-organisms.

A second major challenge to the traditional concept of cell viability has come from the description of a 'viable but non-culturable' (VBNC) state. A major taxonomic subdivision amongst bacteria continues to be the use of the Gram stain providing the distinction: Gram-positive and Gram-negative. Gram-positive organisms constitute a very diverse group also contains a small subset of species that can form a desiccated, meta-bolically dormant and highly heat-resistant stage called the endospore. Endospore forming bacteria such as *C. botulinum* and *B. cereus* are well known food-borne hazards and control measures based around rigorous, moist heat treatment (such as canning) are well established. The VBNC state has been best defined for Gram-negative bacteria[50], but has also been noted among some Gram-positive organisms.

Many important food-borne Gram-negative bacteria such as *Campylobacter*, *Salmonella*, *Vibrio*, and *Escherichia* spp. have been demonstrated to enter the VBNC state. This in normally induced in response to nutrient limitation, but certain thermal and chemical stresses have produced a similar effect. Cells in this state will not form colonies on hitherto appropriate culture media. The media contain all the necessary nutrients to support bacterial growth, yet once the bacteria enter the VBNC state they no longer undergo normal cell replication. Even though the bacteria no longer reproduce they can be demonstrated to be metabolically active using stains for RNA. By definition RNA is only produced by metabolically active bacterial cells since it is the information carrier in protein production and protein production is an absolute requirement for metabolism. Since RNA also has a very short half-life in bacteria, its detection means that cells are displaying metabolic activity. Recovery of cells from a viable but non-culturable state, *i.e.* a restoration of the ability to grow and divide in culture, has also been reported but the signals controlling the process are incompletely understood. The concern is that if we do not know how the entry and exit from this state is effected we have little chance of controlling it, in particular if our current controls are targeted against vegetative organisms that are in a very different physiological state.

Difficulties in accounting for the contribution of sublethally injured cells and viable but non-culturable cells to overall risk assessment has highlighted the limitations of some current methods of microbiological analysis. The realisation that the application of control methods could push vegetative cells into states that we do not understand physiologically and cannot easily be detected by current analytical methods is of concern. This suggests that with some of the advances in control methods outlined below we should also improve methods of microbiological assay, and perhaps move away from heavy reliance on cultural methods to some of the tools afforded by advances in molecular biology. A discussion of this area is beyond the scope of this short article, but recent reviews have identified the gradual transfer of molecular technology from medical to food applications[51,52].

Conclusions

The food industry has come to terms with the control of some long established hazards, *e.g.* group I (proteolytic) strains of C. *botulinum*, C. *perfringens*, Staph. *aureus*, via designed and controlled cooking and temperature control during subsequent storage. However, the nature of microbiological hazards is constantly changing in response to changes in food processing, consumer demands for new and more 'natural' products, changes in purchasing and eating habits and to the introduction of a wider variety of products into traditional markets. Of the more recently identified hazards, *V. parahaemolyticus* and *B. cereus* are increasingly prevalent world-wide, but are still relatively unimportant in the UK, while *C. jejuni/coli* has become the major cause of bacterial gastro-enteritis. Other recent hazards include *L. monocytogenes*, psychrotrophic strains of *Bacillus* spp, *S. enteritidis*, antibiotic-resistant *S. typhimurium*, *V. vulnificus*, *E. coli* O157:H7 and other verocytotoxic strains. Systems that have been designed to protect foods from currently recognised pathogens should be checked for their performance against the most recently identified food-borne pathogens.

The microbiological lessons that have been learned re-inforce the view that the future safety of foods cannot be assured by any realistic amount of end-product testing. It must rely heavily on an integrated strategy combining: (i) a structured approach to understanding hazards and their control, such as HACCP; (ii) the development of specific and rapid methods for identification and characterising microbes; (iii) a full understanding of the factors leading to microbial death, survival and growth, *e.g.* via mathematical modelling; and (iv) control of all the factors affecting microbial survival and growth during processing and through the food-chain.

In many cases, we currently have only a basic knowledge and significant investment in research will be required to provide the information necessary to ensure food safety in a rapidly changing consumer society.

References

1 CAST (Council for Agricultural Science and Technology, USA). *Foodborne Pathogens: Risks and Consequences*. Task Force Report No. 122. (ISSN 0194-4088) CAST, 4420 West Lincoln Way, Ames, Iowa 50014-3447, 1994

2 CAST (Council for Agricultural Science and Technology, USA). *Foodborne Pathogens: Review of Recommendations*. Special Publication No. 22. (ISSN 0194-407X, ISBN 1-887383-14-X)). CAST, 4420 West Lincoln Way, Ames, Iowa 50014-3447, 1998

3 POST (Parliamentary Office of Science and Technology, UK). *Safer Eating: Microbiological Food Poisoning and its Prevention*. POST, 7 Millbank, London SW1P 3JA, UK, 1997

4 WHO (World Health Organization). Foodborne Safety and Foodborne Diseases. *World Health Stat Q* 1997 **50**: 1–154

5 O'Mahoney M, Mitchell E, Gilbert RJ *et al.* An outbreak of foodborne botulism associated with contaminated hazelnut yogurt. *Epidemiol Infect* 1990; **104**: 389–95

6 St Louis ME, Peck SHS, Bowering D *et al.* Botulism from chopped garlic: delayed recognition of a major outbreak. *Ann Intern Med* 1988; **108**: 363–8

7 D'Argenio P, Palumbo F, Ortolani R *et al.* Type B botulism associated with roasted eggplant in oil – Italy, 1993. *Morb Mortal Wkly Rep* 1995; **44**: 33–6

8 Townes JM, Cieslak PR, Hatheway CL *et al.* An outbreak of type A botulism associated with a commercial cheese sauce. *Ann Intern Med* 1996; **125**: 558–63

9 Altekruse SF, Stern NJ, Fields PI, Swerdlow DL. *Campylobacter jejuni* – an emerging foodborne pathogen. *Emerg Infect Dis* 1999; **5**: 28–35

10 Doyle MP, Zhao T, Meng J, Zhao S. *Escherichia coli* O157:H7. In: Doyle MP, Beuchat LR, Montville TJ. (Eds) *Food Microbiology: Fundamentals and Frontiers*. Washington, DC: ASM Press, 1997; 171–91

11 Beuchat LR. Pathogenic microorganisms associated with fresh produce. *J Food Protect* 1996; **59**: 204–16

12 FDA (Food and Drug Administration, USA). *Milk and Cream, Pasteurized.* (21 CFR 131.3b), Code of Federal Regulations. Washington, DC: US Government Printing Office, 1997

13 USDA (United States Department of Agriculture). *Production requirements for cooked beef, roast beef and cooked corned beef.* Federal Register, 48(106): 24314-24318, 1983

14 USDA/FSIS (US Department of Agriculture/Food Safety Inspection Service). *Requirements for the production of cooked beef, roast beef, and cooked corned beef* (9 CFR 318.17). Code of Federal Regulations. Washington, DC: US Government Printing Office, 1997

15 USDA (United States Department of Agriculture). *Heat-processing procedures; cooling instructions, and cooking, handling and storage requirements for uncured meat patties.* Federal Register 58:41138 Docket Number 86-0141F, 1993

16 ACMSF (Advisory Committee on the Microbiological Safety of Food, UK). *Report on Vacuum Packaging and Associated Processes.* ISBN 0 11 321558 4. London: HMSO, 1992

17 Lücke FK, Roberts TA. Control in meat and meat products. In: Hauschild AHW, Dodds L. (Eds) *Clostridium botulinum: Ecology and Control in Food.* New York: Marcel Dekker, 1993; 177–207

18 ECFF. *European Chilled Foods Federation Guidelines.* Paris: ECFF, 1994

19 NFPA. *Guidelines for the Development, Production and Handling of Refrigerated Foods.* National Food Processors Association (US), Microbiology and Food Safety Committee, 1989

20 AFSDAC. *Agriculture Canada – Canadian Code of Recommended Practices for Pasteurised/Modified Atmosphere Packaged/Refrigerated Food.* Agri-Food Safety Division, Agriculture Canada, March, 1990

21 AQIS. Australian Quarantine and Inspection Service, *Code of Hygienic Practice for the Manufacture of Sous Vide Products.* AQIS, Department of Primary Industries and Energy, Australia, 1992

22 France. *Prolongation of Life Span of Pre-cooked Food Modification of Procedures enabling Authorisation to be obtained.* Veterinary Service of Food Hygiene, Service Note DGAL/SVHA/N88/No 8106, 31.5.88, 1988

23 Benelux. *Code for the Production, Distribution and Sale of Chilled Longlife Pasteurised Meals,* 1991

24 Department of Health (UK). *Guidelines on Cook-Chill and Cook-Freeze catering systems.* London: HMSO, 1989

25 CFA. *Guidelines for the Manufacture, Distribution and Retail sale of Chilled Foods,* 2nd edn. London: Chilled Foods Association, 1993

26 USDA (United States Department of Agriculture). *FSIS (Food Safety and Inspection Service) directive: Time/Temperature guidelines for cooling heated products.* FSIS Directive 7110.3, Washington, DC: Food Safety and Inspection Service, US Department of Agriculture, 1988

27 FDA. *Food Code (1993) Recommendations of the United States Public Health Service and Food and Drug Administration.* Springfield, VA: National Technical Information Service, 1993

28 Gaze JE, Brown GD, Gaskell, D, Banks JG. Heat resistance of *Listeria monocytogenes* in homogenates of chicken, beefsteak and carrot. *Food Microbiol* 1989; **6**: 251–9

29 Dainty RH, Edwards RA, Hibbard CM. Spoilage of vacuum-packed beef by a *Clostridium* sp. *J Sci Food Agr* 1989; **49**: 473–86

30 Kalchayanand N, Ray B, Field RA. Characteristics of psychrotrophic *Clostridium laramie* causing spoilage of vacuum-packaged refrigerated fresh and roasted beef. *J Food Protect* 1993; **56**: 13–7

31 Collins MD, Rodriguez UM, Dainty RH, Edwards RA, Roberts TA. Taxonomic studies on a psychrotrophic *Clostridium* from vacuum-packed beef: Description of *Clostridium estertheticum* sp. nov. *FEMS Microbiol Lett* 1992; **96**: 235–40

32 Lawson P, Dainty RH, Kristiansen N, Berg J, Collins MD. Characterization of a psychrotrophic *Clostridium* causing spoilage in vacuum-packed cooked pork: description of *Clostridium algidicarnis* sp. nov. *Lett Appl Microbiol* 1994; **19**: 153–7

33 Dainty RH, Mackey BM. The relationship between the phenotypic properties of bacteria from chill-stored meat and spoilage processes. *J Appl Bacteriol Symp Suppl* 1992; **73**: 103S–14S

34 Bacus JN. Fermented meat and poultry products. In: Pearson AM, Dutson TR. (Eds) *Advances in Meat Research, vol. 2, Meat and Poultry Microbiology.* Westport, CT: AVI Publishing, 1986; 123–64

35 Tompkin RB. Microbiology of ready-to-eat meat and poultry products. In: Pearson AM, Dutson TR. (Eds) *Advances in Meat Research, vol 2, Meat and Poultry Microbiology.*

Westport, CT: AVI Publishing, 1986; 89–121

36 Konisky J. Colicins and other bacteriocins with established modes of action. *Annu Rev Microbiol* 1982; **36**: 125–44

37 Hoover G, Steenson LR. *Bacteriocins of Lactic Acid Bacteria.* New York: Academic Press, 1993

38 Ray B, Daeschel MA. *Food Biopreservation of Microbial Origin.* Boca Raton, FL: CRC Press, 1992

39 Anon. *Nisin preparation: affirmation of GRAS status as a direct human food ingredient.* 21CFR Part 184. Federal Register 53: 11247-11251, 1988

40 Akee T, Rombouts FM, Hugenholtz J, Guihand G, Letellier L. Mode of action of nisin Z against *Listeria monocytogenes* Scott A grown at high and low temperatures. *Appl Env Microbiol* 1994; **60**: 1962–8

41 Ueckert J, Coote PJ, ter Steeg PF. Synergistic antibacterial action of nisin and magainin II amide combined with heat. *J Appl Microbiol* 1998; **85**: 487–94

42 Kalchayanand N, Sikes A, Dunne CP, Ray B. Factors influencing death and injury of foodborne pathogens by hydrostatic pressure pasteurisation. *Food Microbiol* 1998; **15**: 207–14

43 ter Steeg PF, Hellemans JC, Kok AE. Synergistic actions of nisin, sublethal ultrahigh pressure, and reduced temperature on bacteria and yeast. *Appl Env Microbiol* 1999; **65**: 4148–54

44 Baranyi J, Roberts TA. A dynamic approach to predicting bacterial growth in food. *Int J Food Microbiol* 1994; **23**: 277–94

45 Baranyi J, Roberts TA. Mathematics of predictive food microbiology. *Int J Food Microbiol* 1995; **26**: 199–218

46 McClure PJ, Boogard E, Kelly TM, Baranyi J, Roberts TA. A predictive model for the combined effects of pH, sodium chloride and temperature, on the growth of *Brochothrix thermosphacta*. *Int J Food Microbiol* 1993; **19**: 161–78

47 Sutherland JP, Bayliss AJ, Roberts TA. Predictive modelling of growth of *Staphylococcus aureus*: the effects of temperature, pH and sodium chloride. *Int J Food Microbiol* 1994; **21**: 217–36

48 McCarthy SA. Pathogenicity of nonstressed heat-stressed and resuscitated *Listeria monocytogenes*. *Appl Env Microbiol* 1991; **57**: 2389–91

49 Mackey BM., Boogard E, Hayes CM, Barayani J. Recovery of heat injured *Listeria monocytogenes*. *Int J Food Microbiol* 1994; **22**: 227–37

50 Oliver JD, Hite F, McDougald D, Andon NL, Simpson LM. Entry into and resuscitation from the viable but non culturable state by *Vibrio vulnificus* in an estuarine environment. *Appl Environ Microbiol* 1995; **61**: 2624–30

51 Persing DH, Smith TF, Tenover FC, White TJ. (Eds) *Diagnostic Molecular Microbiology: principles and applications.* Washington, DC: ASM Press, 1993

52 Barbour WM, Tice G. Genetic and immunologic techniques for detecting foodborne pathogens and toxins. In: Doyle MP, Beuchat LR, Montville TJ. (Eds) *Food Microbiology: Fundamentals and Frontiers.* Washington, DC: ASM Press, 1997; 710–27

53 ICMSF (International Commission on Microbiological Specifications for Foods). *Microorganisms in Foods 5: Characteristics of Microbial Pathogens.* London: Blackie Academic & Professional, 1996

54 Shapton DA, Shapton NF. *Principles and Practices for the Safe Processing of Foods.* Oxford: Butterworth Heinemann, 1991

Control of bacterial spores

K L Brown

Food Hygiene Department, Campden and Chorleywood Food Research Association, Chipping Campden, Gloucestershire, UK

Bacterial spores are much more resistant than their vegetative counterparts. The most dangerous spore-former is *Clostridium botulinum* which produces a potent neurotoxin that can prove fatal. The most common food poisoning from a spore-former is caused by *C. perfringens*. Other food poisoning spore-formers include *Bacillus cereus, B. subtilis* and *B. licheniformis*. There are a number of non-pathogenic spore-formers including butyric and thermophilic anaerobes that cause significant economic losses to food producers. Some unusual spoilage complaints have been reported, for example, *B. sporothermodurans* in UHT milk, *Alicyclobacillus acidoterrestris* in apple and orange juice and *Desulfotomaculum nigrificans* in hot vending machines. Control of spore-formers requires an understanding of both the resistance and outgrowth characteristics of the spores.

Bacterial spores are much more resistant to heat, chemicals, irradiation and desiccation than their vegetative cell counterparts. The main food poisoning spore-formers are *Clostridium botulinum*, *C. perfringens* (formerly known as *C. welchii*) and *Bacillus cereus*. Occasionally *B. subtilis* and *B. licheniformis* have been implicated in food poisoning incidents. The most common food poisoning in the UK caused by a spore-former is from *C. perfringens*[1]. Between 1985 and 1994, the number of reported cases of *C. perfringens* food poisoning ranged from 446 to 1466 each year, whereas *Bacillus* spp. only accounted for 31 to 418 cases a year. By comparison, in the UK, outbreaks of botulism caused by the deadly *C. botulinum* are very rare with only 10 recorded outbreaks this century[2].

Non-food poisoning spore-formers can also produce spoilage in food products resulting in commercial loss, which can be substantial. Spoilage should be carefully investigated because it may be an indication that there is a fault in the processing or that hygiene standards are insufficient. Today's spoilage outbreak may be tomorrow's food poisoning incident.

Because spore-formers are inherently more resistant than vegetative cells, methods of control need to be chosen carefully. The reader is referred to *ICMSF Book 5* for the most comprehensive recent text on the characteristics and control of food pathogens[3].

Correspondence to:
Dr K L Brown, Food Hygiene Department, Campden and Chorleywood Food Research Association, Chipping Campden, Gloucestershire GL55 6LD, UK

© The British Council 2000

One of the most common methods of control of spore-formers is by heat. The most recent and comprehensive text on thermal processing is that by Holdsworth[4]. The UK Department of Health has also produced guidelines for the safe production of heat preserved foods[5].

Information on control of spore-formers by disinfectants is best obtained from the manufacturers of these chemicals. Formulation of disinfectants is constantly evolving to meet the demands of the food industry and to meet international disinfectant tests. The most widely used disinfectant is probably chlorine, but it is only slowly sporicidal and is readily inactivated by organic matter, although there are organic chlorine release agents which are more effective in the presence of soiling.

UV light is finding increased use in the food industry for the destruction of micro-organisms on surfaces and in water and air. UV lamp technology has improved considerably in the last 8–10 years and it is now possible to obtain very powerful lamps, which can produce significant reduction of spore-formers. Much of the recent work is not yet published and is held by manufacturers of the lamp systems or their customers. Multi-lamp arrays are also being developed to fit around conveyor systems so that the surfaces of product and packaging can be 'sterilised' before transfer to high care areas.

Spore-formers causing food poisoning

Clostridium botulinum

The most important spore-forming pathogen is *C. botulinum* because of the potent neurotoxin that it produces. The strains of *C. botulinum* are divide into seven types, A–G, based on the serological specificity of the toxins. There is also a further division into proteolytic and non-proteolytic strains. Only types A, B, E and F have been implicated in human food-borne botulism[6]. Types C and D produce botulism in birds and cattle, while type G has not been implicated in an outbreak.

In the US, where home canning is common, there were 688 reported outbreaks of botulism between 1899 and 1973 resulting in 978 deaths[7]. Hauschild[6] surveyed botulism outbreaks in 18 countries and found that 60–100% of the recorded outbreaks were from home-prepared foods. Between 1978 and 1991 in the US, types A, B and E accounted for 60%, 13% and 24%, respectively, of the 371 cases of food-borne botulism (Table 1)[8]. Only one case of type F, from home-prepared pig's feet was recorded in the same period.

Products associated with outbreaks of botulism are very diverse and include meat, fish, vegetables, dairy and honey products. The pH of

Table 1 Yearly incidence of botulism in the United States

Year	Foodborne type				Total cases	Infant type			Total cases	Wound type			Total cases	Un-known	Year total
	A	B	E	?		A	B	?		A	B	?			
1978	54	4	0	0	58	20	18	1	39	0	0	0	0	14	111
1979	4	2	2	0	8	13	10	1[a]	24	2	0	1[b]	3	5	40
1980	12	4	2	0	18	31	34	1[c]	66	2	0	0	2	1	87
1981	5	6	9	2	22	40	31	0	71	3	2	0	5	1	99
1982	27	3	0	0	30	29	31	0	60	0	0	1	1	1	92
1983	38	4	1	0	43	33	46	0	79	0	0	0	0	3	125
1984	12	1	4	1	18	42	54	1[b]	97	2	1	0	3	3	121
1985	10	8	14	0	32	36	35	0	71	0	1	0	1	1	105
1986	10	5	8	1[a]	24	53	35	0	88	1	0	2	3	0	115
1987	10	2	3	5	20	42	44	0	86	2	1	0	3	0	109
1988	14	3	26	2	45	32	42	4	78	2	0	0	2	1	126
1989	17	1	5	0	23	28	45	1	74	2	1	1	4	0	101
1990	8	6	8	0	22	29	45	0	74	3	1	0	4	0	100
1991[d]	0	1	7	0	8	21	23	1	45	0	0	0	0	0	53
Total	221	50	89	11	371	449	493	10	952	19	7	5	31	30	1384

Table compiled from summaries of botulism cases reported to CDC[8].
[a]Type F; [b]types A/B; [c]types B/F; [d]1 January – 30 June 1991.

these products is normally above 4.5. However, there were 34 reported outbreaks in the US of food-borne botulism between 1899 and 1975 from acid products including pears, apricots, tomato products, pickles, apple sauce, okra, peaches, huckleberry and blackberries[9]. Spores of *C. botulinum* have been shown to survive for long periods of time at low pH. The lowest pH associated with two cases of botulism in Kentucky was 3.5. In order for *C. botulinum* to grow in products with pH values below 4.5, it is necessary for initial spoilage caused by other micro-organisms to occur first. The initial spoilage organism raises the pH (*e.g.* beneath a pellicle of mould growth) above 4.5 which then allows the spores of *C. botulinum*, which have survived the pasteurisation step, to germinate and produce toxin.

Early researchers, such as Weiss[10] and Esty and Meyer[11], were not aware that *C. botulinum* was unlikely to grow in acid products and, therefore, did many experiments to determine the heat resistance of the spores in fruit products with pH values as low as 2.1. Once pH 4.5 became established in the 1930s as the minimum pH for growth and toxin production, little attention has been paid to resistance of spores at pH values lower than this. Recently, however, there are many examples of pasteurised fruit products being mixed with food components with pH above 4.5 (*e.g.* fruit pulp in dairy desserts, pasteurised fruit pieces mixed with cooked meat toppings). The only recent study into the heat resistance of spores of *C. botulinum* in fruit has been by Smelt[12] who

Table 2 Recorded incidents of food-borne botulism in the UK

Year	Cases	Deaths	Food implicated	*C. botulinum* type
1922	8	8	Duck paste	A
1932	2	1	Rabbit and pigeon broth	?
1934	1	0	Jugged hare	?
1935	5?	4?	Vegetarian nut brawn	A
1935	1	1	Minced meat pie	B
1947	5	1	Macaroni cheese	?
1955	2	0	Pickled fish from Mauritius	A
1978	4	2	Canned salmon from US	E
1987	1	0	Kosher airline meal	A
1989	27	1	Hazelnut yoghurt	B

Compiled from Gilbert *et al*[2].

specifically addressed the elimination of the spores in strawberries which were to be pasteurised and mixed with a sterilised dairy product. The decimal reduction time of spores of proteolytic strains at 90°C ranged from 2.3 to 7.5 min. He concluded that spores of proteolytic *C. botulinum* could not be eliminated by heat without impairing the quality of the strawberries.

The most recent, and largest, outbreak of botulism in the UK in which 27 people were affected and one died was associated with hazelnut yoghurt[13]. This was caused by the failure to apply a botulinum cook to the canned hazelnut used to flavour the yoghurt. This example of botulism from a final product with pH below 4.5 emphasises the need for vigilance at all stages of food manufacturing.

The 10 recorded outbreaks in the UK began in 1922 with the Loch Maree outbreak in Scotland caused by *C. botulinum* type A in potted duck paste (Table 2)[2]. This had been processed at 113.9–115.6°C for 2 h, removed from the steriliser, filled into glass containers which were capped and cooked at 99°C for 40 min. Eight people died in this outbreak. The incidents between 1932 and 1947 all involved home prepared foods. The incident in 1955 involved pickled fish from Mauritius, in 1978 the outbreak was caused by Alaskan canned salmon, in 1987 an airline meal was involved and in 1989 the hazelnut yoghurt incident occurred.

In the US, the most common form of human botulism is infant botulism[14]. Between 1976 and 1989 over 850 laboratory-confirmed hospitalised cases had been reported in the US. The illness results when ingested spores of *C. botulinum* germinate and colonise the large intestine of infants. Most early cases are due to types A and B (proteolytic group 1) strains. Cases have also been attributed to *C. butyricum* producing type F toxin and to *C. barati* producing type E toxin. Infant botulism has been reported in 14 countries. Because honey fed to infants has been identified

Table 3. Wet heat resistance of spores of C. botulinum

Type	Typical D value (min)			Typical z value	Reference
	100°C	121°C	140°C	(°C)	
A proteolytic	29.2*	0.05–0.13	0.001*	8.2–9.1	15
B proteolytic	10.5*	0.13*	0.002	11.0	16
	20.7–23.5				17
B non-proteolytic	0.08*	0.0003*	–	8.6–9.8	18
C mildly or non-proteolytic					19
Terrestrial	3.4*	0.003*	–	10.0–11.5	
Marine	0.6*	0.0002*	–	10.7–10.8	
D mildly or non-proteolytic	–	–	–	–	20[†]
E non-proteolytic	0.03*	0.0002*	–	6.1–8.4	21
F proteolytic	8.8–17.8*	0.14–0.22*	0.003–0.004	9.3–12.1	22
F non-proteolytic	0.0001–0.0002*	–	–	9.5–14.8	23
G proteolytic	1.1–1.3*	0.14–0.19	0.02–0.04*	20.9–27.3	24

*Calculated from published data.
[†]No data has been found for type D but reported[20] to have similar resistance to type C.

as a source of spores of *C. botulinum*, it is not recommended to give honey to infants until they reach one year of age.

The wet heat resistance of spores of *C. botulinum* is summarised in Table 3[15–24]. The reader should also consult *ICMSF Book 5*[3] and Brown[25] for reviews of heat resistance data on *C. botulinum*.

A third type of botulism, wound botulism, caused by germination and outgrowth of spores of *C. botulinum* in wounds accounted for 31 cases of botulism between 1978 and 1991 in the US[8]. A number of cases of wound botulism were a result of intravenous drug use.

C. botulinum can grow and produce toxin with ease in many foods. It is important to ensure that not only are the correct thermal processes and preservative regimens followed, but also that all parts of the food are under control. Several instances of growth of *C. botulinum* in unusual circumstances are cited in *ICMSF Book 5*[3]. These include chopped garlic in oil that was unheated, contained no preservatives and relied solely on refrigeration for safety, preserved peanuts, and 'kapchunka' – a salt-cured, air-dried, whole uneviscerated whitefish. 'Kapchunka' preservation relies on the salt concentration inside all parts of the flesh of the fish reaching an inhibitory level quickly enough to prevent *C. botulinum* growing. Botulism outbreaks have also been reported from potato salad prepared from foil wrapped baked potatoes which had been stored at room temperature after baking and sautéed onions where the spores had survived the frying step and germinated in the anaerobic conditions provided by the layer of margarine on the surface of the onions. Non-proteolytic *C. botulinum* can grow down to

3.3°C and, therefore, presents a risk to chilled foods. The proteolytic strains can grow down to 10°C.

Clostridium perfringens

C. perfringens was the cause of 18,970 cases of food poisoning between 1970–1980 in England and Wales[26] and 982 cases between 1985–1994[1]. It poses a world-wide problem.

Food poisoning from this organism is typically characterised by acute diarrhoea and severe abdominal pain 8–24 h after ingestion of food containing large numbers of vegetative cells. Full recovery within 24–48 h is normal.

C. perfringens is grouped into 5 types, A–E, depending on the exotoxin produced (as distinct to the enterotoxin). Type A is the usual strain associated with food poisoning in the UK and the West. This strain can also cause gas gangrene and septicaemia as well as food poisoning.

In New Guinea, a type of food poisoning called 'pig-bel' is caused by *C. perfringens* type C. During pig roasts at tribal celebrations, spores of this strain germinate and proliferate during the slow cooking and cooling of the meat which is often cooked as whole carcasses in shallow pits in the ground. Consumption of sweet potatoes, which contain a heat stable trypsin inhibitor, at the same time prevents destruction of the bacterial toxin and is believed to be responsible for the number of fatalities from 'pig-bel'.

Spores of *C. perfringens* type A are widespread in the environment and are present in a wide variety of foods including meat, fish, poultry, vegetables, dairy products and dried foods[3]. Outbreaks of food poisoning from *C. perfringens* have often followed consumption of meals prepared for large numbers of people in schools, factories, hospitals and social functions.

An outbreak investigated by the author serves as a typical example. Guests at a wedding reception were served with sliced turkey by the hotel. A number of guests, including the bride and groom and close relatives, became ill later that evening. Only about a third of the guests became ill even though most had eaten turkey. The hotel had cooked two large pieces of turkey roll the previous day. The joints, produced by a local butcher, were formed by pressing pieces of turkey into a roll thus ensuring that any contaminating spores of *C. perfringens* were distributed to the centre. The size of the two rolls of meat and the cooking details were not definitely established but each roll weighed 20 lb and was cooked for 20 min/lb. The cooking temperature was not definitely established either, but due to the size of the roll and the moisture content of the meat, it was calculated that the temperature at the centre could have been anything from 67–117°C at the end of the cooking time. It is not generally appreciated that when products containing a high moisture content are cooked or deep fried, the centre temperature does not rise much above 100°C until the water is driven off. At normal atmospheric pressure, water boils at 100°C whether it is deep fried, oven baked or boiled in a kettle.

After cooking, which was insufficient to kill the spores of C. perfringens, (decimal reduction time up to 17 min at 100°C)[27] the rolls of meat were allowed to cool at room temperature for 1 h, wrapped in cling film and placed in a chiller at 15°C for another hour followed by refrigeration at 0–2°C for 12 h. Simulations of the centre temperatures during cooling demonstrated that they would have been at 15–50°C for 5–6 h. This would have been more than sufficient for each individual surviving spore to germinate and increase to over 2×10^6 cells assuming an average generation time of 17 min (generation times as short as 7 min have been reported[27]). The joints of meat were then removed from the refrigerator, sliced and overlapped on plates for ease of serving. The meat was sprinkled with water, covered with foil and kept 'hot' in a fan oven set at 180°C for up to 2 h before serving. The reason only some of the guests became ill was believed to be because only the centre of one of the two meat rolls was thought to contain sufficient of the organism. Since the slices were served sequentially, most of the guests affected were sitting together. The organism was isolated from some of the turkey roll taken home by one of the guests for her cat. Fortunately for the cat, the meat was sent instead to the local environmental health officer for analysis when its owner succumbed to the food poisoning.

Cooking and cooling the meat in smaller portions, which would have heated and cooled more rapidly, would have significantly reduced the risk of C. perfringens food poisoning. The reheating of the meat slices in the fan oven was not effective because of the thickness of the over-lapping slices. A temperature above 70°C would be necessary to destroy the vegetative bacteria before consumption.

Bacillus cereus, B. subtilis and B. licheniformis

The causes of B. cereus food poisoning are similar in many respects to those of C. perfringens. The conditions that favour the growth of B. cereus include cooking procedures that activate the spores followed by slow cooling and storage of food at 10–50°C[3]. B. cereus and the other food poisoning bacilli, B. subtilis and B. licheniformis, are widespread in the environment. Rice, cereals and spices are commonly contaminated with spores of B. cereus. Following cooking, in the absence of a competitive microflora, the surviving spores germinate and proliferate rapidly. There are two forms of illness produced by B. cereus. One is caused by a diarrhoeal toxin, which is produced during the exponential phase of growth. The onset of diarrhoea occurs 8–24 h after ingestion of large numbers of bacteria or toxin. This toxin is heat sensitive and is inactivated by heating at 56°C for 5 min. The other is caused by an emetic toxin, which is produced during the stationary phase of growth. Emesis occurs 1–6 h after ingestion of the toxin. This toxin is heat stable and can withstand normal cooking procedures[3].

The spores of B. cereus appear to vary widely in heat resistance. However, when the published data are plotted as log decimal reduction or D value against temperature, most of the data clusters together[25] with only the ileal loop 2 strain of Bradshaw et al.[28] standing out as a particularly heat resistant strain. A D value of 2.35 min at 121.1°C was reported[28] for this strain.

B. licheniformis spores are similar in resistance to typical B. cereus spores with D values at 100°C around 4–8 min. B. subtilis spores typically have D values at 121.1°C of approximately 0.5 min. Compilations of thermal resistance data can be found in ICMSF Book 5[3], Holdsworth[4] and Brown[25].

Control of B. cereus, B. subtilis and B. licheniformis depends on adequate heat processing to destroy the spores and rapid cooling of product after cooking. Holding of food at temperatures of 10–50°C will allow the organism to proliferate provided other growth conditions, such as pH, are favourable.

Under dry heat conditions, spores of B. subtilis can be extremely resistant with D values at 160°C of 0.1–3.5 min being reported by various researchers[29].

Spore-formers causing spoilage

Clostridium butyricum, C. beijerinckii and C. pasteurianum

There are several spore-formers which have not been associated with food poisoning but which can produce significant economic spoilage of foodstuff.

Butyric anaerobes, for example, C. butyricum, C. beijerinckii and C. pasteurianum produce gas and butyric odours in canned foods, particularly those with pH values between 3.9 and 4.5 (e.g. tomatoes and pears)[30]. During the storage and ripening of hard cheeses such as Gouda, Edam and Emmentaler, C. butyricum and C. tyrobutyricum can cause spoilage and gas production ('blowing'), the spores often occurring in milk from cows fed silage during winter months. Spores of C. butyricum have been reported to have D values as high as 23 min at 85°C and pH 7[31]. At pH 4.4, the thermal death time may be 10–15 min at 100°C[30].

For destruction of spores of *C. pasteurianum*, it has been suggested that a centre temperature of 95°C should be reached for products with a pH between 4.2 and 4.5 and a centre temperature of 84°C for products with a pH below 4.2[30].

C. beijerinckii is a close relative of *C. butyricum* with D values of 2–4 min at 85°C and pH 7[32].

Control of butyric anaerobes requires thorough washing of the raw material together with pH and process temperature control. Failure to control spore-formers in products with pH values 3.9–4.5 may result not only in spoilage but also a rise in pH which could allow spores of *C. botulinum*, which had survived pasteurisation, to germinate and produce toxin.

Clostridium sporogenes

C. sporogenes is closely related to the proteolytic strains of *C. botulinum*, but produces spores which are approximately 5 times as resistant with D values up to 1.5 min at 121°C[25]. Spoilage from this organism produces typically blown or burst packs with a strong putrefactive odour. If spoilage from *C. sporogenes* is experienced, all suspect packs should be recalled and investigations into the cause of spoilage undertaken. A process fault that allows *C. sporogenes* to survive and proliferate may also have been serious enough to allow spores of *C. botulinum* to survive, germinate and produce toxin.

Bacillus sporothermodurans

This is a mesophilic spore-former which produces highly heat-resistant spores. It was first detected in UHT milk in 1985 in southern Europe and in UHT milk in Germany in 1990[33]. Since then, there have been several reports from other European and non-European countries[34]. The spores survive the heat process and then multiply to a maximum of about 10^5/ml of milk during incubation at 30°C for 5 days, but cause no noticeable spoilage and are non-pathogenic.

The decimal reduction times of spores from 3 dairies ranged from 19–34 s at 121°C[35]. Raw milk must be autoclaved to enrich for the spores and eliminate competitive microflora. According to Meier *et al.*,[35] the spores of *B. sporothermodurans* are more resistant than the spores of many thermophiles.

Clostridium thermosaccharolyticum

The most heat resistant spores are those of *C. thermosaccharolyticum*. D values as high as 195 min at 121°C have been recorded[36]. The author investigated a spoilage outbreak in canned mushrooms caused by heat resistant spores of *C. thermosaccharolyticum* that had grown in the composted forest bark used on the mushroom beds[37]. D values of these spores were 68 min at 121°C.

Spoilage from this organism manifests itself by blown or burst packs with a strong butyric or cheesy odour. The spores survive thermal processing to germinate and grow when the product is stored at elevated temperatures around 30–60°C (*e.g.* in pallets of inadequately cooled cans). Spoilage by *C. thermosaccharolyticum* is not uncommon.

Desulfotomaculum nigrificans

In contrast, spoilage caused by *D. nigrificans*, another thermophile, is now quite rare although, in the 1920s, an entire season's production of canned sweet corn could be lost from this organism. *D. nigrificans* causes 'sulphur stinker' spoilage often resulting in blackened product when the steel in cans reacts with the H_2S produced. D values as high as 55 min at 121.1°C have been recorded[38]. An unusual outbreak of spoilage caused by *D. nigrificans* and *Clostridium thermoaceticum* in Japan was reported by Matsuda *et al.*[39]. The spoilage occurred in canned coffee and 'Shiruko' (a soft drink made from red beans and cane sugar) produced for retail in hot vending machines at temperatures above 50°C.

Bacillus stearothermophilus and B. coagulans

B. stearothermophilus is a common thermophilic spoilage organism that normally produces acid but no gas in spoiled packs that have been held at elevated temperatures around 50–55°C. If readily fermentable sugars are in limited supply, the author has found that this organism can elevate pH. The minimum pH for growth is around 5.3. The D value at 120°C can be as high as 16.7 min[40]. Prevention of spoilage is achieved by holding product below 30–60°C because it is often impracticable to try to process product for long enough to destroy the spores.

Under dry heat conditions at 121°C, the D value of spores of *B. stearothermophilus* can be as high as 936 min[41].

B. coagulans is also a thermophile but differs from *B. stearothermophilus* in being able to grow at pH values down to 4.0[30]. It is less heat resistant having a D-value at 98.9°C of 3.1 min[30]. It produces off-flavours and souring of product during spoilage.

Alicyclobacillus acidoterrestris

Traditionally, pasteurised acidic fruit juices with pH values below 4.0 have been considered unlikely to support the growth of spore-forming bacteria[30,42]. However, in Germany in 1982. a spoilage outbreak in apple juice was caused by an acid tolerant, heat resistant, thermophilic spore-forming bacterium[43]. The organism was identified as a strain of *Alicyclobacillus acidoterrestris* that could grow over the pH range 2–6 and at temperatures between 35–55°C. The decimal reduction time for the spores at 90°C was 15 min. The organism produces a 'disinfectant' or 'antiseptic' taint in apple and orange juice. The most recent reports of spoilage from this organism were in 1994/5 with unusual taint development in aseptically packed orange juice and concentrate in the UK and North America[44].

The most likely cause of contamination of the fruit is from soil contamination during harvesting. The heat resistance of the spores is such that pasteurisation will not guarantee freedom from the organism. Thorough washing of the fruit prior to processing appears to be the only control measure at present. There is no evidence that the organism is pathogenic, and since it does not change the pH of the fruit, there should be no risk of secondary growth of spore-forming pathogens such as *C. botulinum*. Brown[45] has reviewed *A. acidoterrestris* and others in the same genus which have been isolated from hot springs.

Clostridium putrefaciens

In the early 1900s, *C. putrefaciens* was of considerable concern to the ham curing industry. Studies by Roberts and Derrick[46] demonstrated that this organism was able to grow in 4% NaCl + 100 p/m of $NaNO_2$ at pH 7.0 even at 5°C. The spores were not particularly heat resistant however (D-value 8–14 min at 80°C). Modern processing trends are to use lower levels of salt and nitrite, increased pH levels of 6.8–7.0 and chill storage which would tend to favour the growth of *C. putrefaciens*.

Key points for clinical practice

Bacterial spores are resistant to heat, chemicals, freezing, desiccation and irradiation. Resistance can vary widely from species to species. The

Table 4 Growth range temperatures of some spore-formers

Organism	Temperature (°C)			Reference
	Minimum	Optimum	Maximum	
A. acidoterrestris	26	42–53	80	45
B. cereus	3–4	30	48	47
	4	30–40	55	3
	5		50	48
B. coagulans	30	45	60	47
		50–55		42
B. licheniformis	30	–	60	49
B. sporothermodurans	10	–	50	34
B. stearothermophilus	28	55	72	47
B. subtilis	10	28	51	47
	12	43–46	55	49
C. beijerinkii	–	30	–	49
C. botulinum (proteolytic)	10	38–40	48	47
C. botulinum (non-proteolytic)	3.3	25–30	40	3
C. butyricum	10	–	45	49
C. pasteurianum	–	30	–	50
		25-35		42
C. perfringens	12	43–47	50	3
	15		50	27
C. putrefaciens	5	15–22	35	46
	0	20	35	47
C. sporogenes	–	28–30	–	42
	18		45	49
C. thermosaccharolyticum	30	55	71	47
		50–55		42
D. nigrificans	30	55	71	47

most dangerous food poisoning species is *C botulinum* and the most common is *C. perfringens*. *B. cereus*, *B. subtilis* and *B. licheniformis* have also been implicated in food poisoning. *C. perfringens*, *C. botulinum* and *C. sporogenes* can cause deep wound infections and, in the case of the first two, cause wound botulism and gas gangrene. The most common type of botulism is infant botulism. Several non-pathogenic spore-formers can cause significant spoilage in food products. A number of spoilage spore-formers are thermophilic and these proliferate when the food is held at elevated temperatures (30–60°C). Other spore-formers, such as non-proteolytic *C. botulinum*, can grow down to 3.3°C and can, therefore, present a risk to chilled foods. Many foods receive heat treatments that do not eliminate all bacterial spores, and rely upon chilled storage for their shelf-life and safety. Examples of the range of temperatures for growth, including the minimum, are given in Table 4 (*see also* chapter on 'Control of vegetative micro-organisms'). Bacterial spores are several orders of magnitude more resistant under dry heat than wet heat conditions. Control of spore-formers requires an understanding of both the resistance and outgrowth characteristics of the spores.

References

1   Sprenger RA. *Hygiene for Management*. Doncaster: Highfield Publications, 1995
2   Gilbert RJ, Rodhouse JC, Haugh CA. Anaerobes and food poisoning. In: Borriello SP. (Ed) *Clinical and Molecular Aspects of Anaerobes*. Petersfield: Wrighton Biomedical, 1990; 85–9
3   ICMSF. *Microorganisms in Foods 5: Characteristics of Microbial Pathogens*. London: Blackie, 1996
4   Holdsworth SD. *Thermal Processing of Packaged Foods*. London: Blackie, 1997
5   Department of Health. *Guidelines for the Safe Production of Heat Preserved Foods*. London: HMSO, 1994
6   Hauschild AHW. *Clostridium botulinum*. In: Doyle MP. (Ed) *Foodborne Bacterial Pathogens*. New York: Marcel Dekker, 1989; 111–89
7   Center for Disease Control. Botulinum in the United States 1899–1973. In: CDC *Handbook for Epidemiologists, Clinicians and Laboratory Workers*, DHEW Publ. (CDC), 74-8279. Atlanta, GA: US Department of Health, Education and Welfare, 1974
8   Center for Disease Control. *Annual Summaries of Botulism Cases reported to CDC*. Atlanta, GA: US Department of Health, Education and Welfare, 1978–1991
9   Odlaug TE, Pflug IJ. *Clostridium botulinum* and acid foods. *J Food Protect* 1978; **41**: 566–73
10 Weiss H. The thermal death point of the spores of *Bacillus botulinus* in canned foods. *J Infect Dis* 1921; **29**: 362–8
11 Esty JR, Meyer KF. The heat resistance of the spores of *B. botulinus* and allied anaerobes XI. *J Infect Dis* 1922; **31**: 650–63
12 Smelt JPPM. *Heat resistance of Clostridium botulinum in acid ingredients and its significance for the safety of chilled foods*. PhD Thesis, University of Utrecht, The Netherlands 1980
13 O'Mahoney M, Mitchell E, Gilbert RJ *et al*. An outbreak of foodborne botulism associated with contaminated hazelnut yoghurt. *Epidemiol Infect* 1990; **104**: 389–95
14 Arnon SS. Infant botulism. In: Borriello SP. (Ed) *Clinical and Molecular Aspects of Anaerobes*. Petersfield: Wrightson Biomedical, 1990; 41–8
15 Stumbo CR, Murphy JR, Cochran J. Nature of thermal death time curves for PA3679 and *Clostridium botulinum*. *Food Technol* 1950; **4**: 321–6
16 Gaze JE, Brown KL. The heat resistance of spores of *Clostridium botulinum* 213B over the temperature range 120 to 140°C. *Int J Food Sci Technol* 1988; **23**: 373–8
17 Kaplan AM, Reynolds H, Lichtenstein H. Significance of variations in observed slopes of thermal death time curves for putrefactive anaerobes. *Food Res* 1954; **19**: 173–81
18 Gaze JE, Brown GD. *Determination of the heat resistance of a strain of non-proteolytic Clostridium botulinum type B and a strain of type E heated in cod and carrot homogenate over the temperature range 70 to 92°C*. Technical Memorandum No 592. Chipping Campden: Campden and Chorleywood Food RA, 1990
19 Segner WP, Schmidt CF. Heat resistance of spores of marine and terrestrial strains of *Clostridium botulinum* type C. *Appl Microbiol* 1971; **22**: 1030–3
20 Sakaguchi G. Botulism. In: *Progress in Food Safety*. Proceedings of symposium: Progress in our knowledge of foodborne disease during the life of the Food Research Institute; held 28 May 1986, University of Wisconsin-Madison. 1986; 18–34
21 Lynt RK, Solomon HM, Lilly Jr T, Kautter DA. Thermal death time of *Clostridium botulinum* type E in meat of the blue crab. *J Food Sci* 1977; **42**: 1022–5, 1037
22 Lynt RK, Kautter DA, Solomon HM. Heat resistance of proteolytic *Clostridium botulinum* type F in phosphate buffer and crabmeat. *J Food Sci* 1981; **47**: 204–6, 230
23 Lynt RK, Kautter DA, Solomon HM. Heat resistance of non-proteolytic *Clostridium botulinum* type F in phosphate buffer and crabmeat. *J Food Sci* 1979; **44**: 108–11
24 Lynt RK, Solomon HM, Kautter DA. Heat resistance of *Clostridium botulinum* type G in phosphate buffer. *J Food Protect* 1984; **47**: 463–6
25 Brown KL. *Heat resistance of bacterial spores*. PhD Thesis, University of Nottingham, UK, 1992
26 Stringer MF. *Clostridium perfringens* type A food poisoning. In: Borriello S. (Ed). *Clostridium in gastrointestinal disease*. Bocca Raton, FL: CRC Press, 1985

27 Labbe R. *Clostridium perfringens.* In: Doyle MP. (Ed) *Foodborne Bacterial Pathogens.* New York: Marcel Dekker, 1989; 191–234

28 Bradshaw JG, Peeler JT, Twedt RM. Heat resistance of ileal loop reactive *B. cereus* strains isolated from commercially canned food. *Appl Microbiol* 1975; **30**: 943–5

29 Brown KL. Spore resistance and ultra heat treatment processes. *J Appl Bacteriol Symp Suppl* 1994; **76**: 67S–80S

30 Hersom AC, Hulland, ED. *Canned Foods, Thermal processing and Microbiology.* Edinburgh: Churchill Livingstone, 1980

31 Russell AD. *The Destruction of Bacterial Spores.* London: Academic Press, 1982

32 Brown KL. The problems of heat resistant spores in food production. In: Borriello SP. (Ed) *Clinical and Molecular Aspects of Anaerobes.* Petersfield: Wrightson Biomedical, 1990; 91–101

33 Hammer P, Lembke F, Suhren G, Heeschen W. 1. Characterisation of a heat resistant mesophilic *Bacillus* species affecting the quality of UHT-milk. In: Proceedings of the IDF Symposium *Heat Treatments and Alternative Methods.* Vienna, Austria, 6–8 September 1995. Brussels: IDF, 1996; 9–16

34 Pettersson B, Lembke F, Hammer P, Stackebrandt E, Priest FG. *Bacillus sporothermodurans,* a new species producing highly heat-resistant endospores. *Int J System Bacteriol* 1996; **46**: 759–64

35 Meier J, Rademacher B, Walenta W, Kessler HG. 2. Heat-resistant spores under UHT treatment. In: Proceedings of the IDF Symposium *Heat Treatments and Alternative Methods.* Vienna, Austria, 6–8 September 1995. Brussels: IDF, 1996; 17–25

36 Xezones H, Segmiller JL, Hutchings IJ. Processing requirements for a heat tolerant anaerobe. *Food Technol* 1965; **19**: 1001–3

37 Brown KL. Heat resistant thermophilic anaerobe isolated from composted forest bark. In: *Fundamental and Applied Aspects of Spores,* Proceedings of Cambridge Spore Conference. London: Academic Press, 1983; 387–94

38 Donnelly LS, Busta FF. Heat resistance of *Desulfotomaculum nigrificans* spores in soy protein infant formula preparations. *Appl Environ Microbiol* 1980; **40**: 721–5

39 Matsuda N, Masuda H, Komaki M, Matsumoto N. Thermophilic spore-forming strict anaerobes isolated from spoiled canned 'Shiruko' and coffee containing milk. *J Food Hygiene Soc Jpn* 1982; **23**: 480–6

40 Davies FL, Underwood HM, Perkins AG, Burton H. Thermal death kinetics of *Bacillus stearothermophilus* spores at ultra high temperatures. 1. Laboratory determination of temperature coefficients. *J Food Technol* 1977; **12**: 115–29

41 Collier CP, Townsend CT. The resistance of bacterial spores to superheated steam. *Food Technol* 1956; **10**: 477–81

42 Stumbo CR. *Thermobacteriology in Food Processing.* London: Academic Press, 1973

43 Cerny G, Hennlich W, Poralla K. Spoilage of fruit juice by Bacilli: isolation and characterisation of the spoilage organism. *Z Lebens Unters Forschung* 1984; **179**: 224–7

44 Splittstoesser DF, Churey JJ, Lee CY. Growth characteristics of aciduric sporeforming bacilli isolated from fruit juices. *J Food Protect* 1994; **57**: 1080–3

45 Brown KL. New microbiological spoilage challenges in aseptics: *Alicyclobacillus acidoterrestris* spoilage in aseptically packed fruit juices. In: *Proceedings of International Symposium on advances in aseptic processing and packaging technologies,* Copenhagen, Denmark, Sept 11-12, 1995. Ohlsson T. (Ed) Goteborg, Sweden: SIK, 1995

46 Roberts TA, Derrick CM. Sporulation of *Clostridium putrefaciens* and the resistance of the spores to heat, γ-radiation and curing salts. *J Appl Bacteriol* 1975; **38**: 33–7

47 Shapton DA, Shapton NF (Eds) *Principles and Practices for the Safe Processing of Foods.* Oxford: Butterworth-Heinemann, 1991

48 Kramer JM, Gilbert RJ. *Bacillus cereus* and other *Bacillus* species. In: Doyle MP. (Ed) *Foodborne Bacterial Pathogens.* New York: Marcell Dekker, 1989; 22–70

49 Mitscherlich E, Marth EH. *Microbial survival in the environment. Bacteria and rickettsiae in human and animal health.* Berlin: Springer, 1984

50 Townsend CT. Spore-forming anaerobes causing spoilage in acid canned foods. *Food Res* 1939; **4**: 231–7

Control of food-borne viruses

Hazel Appleton

Enteric and Respiratory Virus Laboratory, Central Public Health Laboratory, London, UK

There are two main food-borne virus infections. These are viral gastroenteritis caused by small round structured viruses (SRSV) of the Norwalk group and hepatitis A. Both infections are normally transmitted directly from person-to-person, but on occasions they may also be food-borne or water-borne. Viruses do not multiply or produce toxins in foods, and foods merely act as vehicles for their passive transfer. Foods may be contaminated by infected food-handlers, and outbreaks frequently involve cold foods that require much handling during preparation. Foods may also be contaminated in their growing and harvesting areas by sewage polluted water, and molluscan shellfish have been particularly implicated. PCR and ELISA based methods are being developed for detection and typing of viruses in patients and also in food samples. Sensitive detection methods should facilitate the design of improved food processing methods to ensure virus-free food.

> *She pushed her wheelbarrow*
> *Through streets broad and narrow,*
> *Crying 'cockles and mussels, alive, alive O!'*

According to the song, Molly Malone died of a fever. It is not specified whether this was as a result of consuming her wares of cockles and mussels, but in the earlier part of the twentieth century probably the greatest danger from eating shellfish was typhoid. Now almost all illness arising from the consumption of molluscan shellfish is viral, and indeed the whole story of food-borne viral illness has been very closely linked with shellfish.

There are two main food-borne viral infections, namely viral gastroenteritis and hepatitis A. Since the early 1970s, several different viruses have been discovered which all cause gastroenteritis. Food-borne incidents of viral gastroenteritis are nearly all caused by just one of the viruses, commonly known as small round structured viruses (SRSV) or Norwalk-like viruses. The other well-known gastroenteritis viruses, such as rotavirus and astrovirus, are only rarely implicated in food-borne outbreaks. Food and water-borne outbreaks of hepatitis A are infrequently reported.

Both viral gastroenteritis and hepatitis A are most usually transmitted directly from person-to-person, and food- or water-borne transmission appears to be responsible for only a small proportion of incidents.

Correspondence to:
Dr Hazel Appleton,
Enteric and Respiratory
Virus Laboratory, Central
Public Health Laboratory,
61 Colindale Avenue,
London NW9 5HT, UK

© The British Council 2000

Unlike bacteria, viruses do not multiply or produce toxins in foods. Food or water merely act as vehicles for their passive transfer. The true incidence of food-borne viral transmission is undetermined, but probably grossly under-reported. As a result of the rising numbers of food poisoning reports in recent years, the Advisory Committee on the Micro-biological Safety of Food (ACMSF) was set up. A report from this committee was published in 1998, identifying the problems associated with food-borne viral infections and areas of research required[1].

Routes of contamination

Foods may be contaminated with viruses in two main ways. Firstly, they may be contaminated at source in their growing and harvesting areas, usually by coming into contact with polluted water. Shellfish have been a particular problem and have been implicated in many outbreaks world-wide. Secondly, foods may be contaminated during handling and preparation, often from infected food-handlers.

Shellfish

It is the bivalve molluscs – including oysters, mussels, clams and cockles – that are mainly involved in transmitting viral illness, and in fact most illness associated with these shellfish is viral. In the period 1992–1997, 42 outbreaks associated with consumption of oysters in England and Wales were reported to the PHLS Communicable Disease Surveillance Centre (CDSC). Of these, 17 outbreaks were caused by SRSV and one outbreak by an astrovirus. The remaining 24 outbreaks were of unknown aetiology, but mostly had the characteristic features of viral gastroenteritis. Of 119 oyster-associated outbreaks reported since 1982, only two are known to have been caused by a bacterial pathogen.

The bivalve molluscs live in shallow, coastal and estuarine waters which are frequently polluted with sewage. They feed by filtering particulate matter from the large volumes of water passing over their gills, and this can include potentially pathogenic micro-organisms. Although human viruses do not replicate in shellfish, they can be concentrated within the molluscs to higher concentrations than occur within the surrounding water up to 100-fold. Cockles, mussels and clams are only lightly cooked and frequently oysters are consumed raw.

Fruit and vegetables

There is the potential for fruits, vegetables and salad items to be contaminated with polluted water and sewage sludge during irrigation and fertilisation. Although several outbreaks of viral gastroenteritis have been attributed to salad items, contamination on these occasions is usually thought to have occurred at the time of preparation. Soft fruits believed to have been contaminated at their source, have been implicated in outbreaks of hepatitis A, and there has been one report of viral gastroenteritis due to SRSV and associated with raspberries affecting 300 people in Canada in 1997.

Food-handlers

Viruses causing gastroenteritis and hepatitis A are infectious in very low doses, and thus are spread very easily from infected persons. It is now recognised that outbreaks arising from food contamination by infected food handlers are common occurrences. Cold items, such as sandwiches and salads that require much handling during preparation, are implicated most frequently. Without meticulous attention to personal hygiene and thorough and frequent hand-washing, faecally-contaminated fingers can contaminate food and work surfaces.

Viral gastroenteritis

Viral gastroenteritis is usually regarded as a mild, self-limiting illness lasting 24–48 h. Symptoms commonly include malaise, abdominal pain, pyrexia, diarrhoea and/or vomiting. Onset may be sudden and commence with projectile vomiting. This is a particular hazard where food is being prepared and laid out, as virus can be disseminated over a wide area in aerosol droplets. The viruses are usually transmitted from person-to-person via the faecal–oral route, but may also be spread by contaminated food and water causing common source outbreaks. Viruses account for 6% of food-borne outbreaks and 5% of water-borne outbreaks occurring in England and Wales and reported to CDSC. Secondary person-to-person transmission to close contacts is a characteristic feature of food-borne and water-borne virus outbreaks. Several different types of viruses cause gastroenteritis: the most important include rotavirus, SRSV or Norwalk group viruses, astrovirus and adenovirus types 40 and 41. However, in almost all food-borne outbreaks, where a virus is identified it is an SRSV. Rotavirus and astrovirus are only rarely implicated. Adenovirus has not been associated with food or water-borne transmission.

Small round structured viruses

This group of viruses[2] infects all age groups. There is a variable incubation period from about 12–60 h. It occurs all year round, although in

Table 1 Outbreaks of infectious intestinal disease in England and Wales, 1992–1997

Organism	All outbreaks	Food-borne outbreaks	Waterborne outbreaks
SRSV	1159 (33%)	69 (5.8%)	1 (2.7%)
Rotavirus	97 (2.8%)	1 (0.1%)	0
Astrovirus	18 (0.5%)	2 (0.2%)	1 (2.7%)
Calicivirus	3 (0.1%)	0	0
Salmonella	798 (23%)	656 (55%)	0
Other	621 (18%)	321 (27%)	33 (89%)
Unknown	776 (22%)	145 (12%)	2 (5.4%)
Total	3472	1194	37

Data from PHLS Communicable Disease Surveillance Centre

temperate climates, most infections occur over the winter months. These viruses are responsible for both sporadic cases of gastroenteritis in the community and for outbreaks in schools, hospitals, old peoples' homes, hotels and cruise ships. A national study of infectious intestinal disease in England from 1993 to 1996 has indicated that viruses are the most common cause of infectious intestinal disease in the community with SRSV the most frequently reported organism[3]. From 1992 to 1997, SRSV accounted for one-third of all gastroenteritis outbreaks reported to CDSC and the number of outbreaks of SRSV exceeded the number of outbreaks of salmonella. Unlike the salmonella outbreaks, however, only 6% of the SRSV outbreaks were known to be food- or water-borne (Table 1).

The virus was discovered in 1972 by electron microscopy (Fig. 1). The

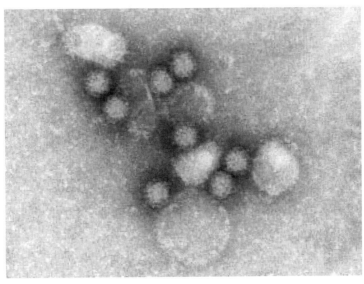

Fig. 1 Electron micrograph of SRSV. The virus particles have an amorphous surface and ragged spikey edge. Magnification x250,000.

name small round structured virus describes the morphology and has been used in the UK. In the US, the term Norwalk-like virus has been used. The first virus originated from an outbreak in the town of Norwalk in the US, and became the prototype of the group.

SRSVs cannot be cultured and until recently detection relied on electron microscopy. This is a time-consuming technique and is not conducive to examining large numbers of specimens. It is also insensitive: it cannot be used for examining food samples and usually virus can only be detected in clinical samples if collected within 48 h of onset of symptoms. More recently, methods of detection have been developed based on PCR assays. Virus can be detected for up to a week after onset in patients, although it is not clear whether this is infectious virus. PCR assays are sensitive enough to detect virus in shellfish, environmental samples and other foods. Such tests are only available in specialised laboratories at present and cannot be used for routine testing of food samples. There is great diversity within the SRSV group[4] and current PCR tests do not detect all strains. Hence, electron microscopy is still necessary for the investigation of some outbreaks.

The SRSVs form a complex group of viruses. They have formally been classified with the *Caliciviridae* and now are often referred to as human caliciviruses. They are split into three broad genogroups. Two groups have the morphology of SRSVs and the third group has the classical morphology of a calicivirus and a genomic arrangement distinct from the other two groups. There are several serotypes which broadly correspond with the genotypic groups. Immunity is complex and short-lived. Persons can be infected repeatedly with the same strain. The incidence is grossly under-reported, partly due to the mild nature of the infection and partly from the difficulty in detecting and identifying the virus (Table 2).

Viral antigen has been produced by expression of virus capsids in insect cells or yeast cells, and is providing material for development of ELISA-based detection tests[5]. However, these only select for a very few strains and are not available for routine use at present.

Rotavirus

Rotaviruses[6] mainly infect young children. It is estimated that they may cause 1 million deaths a year in children under 5 years of age, mostly in

Table 2 Under-reporting of food-borne virus outbreaks

SRSV	Short incubation period of 12–60 h. But mild illness – hence not reported. Virus only readily detected for 48 h from onset
Hepatitis A	Incubation period 3–6 weeks hence difficult to identify food source

non-industrialised countries. In industrialised countries deaths are relatively rare, but rotavirus gastroenteritis is the most frequent reason for admission of young children to hospital. Food-borne and particularly water-borne spread are probably a significant mode of transmission in non-industrialised countries, but in industrialised countries reports are rare (Table 1). Although rotavirus has been detected in shellfish, so far there have been no reports of illness from this source.

Astrovirus

The astroviruses[2] form a morphologically distinct group of viruses, and are named from the five or six point star seen by electron microscopy on the surface of some particles. Astroviruses are normally associated with gastroenteritis in young children, often under 1 year of age. Adults are infected infrequently, although outbreaks have been reported in the elderly. Astroviruses have been seen in some adults following the consumption of shellfish or contaminated water, but these incidents appear comparatively rare (Table 1).

Parvovirus

Small round viruses measuring 20–26 nm in diameter and with the characteristics of parvoviruses[2] have been observed in outbreaks of gastroenteritis, but their role as causative agents in humans remains uncertain. Parvoviruses do cause other illnesses in humans and are an important causes of gastroenteritis in some animal species.

Parvoviruses have been observed in school outbreaks of winter vomiting disease and in a number of outbreaks associated with the consumption of shellfish. Parvovirus-like particles have been detected occasionally in shellfish that have been implicated in illness and where similar virus has been found in patients. Reports of parvovirus in association with gastroenteritis are infrequent and there have been few studies on the nature and role of these viruses.

Hepatitis

There are two types of enterically transmitted hepatitis – hepatitis A and hepatitis E[7].

Hepatitis A

Food- and water-borne outbreaks of hepatitis A have been recognised for over 40 years, but are infrequently reported. Between 1992 and 1997, 228 outbreaks occurring in England and Wales were reported to CDSC, but only one of these was known to be food-borne. That outbreak was associated with shellfish. The incubation period is 2–6 weeks making it difficult to associate the source of infection with a particular food item, or even recognise an outbreak (Table 2). Like viral gastroenteritis, transmission is via the faecal–oral route, although with hepatitis the main site of viral replication is the liver.

The epidemiology of food-borne hepatitis A is similar to that of viral gastroenteritis. Contaminated shellfish have been the cause of many outbreaks world-wide. In one notable outbreak in Shanghai in 1988, over 300,000 people were infected after eating inadequately cooked clams. Cases of viral gastroenteritis were also reported in the proceeding month indicating the gross sewage pollution of the shellfish waters. Outbreaks are not just confined to non-industrialised countries, but also continue to be reported from Europe, North America and Australia. Soft fruits, particularly strawberries and raspberries, and lettuce contaminated at source have been implicated in outbreaks. Some outbreaks have originated from infected food-handlers. Virus excretion may commence up to a week before symptoms are apparent, making control difficult.

There is only one serotype of hepatitis A. Once infected immunity is life-long. An effective vaccine is available, but is not used widely. Incidence in industrialised countries has fallen in recent years and hence a susceptible population has built up. As endemic infection declines, it is possible that an increase in food-borne outbreaks will be seen.

Hepatitis E

Hepatitis E, has been associated with large water-borne outbreaks in some non-industrialised countries, notably in Asia, Africa and Central America. Food-borne transmission has been suggested, but not proved conclusively. Illness appears more severe than hepatitis A, particularly in pregnant women where a death rate of 17–33% has been observed. Secondary person-to-person transmission is estimated at only 0.7–8%. The primary source of infection appears to be contaminated water rather than person-to-person spread. Hence, control should be directed at improving the quality of water supplies. Cases in the UK are reported infrequently and are mainly imported from endemic areas.

Tick-borne encephalitis

Tick-borne encephalitis[8] is possibly the only known viral zoonosis that is transmitted via food. It occurs in Eastern Europe. Goats, sheep and cattle bitten by infected ticks become infected with the virus which is then shed in their milk. Outbreaks have occurred from the consumption of raw milk or products made from unpasteurised milk. These incidents are fortunately rare, because of the limited distribution of the appropriate ticks.

Virus survival

Gastroenteritis viruses and hepatitis viruses survive extremely well in the environment. There is little precise information on the stability of SRSVs since they cannot be cultured. Most information comes from epidemiological observations and limited studies of infectivity in volunteers[2]. Some strains of hepatitis A and rotavirus have been cultured in the laboratory and there have been a small number of experimental studies on their stability[6,7]. Of all the enteric viruses, however, SRSVs and hepatitis A virus seem to be the most resistant to inactivation. Observations and studies on readily culturable enteroviruses, such as poliovirus and Coxsackie viruses cannot be used to predict the survival of SRSV or hepatitis A virus.

Viruses that infect via the gastrointestinal tract are acid stable. Hence they survive food processing and preservation conditions designed to produce the low pH that inhibits bacterial and fungal spoilage organisms (*e.g.* pickling in vinegar and fermentation processes that produce foods such as yoghurt). Outbreaks of viral gastroenteritis have been associated with cockles pickled in brine and vinegar. Both SRSVs and hepatitis A virus retain infectivity after exposure to acidity levels below pH 3.

Most viruses remain infectious after refrigeration and freezing. Frozen foods that have not received further cooking have been implicated in a number of incidents of both viral gastroenteritis and hepatitis A. Gastroenteritis viruses and hepatitis viruses are inactivated by normal cooking processes, but are not always inactivated in shellfish given only minimal heat treatment. Both SRSVs and hepatitis A virus retain infectivity after heating to 60°C for 30 min. It is uncertain that they would be inactivated completely in many pasteurisation processes.

These viruses survive on inanimate surfaces, on hands and in dried faecal suspensions. Lingering outbreaks have occurred in hospitals, in residential homes and on cruise ships, probably as a result of environmental contamination. SRSVs have been detected by PCR in environmental swabs from hospital lockers and hotel carpets supposedly cleaned after incidents of vomiting[9].

There are conflicting reports on the effectiveness of disinfectants. Chlorine-based disinfectants are usually considered the most effective against enteric viruses. However, SRSVs and hepatitis A appear resistant to levels of chlorine present in drinking water, equivalent to free residual chlorine of 0.5–1 mg/l. SRSVs are inactivated by 10 mg chlorine/l, which is the concentration used to treat a water supply after a contamination incident. In the US, a level of 5 mg chlorine/l with a contact time of 1 min is recommended for inactivation of hepatitis A. Sodium hypochlorite, 2% glutaraldehyde and quarternary ammonium compounds with hydro-chloric acid have been shown to reduce the infectivity of hepatitis A virus, but there are no comparative data for SRSVs. Clearly, there is a need for further studies on disinfection of these persistent organisms.

Control

A major factor in the contamination of food and water is sewage pollution. Ideally, there would be no sewage discharge into the coastal waters and rivers, thus preventing contamination of shellfish growing areas. Sewage sludge is applied to agricultural land, with the benefit that useful plant nutrients and organic matter are recycled to the soil. The UK government is proposing more stringent controls for harvesting vegetables from land where conventionally processed sewage sludge is applied and that spread of untreated sewage sludge on agricultural land should cease by the year 2001. Viruses from sewage deposited on land do not bind with soil particles and can enter ground waters, leading to contamination of water sources. Hepatitis A virus has been recovered from a ground water source associated with an outbreak.

Shellfish

Pollution of coastal waters is unfortunately a reality, and shellfish harvested from all but the cleanest waters are required to undergo treatment as laid down in the *European Union Directive on Shellfish Hygiene*[10].

Some molluscs, such as cockles, are subject to a brief heat treatment by boiling or steaming. Thorough cooking will destroy contaminating viruses, but also cause shrinkage of the shellfish meat rendering it tough and unpalatable. Many outbreaks have resulted from consumption of inadequately cooked shellfish. Heat treatment studies in the UK led to recommendations, in 1988, that the internal temperature of shellfish meat should be raised to 90°C and be maintained for 1.5 min[11]. These conditions are known to inactivate hepatitis A virus, but still achieve a commercially acceptable product. Continued surveillance has shown that there have been no recorded incidents of viral illness – either hepatitis A or viral gastroenteritis – from shellfish treated according to these recommendations. More recent laboratory studies have indicated that these conditions will also readily inactivate SRSVs[12].

Some shellfish taken from polluted water are treated by relaying and depuration. This particularly applies to oysters that may be eaten raw. Relaying involves moving shellfish from their original growing site to an area of cleaner water, where the are left for several weeks or months. The level of microbial contamination in the shellfish falls as micro-organisms are washed out during the normal feeding process. Depuration depends on the same principle, but the shellfish are placed in land-based tanks, usually for about 48 h. *Eschericha coli*, the usual indicator of contamination, is virtually eliminated during this period, but viruses can remain for several weeks. There is no guarantee that shellfish that appear safe in bacteriological tests are necessarily free of viruses and, at present, there is no satisfactorily indicator system for viruses.

Detection of viruses in shellfish is technically difficult. Extraction of infectious virus or viral RNA is a complex and unreliable procedure. SRSVs and hepatitis A virus have been detected in shellfish implicated in outbreaks or harvested from polluted beds[13], but routine testing for viruses in shellfish is not feasible.

Food-handlers

The other major source of contamination is from infected persons handling and preparing food. Persons with symptoms should be excluded from food handling. However, food-handlers with only very minimal symptoms have been implicated in transmission of SRSVs. Recommendations[14] that food-handlers should be allowed to return to work 48 h after symptoms have ceased appear to work satisfactorily. These recommendations were based on the rapid decrease in virus excretion observed by electron microscopy. Using more sensitive PCR assays, SRSVs can be detected for longer periods than by electron microscopy and, in some instances, for up to a week after onset of symptoms. It is not clear if persons shedding virus detectable by PCR are infectious, but recommendations on how long to exclude people from work needs to be kept under review.

If vomiting occurs, virus can be spread over a wide area in aerosol droplets. Uncovered food, that is not to receive further cooking, should be discarded. The environment should be thoroughly cleaned, including work surfaces, sinks and door handles.

Control of food-borne viral illness largely depends on strict attention to normal good hygienic practice in the kitchen and serving areas. Salad items, fruits and raw vegetables should be washed thoroughly. Cross contamination from uncooked shellfish should be regarded as a potential hazard.

The future

The key element in reducing food-borne spread of viruses is continued surveillance and awareness. Meticulous attention to good food-handling practices and education, to prevent people with even the mildest symptoms handling food, is essential. Development of sensitive and easily-used detection tests are required for estimating the extent of food-borne viral infections and their control. Sensitive detection tests will give more accurate estimates on the length of time a person excretes virus and hence better informed advice can be formulated on factors such as how long food handlers should be excluded from work.

Expression of recombinant virus capsids in yeast and insect cells has the potential to provide large quantities of non-infectious viral antigen. These antigens are already being used in a few laboratories for the development of ELISA-based diagnostic assays and commercial kits for detecting a wide range of SRSVs are already being evaluated. It is likely that user-friendly diagnostic tests for specimens from patients soon will be widely available. Routine detection of virus contaminants in foods is more difficult. Current methods for extraction of viruses from shellfish are inefficient and unsatisfactory. Extraction of viruses from other types of food, where there is just surface contamination, does not present such a challenge, but the number of virus particles present in food, as compared to specimens from patients, is very low and available detection tests may not always be sufficiently sensitive.

Recombinant capsid proteins provide a relatively safe, non-infectious source of viral antigens. These antigens could be used for assessing and improving food-processing methods including depuration conditions for shellfish. They could also be used, for instance, in assessing the efficacy of washing salads, vegetables and fruit for the ready-to-eat market.

Vaccine for hepatitis A is already available and consideration is being given to licensing of rotavirus vaccines. No vaccines have been developed for SRSVs. Recombinant capsid antigens of SRSVs expressed by baculovirus or yeast cells can be purified in large quantities. They are highly immunogenic and stable at low pH, which offers the potential for development of vaccines. Studies to express SRSV capsid antigens in transgenic plants, such as tobacco leaves and potato tubers, are underway[15]. It has been shown that these antigens are immunogenic in mice, thus offering further potential for the development of oral vaccines.

References

1 Advisory Committee on the Microbiological Safety of Food. *Report on Food-borne Viral Infections*. London: The Stationery Office, 1998

2 Appleton H. Norwalk virus and the small round viruses causing food-borne gastroenteritis. In: Hui YH, Gorham JR, Murrell KD, Cliver DO. (Eds) *Food-borne Diseases Handbook, vol 2: Diseases caused by Viruses, Parasites and Fungi* (2nd edn in press). New York: Marcel Dekker, 1994; 57–79

3 Wheeler JG, Sethi D, Cowden JM *et al*. Study of infectious intestinal disease in England: rates in the community, presenting to general practice, and reported to national surveillance. *BMJ* 1999; **318**: 1046–50

4 Norcott JP, Green J, Lewis D, Estes MK, Barlow KL, Brown DWG. Genomic diversity of small round structured viruses in the United Kingdom. *J Med Virol* 1994; **44**: 280–6

5 Jiang X, Matson DO, Cubitt WD, Estes MK. Genetic and antigenic diversity of human caliciviruses (HuCVs) using RT-PCR and new EIAs. *Arch Virol Suppl* 1996; **12**: 251–62

6 Sattar SA, Springthorpe VS, Ansari SA, Rotavirus. In: Hui YH, Gorham JR, Murrell KD, Cliver DO. (Eds) *Food-borne Diseases Handbook, vol 2: Diseases caused by Viruses, Parasites and Fungi* (2nd edn in press). New York: Marcel Dekker, 1994; 81–111

7 Cromeans T, Nainan OV, Fields H, Favorov MO, Margolis HS. Hepatitis A and E viruses. In: Hui YH, Gorham JR, Murrell KD, Cliver DO. (Eds) *Food-borne Diseases Handbook, vol 2: Diseases caused by Viruses, Parasites and Fungi* (2nd edn in press). New York: Marcel Dekker, 1994; 1–56

8 Gresikova M. Tickborne encephalitis. In: Hui YH, Gorham JR, Murrell KD, Cliver DO. (Eds) *Food-borne Diseases Handbook, vol 2: Diseases caused by Viruses, Parasites and Fungi* (2nd edn in press). New York: Marcel Dekker, 1994; 113–35

9 Green J, Wright PA, Gallimore CI, Mitchell O, Morgan Capner P, Brown DWG. The role of environmental contamination with small round structured viruses in a hospital outbreak investigated by reverse-transcriptase polymerase chain reaction assay. *J Hosp Infect* 1998; **39**: 39–45

10 Council of the European Communities (1991). Council Directive of 15 July 1991 laying down the health conditions for the production and placing on the market of live bivalve molluscs (91/492/EEC). *Off J Eur Communities* 1991; **L268**: 1–14

11 Millard J, Appleton H, Parry J. Studies on heat inactivation of hepatitis A virus with special reference to shellfish. *Epidemiol Infect* 1987; **98**: 397–414

12 Slomka MJ, Appleton H. Feline calicivirus as a model system for heat inactivation studies of small round structured viruses in shellfish. *Epidemiol Infect* 1998; **121**: 401–7

13 Green J, Hensilwood K, Gallimore CI, Brown DWG, Lees DN. A nested reverse transcriptase PCR assay for detection of small round structured viruses in environmentally contaminated molluscan shellfish. *Appl Environ Microbiol* 1998; **64**: 858–63

14 Viral Gastroenteritis Sub-Committee of the PHLS Virology Committee. Outbreaks of gastroenteritis associated with SRSVs. *PHLS Microbiol Digest* 1993; **10**: 2–8

15 Ball JM, Estes MK, Hardy ME, Conner ME, Okpekun AR, Graham DY. Recombinant Norwalk virus-like particles as an oral vaccine. *Arch Virol Suppl* 1996; **12**: 243–9

Toxigenic fungi and mycotoxins

J I Pitt

Food Science Australia, North Ryde, New South Wales, Australia

Growth of commonly occurring filamentous fungi in foods may result in production of toxins known as mycotoxins, which can cause a variety of ill effects in humans, from allergic responses to immunosuppression and cancer. The most important mycotoxins are aflatoxins, ochratoxin A, fumonisins, trichothecenes and zearalenone. Aflatoxins are potent carcinogens and, in association with hepatitis B virus, are responsible for many thousands of human deaths per annum, mostly in non-industrialised tropical countries. Ochratoxin A is a probable carcinogen, and may cause urinary tract cancer and kidney damage in people from northern and eastern Europe. Fumonisins appear to be the cause of oesophageal cancer in southern Africa, parts of China and elsewhere. Trichothecenes are highly immunosuppressive and zearalenone causes oestrogenic effects in animals and man. Currently available records and statistics do not reflect the major role played by mycotoxins in mortality attributable to food-borne micro-organisms.

Only in the last 30 years has it become clear that commonly occurring fungi growing in foods and feeds may produce toxins, known as mycotoxins. These toxins have caused major epidemics in man and animals during historical times. The most important epidemics have been: ergotism, which killed hundreds of thousands of people in Europe in the last millennium[1]; alimentary toxic aleukia (ATA), which was responsible for the death of at least 100,000 Russian people between 1942 and 1948[2]; stachybotryotoxicosis, which killed tens of thousands of horses in the USSR in the 1930s[3]; and aflatoxicosis, which killed 100,000 young turkeys in the UK in 1960 and has caused death and disease in other animals, and probably in man as well[4].

Mycotoxins are secondary metabolites, *i.e.* they appear to have no role in the normal metabolism involving growth of the fungus. Many are bizarre molecules, with structures ranging from single heterocyclic rings with molecular weights of scarcely 50 Da, to groups of irregularly arranged 6 or 8 membered rings with total molecular weights greater than 500 Da. Such small molecules induce no response in the human immune system. A major potential danger of mycotoxins in the human diet, therefore, resides in our inability to detect them biologically.

Correspondence to:
Dr J I Pitt, Food Science
Australia, PO Box 52,
North Ryde,
NSW 2113, Australia

© The British Council 2000

Mycotoxins have four basic kinds of toxicity: acute, chronic, mutagenic and teratogenic. The most commonly described effect of acute mycotoxin poisoning is deterioration of liver or kidney function, which in extreme cases may lead to death. However, some mycotoxins act primarily by interfering with protein synthesis, and produce effects ranging from skin sensitivity or necrosis to extreme immunodeficiency. Others are neurotoxins, which in low doses may cause sustained trembling in animals, but at only slightly higher doses cause brain damage or death.

Long-term effects of low levels of mycotoxin ingestion are also varied. The prime chronic effect of many mycotoxins is the induction of cancer, especially of the liver. Some toxins affect DNA replication, and hence can produce mutagenic or teratogenic effects[1,4,5].

The symptoms of mycotoxicoses are almost as diverse as the chemical structures of the compounds themselves. Some compounds may elicit few symptoms until death results, while others may produce severe effects including skin necrosis, leucopoenia and immunosuppression. Doses producing chronic disease are usually far below those responsible for acute effects, and so long-term effects such as cancer or tumour induction are undetected at the time of ingestion and, indeed, may remain so until disease is quite advanced.

Many of the toxigenic fungi are ubiquitous and, in some cases, apparently have a strong ecological link with human food supplies. The natural fungal flora existing in conjunction with food production is dominated by three genera: *Aspergillus*, *Fusarium* and *Penicillium*. *Fusarium* species are destructive pathogens on cereal crops and other commodities, and produce mycotoxins before, or immediately after, harvest. Certain species of *Aspergillus* and *Penicillium* are also plant pathogens or commensals, but these genera are more commonly associated with commodities and foods during drying and storage. The most significant toxigenic species and mycotoxins are described below.

Aflatoxins

Aflatoxins are both acutely and chronically toxic to animals, including man, causing acute liver damage, liver cirrhosis, induction of tumours and teratogenic effects[6]. The four major naturally produced aflatoxins are known as aflatoxins B_1, B_2, G_1 and G_2. 'B' and 'G' refer to the blue and green fluorescent colours produced by these compounds under UV light on thin layer chromatography plates, while the subscript numbers 1 and 2 indicate major and minor compounds, respectively. When aflatoxin B_1 and B_2 are ingested by lactating cows, a proportion (about 1.5%[7]) is hydroxylated and excreted in the milk as aflatoxins M_1 and

M_2, compounds of lower toxicity than the parent molecules, but significant because of the widespread consumption of cows' milk by infants. Because of their high toxicity, low limits for aflatoxins in foods and feeds have been set by many countries. Under recent agreements, 15 µg/kg of total aflatoxins is likely to become the maximum level permitted in all food commodities in world trade.

Acute toxicity of aflatoxins to humans has been observed only rarely[8]. In 1974, an outbreak of hepatitis that affected 400 Indian people, of whom 100 died, almost certainly resulted from aflatoxins[9]. The outbreak was traced to maize heavily contaminated with *A. flavus*, and containing up to 15 mg/kg of aflatoxins. Consumption of toxin by some of the affected adults was calculated to be 2–6 mg in a single day. It can be concluded that the acute lethal dose for adult humans is of the order of 10–20 mg.

Aflatoxin B_1 has been demonstrated in animal species to be the most potent liver carcinogen known. Human liver cancer has a high incidence in central Africa and parts of Southeast Asia, so a link with aflatoxins appears likely. Studies in several African countries and Thailand showed a correlation between the logarithm of aflatoxin intake and the occurrence of primary human liver cancer[10]. However, studies in areas of the US where dietary aflatoxin is appreciable indicated that aflatoxins are unlikely to contribute significantly to the incidence of liver cancer in the US[11].

The resolution of this conflict is now apparent: hepatitis B virus is also a liver carcinogen. Aflatoxins and hepatitis B are co-carcinogens, and the probability of people developing cancer of the liver is much higher in areas where both aflatoxins and hepatitis B are prevalent[12]. Considerable evidence exists that high aflatoxin intakes are causally related to high human liver cancer incidence[13,14]. Aflatoxin B_1 is considered to be a class 1 human carcinogen[15].

Levels of aflatoxins in some tropical foods[16] and blood samples[17] are sometimes unacceptably high. Based on the data of Pitt and Hocking ([16] and unpublished), it has been estimated that the number of deaths from liver cancer due to aflatoxin in Indonesia alone exceeds 20,000 per annum[18].

From the medical viewpoint, the recent discovery that aflatoxins appear to be immunosuppressive is also important. Other effects observed include an influence on protein energy metabolism, haemoglobin levels and effectiveness of vaccines[17]. Increased susceptibility to disease among people likely to have low resistance due to nutritional and environmental factors can only add to the toll.

Aflatoxins are produced in nature only by *Aspergillus flavus*, *A. parasiticus* and a recently described species, *A. nomius*. *A. flavus* is ubiquitous. Since the discovery of aflatoxins, it has become the most widely reported food-borne fungus, reflecting its economic and medical importance and ease of recognition, as well as its universal occurrence. *A. parasiticus* is apparently less widely distributed[19], but the extent of its occurrence may be obscured by the tendency for *A. flavus* and *A. parasiticus* to be reported only as *A. flavus*. *A. nomius* is not of practical importance.

A. flavus and *A. parasiticus* have a particular affinity for nuts and oilseeds. Peanuts, maize and cotton seed are the three most important crops affected. Early work assumed that invasion was primarily a function of inadequate drying or improper storage, and these factors are certainly important in the occurrence of aflatoxins in the humid tropics. However, in temperate zones, invasion of these crops by *A. flavus* before harvest is of prime importance. Invasion of peanuts occurs as a result of drought stress and related factors[20]. Preharvest invasion in maize is partly dependent on insect damage to cobs, but the fungus can also invade down the silks of the developing ears[21]. Most other nuts are also susceptible to invasion[22].

Cereals are a common substrate for growth of *A. flavus* but, unlike the case of nuts and oilseeds, small grain cereal spoilage by *A. flavus* is almost always the result of poor handling. Aflatoxin levels in small grains are rarely significant[6]. Spices sometimes contain *A. flavus*[22], and aflatoxin levels may be high.

In industrialised countries, stringent sorting and clean up procedures are used to reduce aflatoxins to low levels in foods with a perceived risk. For peanuts, where fungal growth is usually accompanied by discolouration of the kernel, this includes the use of sophisticated colour sorting equipment. Statistically based sampling, the drawing of large samples, homogenising before subsampling and standardised aflatoxin assays are used to ensure that susceptible crops and foods meet the stringent requirements of health laws in both exporting and importing countries. Non-industrialised countries are often less fortunate. Established patterns of local consumption, where substandard nuts and maize may be consumed without any form of sorting or inspection, mean that aflatoxin ingestion remains far too high in many countries, especially in rural areas.

Ochratoxin A

Ochratoxin A is an acute nephrotoxin, with oral LD_{50} values of 20 mg/kg in young rats and 3.6 mg/kg in day-old chicks. It is also lethal to mice, trout, dogs and pigs[23]. Necroses of the renal tubules and periportal liver cells have been the main pathological changes observed after fatal doses. Ochratoxin A has immunosuppressive, embryonic, and probably carcinogenic effects. Ochratoxin A plays a major role in the aetiology of nephritis (kidney disease) in pigs in Scandinavia[24], and indeed in much of northern Europe. This a serious animal health problem.

Because ochratoxin A is fat soluble and not readily excreted, it accumulates in the depot fat of affected animals, and from there is ingested by humans eating pork. A second source is bread made from barley or wheat containing the toxin. Ochratoxin A has been found in human blood over wide areas of Europe, with levels up to 35 µg/kg reported[25], and in human milk at similar concentrations[26]. Although clear evidence of human disease is still elusive, such levels indicate a widespread problem with ochratoxin A in Europe.

Ochratoxin A was originally described as a metabolite of *A. ochraceus*[27], a species with natural habitats in drying or decaying vegetation, seeds, nuts and fruits. *A. ochraceus* and closely related species are widely distributed in dried foods of various kinds[22]. Nuts are also a major source. Although *A. ochraceus* has been isolated from a wide range of cereals, records are rather infrequent[22]. It may be an important source of ochratoxin A in green coffee beans, however.

Ochratoxin A was also reported to be produced by *Penicillium viridicatum*[28], and this view prevailed for more than a decade. Eventually it became clear that isolates regarded as *P. viridicatum* but producing ochratoxin were correctly classified in a separate species, *P. verrucosum*[29]. *P. verrucosum* has been reported almost exclusively in grain from temperate zones. It is associated with northern European barley and wheat, and has also been isolated quite frequently from meat products in Germany and other European countries. It does not appear to be common elsewhere[29].

Occasionally, isolates of the common species *Aspergillus niger* can produce ochratoxin A[30]. However, the closely related *A. carbonarius* is a more common producer[31,32], and a much more important source of ochratoxin A. These species are widespread in tropical foods[33,34], and survive sun drying. *A. carbonarius* is an important source of ochratoxin A in dried vine fruits, wines and probably coffee. The impact on human health of ochratoxin A from this species has not yet been assessed.

Fumonisins

Fumonisins were discovered in the late 1980s[35,36] as the result of many years of study of the disease known as equine leucoencephalomalacia (LEM). Fumonisins consist of a 20 carbon aliphatic chain with two ester linked hydrophilic side chains, resembling sphingosine, an essential phospholipid in cell membranes. The toxic action of fumonisins appears to result from competition with sphingosine in sphingolipid metabolism[37.]

Symptoms of fumonisin toxicity vary widely with animal type, dosage and toxigenic fungal isolate. The best defined disease, LEM, is characterised by liquefactive necrotic lesions in the white matter of the cerebral hemispheres of horses and other equine species. Marked neurotoxicity is evident, with aimless walking and loss of muscle control followed by death, which usually occurs about 2 weeks after toxin ingestion.

The effect of fumonisins on humans has not been fully established, but much evidence suggests a role in human oesophageal cancer. Maize is the major staple food in areas of the Transkei in southern Africa where oesophageal cancer is endemic, and the most striking difference between areas of low and high incidence was the much greater infection of maize by *F. moniliforme* in the high incidence areas[38]. A similar situation occurs in parts of China with an exceptional incidence of oesophageal cancer[39]. The International Agency for Research on Cancer[15] found that fumonisin B_1 was a possible human carcinogen, but was neither mutagenic nor genotoxic. It alters the capacity of cells to proliferate[37,40].

The major producer of fumonisins are *Fusarium moniliforme* and closely related species, which are endemic in maize throughout the world. Maize is the only significant source of these compounds[22].

Trichothecene toxins: deoxynivalenol and nivalenol

Deoxynivalenol (DON; also known as vomitoxin) and nivalenol are among the many trichothecene mycotoxins produced by *Fusarium* species[41]. DON causes vomiting and feed refusal in pigs at levels near 8 mg/kg of feed[42]. It was responsible for a large-scale human toxicosis in India in 1988, and human toxicoses have also been reported from China, Japan and Korea[43]. Symptoms in humans include anorexia, nausea, vomiting, headache, abdominal pain, diarrhoea, chills, giddiness and convulsions[44].

Along with other trichothecenes, deoxynivalenol and nivalenol cause a variety of immunological effects in laboratory animals, leading to increased susceptibility to all kinds of microbial diseases[45]. These toxins do not appear to be carcinogenic, but may act synergistically with aflatoxins[15].

The major source of these toxins is *F. graminearum*, a species endemic in wheat and other cereals throughout the world[22].

Zearalenone

Zearalenone is an oestrogenic toxin, also produced by *F. graminearum* and closely related species. The effect of zearalenone in animals is a well-defined syndrome. Maize, barley and wheat grains infected with *F. graminearum* and containing zearalenone cause genital problems in domestic animals, especially pigs. Symptoms include hyperaemia and oedematous swelling of the vulva in prepubertal gilts, or, in more severe cases, prolapse of the vagina and rectum. Reproductive disorders in sows include infertility, fetal resorption or mummification, abortions, reduced litter size and small piglets. Male pigs are also affected: atrophy of testes, decreased libido and hypertrophy of the mammary glands are all well documented[46]. Zearalenone has been implicated in several incidents of precocious pubertal changes in children[47].

Conclusions

Mycotoxins are much more wide-spread and of much more concern in human food supplies than was believed a decade ago. The documentation of excessive levels of aflatoxin in foods and blood samples from people in non-industrialised countries, along with the synergistic effects of hepatitis B, mean that these toxins are a significant cause of death in parts of Africa and Southeast Asia at least. The detection of ochratoxin A in a wider range of foods than was previously supposed, and in the blood of many people, has raised awareness that this toxin is widespread. The realisation that many mycotoxins, including aflatoxins, fumonisins and trichothecenes, are immunosuppressive has wide implications for the ability of human populations to resist disease. It is very likely that mycotoxins play a significant role in the perceived poorer health of many tropical people. Food-borne bacteria rightly are a major cause for concern to human health, but it is difficult to escape the conclusion that mycotoxins in foods are responsible for much higher numbers of human deaths than are food-borne bacteria.

References

1   Smith JE, Moss MO. *Mycotoxins: Formation, Analysis and Significance*. Chichester, UK: Wiley, 1985
2   Joffe AZ. *Fusarium poae* and *F. sporotrichioides* as principal causal agents of alimentary toxic aleukia. In: Wyllie TD, Morehouse LG. (Eds) *Mycotoxic Fungi, Mycotoxins, Mycotoxicoses: an Encyclopedic Handbook,* vol. 3. New York: Marcel Dekker, 1978; 21–86
3   Moreau C. Moulds, Toxins and Food. Chichester, UK: Wiley, 1979
4   Rodricks JV, Hesseltine CW, Mehlman MA. (Eds) *Mycotoxins in Human and Animal Health*. Park Forest South, IL: Pathotox, 1977
5   Ueno Y. (Ed) *Trichothecenes – Chemical, Biological and Toxicological Aspects*. Amsterdam: Elsevier, 1983
6   Stoloff L. Aflatoxins – an overview. In: Rodricks JV, Hesseltine CW, Mehlman MA. (Eds) *Mycotoxins in Human and Animal Health*. Park Forest South, IL: Pathotox, 1977; 7–28

7   Frobish RA, Bradley BD, Wagner DD, Long-Bradley PE, Hairston H. Aflatoxin residues in milk of dairy cows after ingestion of naturally contaminated grain. *J Food Protect* 1986; **49**: 781–5

8   Shank pop pop pop pop. Mycotoxicoses of man: dietary and epidemiological considerations. In: Wyllie TI Morehouse LG. (Eds) *Mycotoxic Fungi, Mycotoxins, Mycotoxicoses, an Encyclopedic Handbook*. Vol. 1. *Mycotoxigenic Fungi*. New York: Marcel Dekker, 1977; 1–12

9   Krishnamachari KAVR, Bhat RV, Nagarajan V, Tilak TBG. Investigations into an outbreak of hepatitis in parts of Western India. *Indian J Med Res* 1975; **63**: 1036–48

10   Van Rensburg SJ. Role of epidemiology in the elucidation of mycotoxin health risks. In: Rodricks JV, Hesseltine CW, Mehlman MA. (Eds) *Mycotoxins in Human and Animal Health*. Park Forest South, IL: Pathotox, 1977; 699–711

11   Stoloff L. Aflatoxin as a cause of primary liver-cell cancer in the United States: a probability study. *Nutr Cancer* 1983; **5**: 165–86

12   Campbell TC. Mycotoxins. In: Wynder EE. (Ed) Environmental Aspects of Cancer: the Role of Macro and Micro Components of Foods. Westport, CT: Food and Nutrition Press, 1983; 187–97

13   Peers F, Bosch X, Kaldor J, Linsell A, Pluumen M. Aflatoxin exposure, hepatitis B virus infection and liver cancer in Swaziland. *Int J Cancer* 1987; **39**: 545–53

14   Groopman JD, Cain LG, Kensler TW. Aflatoxin exposure in human populations: measurements and relation to cancer. *CRC Crit Rev Toxicol* 1988; **19**: 113–45

15   International Agency for Research on Cancer. *Some naturally occurring substances: food items and constituents, heterocyclic aromatic amines and mycotoxins*. Monograph 56. Lyon, France: International Agency for Research on Cancer, 1993

16   Pitt JI, Hocking AD. Current knowledge of fungi and mycotoxins associated with food commodities in Southeast Asia. In: Highley E, Johnson GI. (Eds) Mycotoxin Contamination in Grains. Canberra: Australian Centre for International Agricultural Research. *ACIAR Technical Reports*, 1996; **37**: 5–10

17   Miller JD. Food-borne natural carcinogens: issues and priorities. *Afr Newslet Occup Health Safety* 1996; **6 (Suppl. 1)**: S22–8

18   Lubulwa ASG, Davis JS. Estimating the social cost of the impacts of fungi and aflatoxins in maize and peanuts. In: Highley E, Wright EJ, Banks HJ, Champ BR. (Eds) Stored Product Protection. Wallingford, UK: CAB International, 1994; 1017–42

19   Klich MA, Pitt JI. Differentiation of *Aspergillus flavus* from *A. parasiticus* and other closely related species. *Trans Br Mycol Soc* 1988; **91**: 99–108

20   Cole RJ, Hill RA, Blankenship PD, Sanders TH, Garren H. Influence of irrigation and drought stress on invasion of *Aspergillus flavus* in corn kernels and peanut pods. *Dev Ind Microbiol* 1982; **23**: 299–326

21   Lillehøj EB, Kwolek WF, Horner ES et al. Aflatoxin contamination of preharvest corn: role of *Aspergillus flavus* inoculum and insect damage. *Cereal Chem* 1980; **57**: 255–7

22   Pitt JI, Hocking AD. Fungi and Food Spoilage, 2nd edn. London: Blackie , 1997

23   Scott PM. *Penicillium* mycotoxins. In: Wyllie TD, Morehouse LG. (Eds) Mycotoxic Fungi, Mycotoxins, Mycotoxicoses, an Encyclopedic Handbook. Vol. 1. Mycotoxigenic Fungi. New York: Marcel Dekker, 1977; 283–356

24   Krøgh P, Hald B, Englund P, Rutqvist L, Swahn O. Contamination of Swedish cereals with ochratoxin A. *Acta Pathol Microbiol Scand, Sect B*. 1974; **82**: 301–2

25   Castegnaro M, Plestina R, Dirheimer G, Chernozemsky IN, Bartsch H. (Eds) *Mycotoxins, Endemic Nephropathy and Urinary Tract Tumours*. IARC Scientific Publications No. 115. Lyon, France: World Health Organization/International Agency for Research on Cancer, 1991

26   Bretholtz-Emanuelsson A, Olsen M, Oskarsson A, Palminger I, Hult K. Ochratoxin A in cow's milk and human milk with corresponding human blood samples. *J AOAC Int* 1993; **76**: 842–6

27   Van der Merwe KJ, Steyn PS, Fourie L, Scott DB, Theron JJ. Ochratoxin A, a toxic metabolite produced by *Aspergillus ochraceus* Wilh. *Nature* 1965; **205**: 1112–3

28   Van Walbeek W, Scott PM, Harwig J, Lawrence JW. *Penicillium viridicatum*. Westling: a new source of ochratoxin A. *Can J Microbiol* 1969; **15**: 1281–5

29   Pitt JI. *Penicillium viridicatum, Penicillium verrucosum* and production of ochratoxin A. *Appl Environ Microbiol* 1987; **53**: 266–9

30   Abarca ML, Bragulat MR, Castella G, Cabanes FJ. Ochratoxin A production by strains of *Aspergillus niger* var. *niger*. *Appl Environ Microbiol* 1994; **60**: 2650–2

31 Varga J, Kevei E, Rinyu E, Téren J, Kozakiewicz Z. Ochratoxin production by *Aspergillus* species. *Appl Environ Microbiol* 1996; **62**: 4461–4

32 Heenan CN, Shaw KJ, Pitt JI. Ochratoxin A production by *Aspergillus carbonarius* and A. niger isolates and detection using coconut cream agar. *J Food Mycol* 1998; **1**: 67–72

33 Pitt JI, Hocking AD, Bhudhasamai K, Miscamble BF, Wheeler KA, Tanboon-Ek P. The normal mycoflora of commodities from Thailand. 1. Nuts and oilseeds. *Int J Food Microbiol* 1993; **20**: 211–26

34 Pitt JI, Hocking AD, Miscamble BF et al. The mycoflora of food commodities from Indonesia. *J Food Mycol* 1998; **1**: 41–60

35 Bezuidenhout SC, Gelderblom WCA, Gorst-Allman CP et al. Structure elucidation of fumonisins, mycotoxins from *Fusarium moniliforme*. *J Chem Soc Chem Commun* 1988; 743–5

36 Marasas WFO, Kellerman TS, Gelderblom WCA, Coetzer JAW, Thiel PG, van der Lugt JJ. Leukoencephalomalacia in a horse induced by fumonisin B_1 isolated from *Fusarium moniliforme*. *Onderspoort J Vet Res* 1988; **55**: 197–203

37 Riley RT, Wang E, Schroeder JJ et al. Evidence for disruption of sphingolipid metabolism as a contributing factor in the toxicity and carcinogenicity of fumonisins. *Nat Toxins* 1996; **4**: 3–15

38 Marasas WFO, Wehner FC, van Rensburg SJ, van Schalkwyk DJ. Mycoflora of corn produced in human esophageal cancer areas in Transkei, southern Africa. *Phytopathology* 1981; **71**: 792–6

39 Chu FS, Li GY. Simultaneous occurrence of fumonisin B_1 and other mycotoxins in moldy corn collected from the People's Republic of China in regions with high incidence of esophageal cancer. *Appl Environ Microbiol* 1994; **60**: 847–52

40 Gelderblom WCA, Snyman SD, Abel S et al. Hepatotoxicity and carcinogenicity of the fumonisins in rats: a review regarding mechanistic implications for establishing risk in humans. In: Jackson LS, DeVries JW, Bullerman LB. (Eds) *Fumonisins in Food*. New York: Plenum, 1996: 251–64

41 Miller JD, Trenholm HL. (Eds) Mycotoxins in Grain. St Paul, MN: Eagan, 1996

42 Williams KC, Blaney BJ, Magee MH. Responses of pigs fed wheat naturally infected with *Fusarium graminearum* and containing the mycotoxins 4-deoxynivalenol and zearalenone. *Aust J Agric Res* 1989; **40**: 1095–105

43 Beardall JM, Miller JD. Diseases in humans with mycotoxins as possible causes. In: Miller JD, Trenholm HL (Eds) *Mycotoxins in Grain*. St Paul, MN: Eagan, 1994; 487–540

44 Yoshizawa T. Red-mold diseases and natural occurrence in Japan. In: Ueno Y. (Ed) *Trichothecenes – Chemical, Biological and Toxicological Aspects*. Amsterdam: Elsevier, 1983; 195–209

45 Pestka J, Bondy GS. Immunotoxic effects of mycotoxins. In: Miller JD, Trenholm HL. (Eds) *Mycotoxins in Grain*. St Paul, MN: Eagan, 1994; 339–58

46 Marasas WFO, Nelson PE, Tousson TA. *Toxigenic Fusarium Species: Identity and Mycotoxicology*. University Park, PA: Pennsylvania State University Press, 1984

47 Kuiper-Goodman T, Scott PM, Watanabe H. Risk assessment of the mycotoxin zearalenone. *Regul Toxic Pharmacol* 1987; **7**: 253–306

Parasites

Christine A Northrop-Clewes* and Christopher Shaw†

*Northern Ireland Centre for Diet and Health and †Applied Biological and Chemical Sciences, University of Ulster, Coleraine, County Londonderry, UK

Ill health related to food-borne infection transcends all geographical, political and cultural boundaries. The incidence of food-borne diseases continues to adversely affect the health and productivity of populations in most countries, especially non-industrialised ones. However, since the 1950s, the emphasis in the industrialised world had shifted away from addressing public health problems, to problems of chemical contaminants *etc.*, but recently food-borne infections have again become of increasing concern to governments and the food industry. Improvements in international transportation means food can be distributed throughout the world, but so can the parasitic pathogens which contaminate foods. Alternatively, tourists are being affected abroad and possibly transmitting the pathogen to others at home. Thus, an increasing number of food-related illnesses are international in scope. In this review parasitic contamination of foods of animal origin, particularly meat and fish, will be discussed together with potential problems associated with water and unwashed fruits and vegetables.

A predominant misconception is that parasites are a problem found only in tropical and third world countries, but nothing could be further from the truth. However, people who live in affluent modern society fail to appreciate the biological importance of parasites because they are so rarely encountered in everyday life. The World Health Organization (WHO) categorises parasites among the six most harmful infective diseases of man and parasitic infections outrank cancer as the number one killer in the world. Parasites can be contracted by eating contaminated under-cooked beef, pork, fish or other flesh foods, walking barefoot on infected soil, by being bitten by flies or mosquitoes, eating unclean raw fruits and vegetables or drinking infected water. There is an increased danger of contracting parasites when travelling to tropical and/or non-industrialised countries and the rise in immigration of people from areas of infection also contributes to the risk.

Correspondence to:
Dr Christine A Northrop-Clewes, Northern Ireland Centre for Diet and Health, University of Ulster, Coleraine BT52 1SA, UK

Definition of a parasite

The definition of a parasite (literally *para* – beside, *sitos* – food) is any organism that derives benefit from living in or on another organism (the

© The British Council 2000

host) at a cost to the host. The cost may be anything from using small amounts of the host's food to causing a fatal illness. The highest costs are paid in the tropics and sub-tropics where parasites present a continual and unacceptable threat to the well-being of millions of people. The cost of harbouring parasites in terms of human misery and economic loss is incalculable. Parasites are also a major cause of mortality and reduced reproductive success among domesticated animals and crops and one of the main concerns in agriculture is the control of parasites that can wipe out crops and livestock.

Helminths

The vast majority of metazoan parasites of vertebrates are representatives of two phyla, the acoelomate Platyhelminthes and the pseudocoelomate Nematoda. The most commonly used term to describe these parasites, 'helminths' includes all the cestodes and digeneans of the former group and all members of the latter. Of the four classes of entirely parasitic platyhelminthes, only the cestodes and digeneans cause important diseases in man and his livestock. The monogeneans of fish can cause serious losses in stocks kept under high-density fish farming conditions. Helminths are common and ubiquitous parasites of man and the causative agents of a list of terrible debilitating, deforming and fatal diseases of humans and their domesticated animals. Table 1 provides an outline classification of the helminth groups and the important genera that infect man. There are about 20 species of helminths which are natural parasites of man, but many others cause zoonoses, *i.e.* infections of animals that also infect man[1].

Table 1 Brief outline classification of helminths parasitic in vertebrates

Phylum: Platyhelminthes (flatworms)

Class 1	Monogenea	
Class 2	Cestoda (tapeworms) (*Diphyllbothrium, Taenia, Echinococcus*)	
Class 3	Aspidogastrea	
Class 4	Digenea (flukes or trematodes) (*Fasciolopsis, Fasciola, Paragonimus*)	

Phylum Nematoda (roundworms)

Order 1	Rhabditida (*Strongloides*)
Order 2	Strongylida (*Necator, Ancylostoma, etc.*)
Order 3	Ascaridida (*Ascaris, Toxocara, etc.*)
Order 4	Oxyurida (*Enterobius*)
Order 5	Spirurida (*Dracunculus, Wuchereria, Brugia, Loa, Onchocerca*)
Order 6	Enoplida (*Trichinella, Trichuris*)

Examples of important genera that infect man are listed in brackets. Adapted from Whitfield[1].

Prevalence of helminths

It is estimated that 3.5 billion (3.5 x 10^9) people are infected with intestinal parasites of which 450 million are ill and the numbers of people infected is increasing in all WHO regions[2]. It is projected that by the year 2025, about 57% of the population in developing countries will be urbanised and, as a consequence, a large number of people will be living in shanty towns where parasites like *Ascaris lumbricoides* and *Trichuris trichuria* will find favourable conditions for transmission[2]. Helminths have been classified as a public health problem in Central and South America, Africa, Asia and the Middle Eastern Crescent and are reported as being transmitted in the US, Spain, Portugal, Greece, Italy, Australia, Turkey and Eastern Europe[3]. However, very little information has been published on current levels of infection in the former Soviet Union and Eastern Europe[4].

Unlike viruses, bacteria and protozoa (microparasites), which are small and possess the ability to multiply directly and rapidly within the host, helminths (macroparasites) are much larger and do not multiply within the human body, one notable exception being *Strongyloides stercoralis* in immunocompromised people. Because of the necessity to have an intermediate host, helminth diseases do not have a sudden acute crisis but tend to be chronic conditions, where the pathology of the disease is positively correlated with the burden of parasites harboured by the host[5].

THE GUERRILLA WORM

Helminths are unique among infectious agents – they do not, as a rule, multiply in the human body. Instead, they appear to follow the prospects of guerrilla warfare as outlined by Chairman Mao, repeatedly infiltrating host defences as individuals or as small groups and gradually building up into larger forces; warfare is usually by attrition and is often prolonged[6].

The individual parasite provides the basic unit of study and it is, therefore, desirable to measure the number of parasites within the host by direct (*e.g.* worm expulsion by chemotherapeutic agents) or indirect (*e.g.* egg or cyst output in the faeces of the host) methods. For most of the common human helminth infections there is a marked over-dispersion or aggregation within their host population, *i.e.* where many hosts harbour a few parasites and a few hosts harbour large numbers of parasites. Prevalence data indicate the proportion of individuals infected but do not give any idea of the number of worms harboured. The marked non-linearity of the relationship between prevalence and intensity is a statistical consequence of the over-dispersed pattern of intensity. For most helminth species, the initial rise in intensity with age mirrors that of prevalence but occurs at a slightly slower rate. For example, the maximum prevalence of *Ascaris lumbricoides* is usually reached before the age of 5 years, but the maximum worm burden is usually found in children aged 5–10 years.

Food safety

Food safety, regardless of the specific food product, should be of paramount concern to everyone. All countries need to ensure that national food supplies are safe, of good quality and available in adequate amounts at affordable prices to safeguard good nutrition and health for all population groups. Parasitic diseases represent one potential health risk from foods.

Tropical infectious diseases not only constitute the leading threat to health for the growing world population who live in tropical areas but also pose a threat to all areas of the world. Rapidly increasing globalisation of travel and trade means that tropical diseases that were once distant and unimportant are now on the doorstep of the industrialised countries. Tourism has now replaced agriculture as the biggest industry in the world with 50 million people travelling from Europe, US, Canada, Japan, Australia, and New Zealand to Asia, Africa, Latin America, the South Pacific islands and parts of Eastern Europe where food, water and vector-borne infections pose significant health risks. In addition, the food industry now sources fruit and vegetables increasingly in non-industrialised countries and many of these products are eaten with minimal processing/cooking in the home. To improve the health of the disadvantaged and protect the people of the industrialised countries, the best of modern medicine, research and public health must be applied to the understanding and control of tropical diseases that remain the leading causes of disability and mortality around the world[7].

Meat

The public health and economic impact of meat-borne parasitic zoonoses is considerable in terms of morbidity and even mortality in man. In addition, reduced productivity in animals and condemnation of parasitised meat is still a significant problem and in some countries the infection rates of cattle with *Cysticercus bovis* (the cysticercus of *Taenia saginata*) have increased. A European committee was recently set up to develop new tools for the diagnosis and control of the infection. Current techniques are unsatisfactory, as there is only a 30% detection rate in animals carrying low numbers of cysticerci. New recombinant antigens are becoming more sensitive for detecting antibodies against cysticerci in cattle, but problems still persist in detecting low level infections[8]. Scientists in Scotland believe that immunodiagnostic techniques could be used on a herd basis to determine whether the herd is free of cysticerci or not[8].

What are the initial sources of infection? This question is problematic. The increase in foreign travel and becoming infected abroad are often blamed, but the maintenance of the life cycle depends on human sewage reaching pasture. Direct contamination from farm workers is one possibility, but proglottides can survive in sewage and eggs may pass into sewage sludge which is regularly spread as fertiliser. However, usually only a few cows in a herd become infected. Herring gulls feed widely and regularly around sewage farms eat the proglottides, which breakdown during digestion but the eggs survive and are deposited onto pasture in the gull's faeces in discontinuous and concentrated aggregations, which might explain scattered infections in herds[9].

Contamination of meat with tapeworms

The cosmopolitan distribution of *Taenia saginata*, the beef tapeworm, is due to the practice of eating beef which is raw or under-cooked and there are an estimated 45 million cases world-wide. In this way, infective cysticercus larvae (about 8 mm in length) found in the muscles of cows, are ingested. Once ingested, the larvae evert their hooked scoleces, attach and grow. The adult tapeworms are located in the ileum with their scolex (head end) embedded in the mucosa and the rest of the organism, up to 5 m in length, hanging free in the lumen. Posterior segments (proglottides) filled with eggs are passed out with the faeces. The eggs once ingested by cattle hatch to release hexacanth larvae in the duodenum. The larvae penetrate the gut wall and reach voluntary muscles via the blood stream and within 10–12 weeks transform into the infective cysticercus larvae in the muscle[1]. Once man ingests the under-cooked or raw beef muscle the whole life cycle begins again.

Taenia solium is the pork tapeworm and is less widely distributed than *T. saginata* with an estimated 3 million cases. *T. solium* is very similar in morphology and life-cycle characteristics to *T. saginata* and man is the only definitive host for both species. *T. solium* is found where pork and pork products are eaten raw or under-cooked.

Effective meat inspection should remove infected carcasses from the human food chain, but if the levels of infection are relatively low, the infection might be missed (see above). However, in many countries, none of these measures are in place and tapeworm infections are common. Even in Britain there has been an increase in *T. saginata* cases recently, although *T. solium* does not appear to be a problem. There is little risk if meat is thoroughly cooked or subject to prolonged deep freeze storage, at −10°C or below, which kills the cysticercus larvae of both tapeworms. In Europe, eating steak tartare or rare steak means tapeworm infection is an affliction of the affluent, as they are more likely to afford the raw material. In developing countries, it is the poor who cannot afford the cost of the fuel to cook their meat who are most at risk!

Contamination of meat with tissue nematodes

Trichinellosis, caused by *Trichinella spiralis*, is a cosmopolitan disease, which has a very low vertebrate host specificity. Short-lived adult infections in the small intestine of a wide range of carnivorous and omnivorous mammals give rise to a large number of invasive larvae (2000/female) which migrate via the blood stream to voluntary muscles throughout the bodies of the host animal. Once in the muscle they encyst. The cysts are the infective stages that can be transmitted to any new host when the flesh is eaten. Human infection is contracted by eating raw or under-cooked pork or pork products containing encysted larvae. Domestic pigs provide the main source of human infections in all areas except Africa where the wild boar, bears, bushpigs or warthogs transmit the disease and in the far north among the Eskimos where polar bears are most important. In the recent *International Commission on Trichinellosis Country Status Report (1995–97)*, 10,000 cases of trichinellosis were reported world-wide, of which 167 were in Western Europe and 7213 were in Eastern Europe. In addition, Switzerland and Norway revealed *Trichinella* infections in foxes (1.3% and 7.5%, respectively) but no infections in domestic pigs. Identification of *Trichinella* in wild animals is important as they may act as reservoir hosts[10].

The adult *T. spiralis* is a small worm living partially embedded in the mucosa of the ileum, where it gives rise to some gut damage. However, important pathology occurs when the larvae migrate to and encyst in the muscles, when in heavy infections a diverse range of symptoms from vomiting and diarrhoea to high fever and muscle pain appear.

LIVERPOOL
JOHN MOORES UNIVERSITY
AVRIL ROBARTS LRC
TITHEBARN STREET
LIVERPOOL L2 ___
TEL. 0151 231 4___

Water

Nematode contamination of water

Dracunculiasis, guinea worm disease, is confined to rural communities in East, Central and West Africa, India, Pakistan and the Arabian peninsula. Human infections occur when people drink water contaminated with copepods (crustaceans) containing infective larvae. Ingested larvae penetrate the intestinal wall and spend about 12 weeks in subcutaneous tissues. After mating, the female worm moves down the body reaching an ankle or foot about 8–10 months after the original infection. Here the female, containing up to 1 million eggs, induces a blister in the human host, which subsequently bursts enabling large numbers of actively swimming larvae to leave the lesion each time it is immersed in water[1].

Safe drinking water would eradicate the disease from the world and, in 1991, the 44th World Health Assembly declared the goal of eradicating dracunculiasis by the end of 1995. By 1996, there were less than 153,000 cases, 78% of which were notified in Sudan[10]. Transmission is easily interrupted by simple measures such as provision of safe water supplies and where it is not possible to provide safe water, control is by health education, by provision of filters (even an old T-shirt will do!) and by treatment of ponds with insecticides. Hopefully *Dracunculus medinensis* is an endangered species that will disappear without a whisper of protest!

Salad vegetables

Contamination of salad vegetables with roundworms

Ascaris lumbricoides, 'the large roundworm' of man, is one of the commonest and most wide-spread of human infections with an estimated 1300 million cases (24% prevalence) world-wide. It is found in all tropical, sub-tropical and temperate regions where standards of hygiene are low. The mortality rate from ascariosis is low, 2 per 100,000 people (total 60,000 deaths/year) but, due to the high prevalence rate, it is regarded as a serious public health problem[2]. Infection follows the ingestion of salad vegetables contaminated with embryonated eggs. Following ingestion, the hatched larvae penetrate the intestinal wall and are carried to the lungs where they may cause pneumonitis with numerous lesions and perhaps blood-stained sputum. The maturing larvae ascend the trachea and are swallowed to re-enter the ileum. Adult worms in the small intestine are long-lived (maximum survival 7 years) and in high density can cause obstruction. Worms can migrate out of the gut into the bile duct, pancreatic duct, oesophagus or mouth. However, in general, ascariosis probably causes little ill-health to the host except for the rare occasions when it does cause obstruction of the intestine or bile duct.

Trichuris trichuria is the causative agent of whipworm infection, an infection which is often found in the same areas as ascariosis. It is estimated that there are 902 million cases world-wide (17% prevalence). *Trichuris* spp. larvae do not migrate after hatching but moult and mature in the intestine. Adults are not as large as *A. lumbricoides.* Symptoms range from inapparent through vague digestive tract distress to emaciation and mucoid diarrhoea. Toxic and allergic symptoms may also appear.

The eggs of both *A. lumbricoides* and *T. trichuria* are found in insufficiently treated sewage-fertiliser and in soils where they may contaminate crops grown in soil or fertilised with sewage. Humans are infected when such produce is consumed raw. The eggs of these roundworms are 'sticky' and may be carried to the mouth by hands, inanimate objects or foods, transmission may also be caused by contamination of a wide variety of foods by infected food-handlers. Prevention of infection is by thorough washing of salad vegetables, improved hygiene practices of food-handlers and at the source of salad production by an improvement in standards of sanitation.

Eggs of *Ascaris* spp. have been detected on fresh vegetables in industrialised countries but no major outbreaks have occurred, although individual cases do occur.

Contamination of salad products with liver flukes

The sheep and cattle fluke, *Fasciola hepatica,* is endemic in many parts of the world and causes some human infections in South America, Cuba, North Africa and Western Europe including the UK and France. Most human infections come from the ingestion of watercress, lettuce or radishes in salads contaminated with metacercarial cysts. Following ingestion, the young worms penetrate the gut wall then eat their way to the bile ducts causing necrosis and inflammatory reactions *en route.* Early symptoms consist of abdominal pain, nausea, fever and hepatomegaly.

Human liver flukes are discussed later (fish and shellfish).

Fish and shellfish

A multitude of parasites has been reported in aquatic food products but only a few are capable of infecting humans. A total of 50 species of helminth parasites have been implicated as producing zoonotic infections resulting from eating raw or under-cooked aquatic foods such as fish, crabs, crayfish, snails and bivalves[12]. Fish or crustacean-borne trematodes infect about 39 million people and another 550 million are at risk[8]. Examples of common raw seafood dishes known to transmit parasitic zoonoses are Japanese sushi, sashimi, and salad (contains raw fish), Hawaiian lomi lomi salmon, tako poki (Cephalopod dish), palu (meat from a fish head and visceral organs allowed to ripen in a closed container), Dutch green herring, Scandinavian gravalax, Latin American ceviche (fillets marinated in lime juice), Philippine bagoong (uncooked fish viscera) and Pacific island poisson cru (fish fillets marinated in coconut juice)[12].

Contamination of fish with nematodes and liver flukes

The increasing exploitation of the marine environment by humans, changes in dietary habits incorporating 'natural' seafood dishes, tendencies to reduce cooking times when preparing seafood products all increase the chances of becoming infected with helminth parasites. Most helminth zoonoses are rare and cause little damage; however, some are more prevalent and pose serious potential health hazards. For example, in Japan in 1987, there were 4882 reported cases of anisakiasis (a severe gastric upset), caused by larvae in sushi or sashimi. The nematodes attach to or penetrate the intestinal lining but as humans are not a suitable host, the larvae will not live longer than 7–10 days in the human digestive tract[13]. A more serious problem is caused by the human liver flukes, *Clonorchis sinensi* and *Opisthorchis viverrini,* in South–East Asia. *O. viverrini* is the leading cause of food-borne parasitic disease in Thailand, Laos and Vietnam where it affects more than 8 million people. In Thailand, data from a liver fluke control operation in 1996 showed the country-wide prevalence of opisthorchiasis to be 21.5%. Opisthorchiasis is transmitted as a result of consuming raw or insufficiently cooked freshwater cyprinoid fish (carp). Economically, the estimated wage loss in Thailand may be as high as Baht 1620 million (~£27 million, if Baht 59 = £1) and the direct cost of medical care may be as high as Baht 495 million (~£8 million) per year[14].

Contamination of fish with tapeworms

Diphyllobothrium latum, the broad fish tapeworm, found in Northern Europe, is transmitted when raw, undercooked or lightly smoked fish (*e.g.* pike or salmon) containing viable plerocercoids are eaten. In many cases, human infections largely go unnoticed because of the non-specific symptoms such as intestinal discomfort, nausea and diarrhoea. However, in some *D. latum* infections, the parasite cleaves and selectively takes up vitamin B_{12} competing with the host for the vitamin, so that, in heavy infections, the parasite might take all available dietary vitamin B_{12} and in more susceptible people this can lead to megablastic anaemia[15].

In regions with poor sanitation where untreated sewage is released directly into rivers or lakes, infected fish with high prevalence and intensity rates are common. Effective control measures include cooking fish properly or freezing fish below −12°C for a minimum of 24 h. In addition, properly treated and managed sewage is also important.

Contamination of crustaceans with parasites

Over 20 million people are infected with the lung fluke, *Paragonimus*, the treatment of which is currently unsatisfactory. Eggs from the adults are passed out in human faeces and once in fresh water, the larvae burst out of the eggs and enter a suitable snail host. A free-living stage, the cercaria, emerges from the snail and penetrates a freshwater crustacean (crab or crayfish). When the crustaceans are eaten uncooked, the meta-cercarial larvae excyst and reach the lungs after passing through the intestinal wall and diaphragm. The developing worms in the lungs provoke inflammatory and granulomatous reactions, forming a cyst with an opening into a bronchiole. The majority of infections are asymptomatic; but, in heavier infections, there is a dry cough, chest pain, dyspnoea and haemoptysis. Control of the parasite can be achieved by cooking the crustaceans before consumption, alternatively, the sanitary disposal of human faeces will reduce transmission.

Seafood safety

World-wide, the majority of seafood zoonoses used to occur along coastal regions where seafood products were commonly consumed but continual improvements in transportation, technology and food handling allow fresh seafood to be shipped throughout the world and further inland. In 1993, the UK imported 684,000 tons of fish for direct human consumption and 1,381,000 tons for animal feed and other purposes[16]. Reports of imported seafood contaminated with viable parasites are known; therefore, marine foods on a global scale must be considered by government regulatory agencies to ensure a safe seafood supply.

Health authorities in the past focused on the safety of their own fisheries and seafood products and problems associated with marine products imported from other countries were of little concern. However, this approach to seafood safety was not prudent because parasites do not honour national borders. The strengthening of national food control infrastructures, in particular in non-industrialised countries, the need for harmonisation of food control at international levels, the need for collection and exchange of data on food control and contamination issues are essential elements to ensure food safety in the world.

Fish farming – food for the future?

Potential problems

Aquaculture is important to the world's fishery system. Both import and export markets for aquaculture products will expand and increase, as over-fishing of wild stock will necessitate supplementation and replenishment through aquaculture. However, future aquaculture development will require an integrated public health approach to ensure that it does not cause unacceptable risks to public or environmental health and negate its potential economic and nutritional benefits[17].

A common practice in many developing countries is the creation of numerous small fishponds. This approach greatly increases the overall aggregate shoreline causing higher densities of mosquito larvae and cercaria. Centralised planning for new freshwater and marine aquaculture sites should include discussions about optimal conditions on issues such as disease transmission (*e.g.* from fish-to-fish and fish-to-man), water supply, irrigation and power generation. Ignorance of the hazards associated with the use of untreated animal or human waste in aquaculture ponds to increase production also has tremendous health implications, for example, in China, where the two liver flukes, *Clonorchis sinensi* and *Opisthorchis viverrini,* are common, human faeces were commonly used to enrich ponds containing the host fish, but in recent years the faeces have been stored or treated before use. In addition, food growers have traditionally used cultured species in waste water fed ponds and grown secondary vegetable crops in waste water and sediment material in integrated aquaculture operations. The potential for transmission of human pathogens to the cultured species and secondary vegetable crops was rarely considered.

Disease control in aquaculture

Procedures to help protect humans from aquaculture-associated risks include better education and training of aquaculture staff and FAO and WHO recommend that the hazard analysis and critical control points (HACCP) concept be applied to fresh water aquaculture programmes to control food-borne digenetic trematode infections in humans. A study in Vietnam used 2 ponds, one in which fish were cultured according to HACCP principles and one used conventional local aquaculture practices. Water supply, fish fry, fish feed and pond conditions were identified as critical control points. Results showed 45% of control pond fish were infected with *Clonorchis sinensis* metacercaria while the fish monitored according to HACCP principles were free of trematode infection. Similarly, the application of the HACCP principles to freshwater aquaculture ponds in Thailand and Laos to control *Opisthorchis viverrini* infection were also successful[17].

The organic food revolution in industrialized countries – the hidden menace

In parallel with increasing public anxiety over the emergence of genetically-modified foods in industrialised countries has been a trend towards ever increasing public demand for organically-grown produce. In commercial response, most, if not all, of the major food retailers in the UK have now a stated policy of removal of genetically-modified foods from their shelves with an increase in capacity for organic produce. While such trends may appear to be eco-friendly on face value, there are potential hidden dangers for consumers. Over the past 20 years, the use of artificial fertilisers on farmland to facilitate an intensive agriculture focused on the rapid production of uniform products for mass consumption has led to a massive reduction in the use of organic manures on the land. During the same time period, intensive usage of anthelmintics in domestic livestock for the same purpose of maximising productivity has led to massive reductions in parasite burdens. Taking both factors into account, one can see the reason for the virtual elimination of parasitic disease as a major clinical problem in industrialised countries. However, changing practices for economic or social reasons can provide parasites with new opportunities for transmission which they will exploit with gusto. After all, this is what evolution has gifted parasites to do. While little evidence exists of the nutritive benefits of organic produce, the change from the relative sterility of inorganic farming to an organic culture system may turn back the pages of history to the time when parasitic disease in the population was the norm. After all, it is a fact that under natural conditions, all vertebrates (including man) are probably universally infected with at least one helminth parasite – is this really to where we wish to return? How many of us who live in the countryside or who drive through such *en route* to our places of employment have not been subjected to mighty olfactory attack as farmers spread 'muck' on their fields? Such spreadings usually have large flocks of attendant gulls, many of which defecate over a wide area including in our parks, playing fields and reservoirs. The factors are thus already in place for the resurgence of helminth parasitic disease – one can be sure that it remains a matter of when, rather than if, this will occur.

Anthelmintic resistance

The picture of impending doom which has been painted would be somewhat moderated if society had in its possession a broad and effective arsenal of chemotherapeutic agents (anthelmintics) for the treatment of parasitic infection. It is a sobering thought that virtually all anthelmintic discovery programmes in multinational pharmaceutical companies are directed towards finding drugs of efficacy, not in man, but rather in his domestic pets and livestock. The curious reason for this is market driven. Put simply, industrialised countries can afford to spend vast sums on anthelmintics for veterinary purposes with little need for human clinical application. Non-industrialised countries, while having a greater veterinary problem but more importantly, a crippling human clinical problem, cannot afford the costs of new pharmaceuticals which have to be priced to cover development costs as well as procure profits. The economic reasons for this state of affairs undoubtedly presents the parasites with yet another potential avenue of exploitation. In common with antibiotics, whose wide-spread usage has led to virtual universal resistance acquisition in bacteria, anthelmintics used with equal abandon in domestic livestock have initiated resistance in many highly pathogenic helminths. Levamisole-resistant strains of *Strongyloides* and *Haemonchus* are now widespread in Australian and New Zealand sheep and praziquantal and oxamniquine resistant schistosomes are now found in humans in Africa and Brazil, respectively. First generation anthelmintics, such as the benzimidazoles, are now all but useless due to selection of allelic variants of the β-tubulin gene which confer resistance. The picture painted, as with antibiotic resistant bacteria, is one of impending defeat by the enemy in the absence of effective defensive weaponry. For this reason, industrialised countries should reflect much more carefully on the potential effects of radical change in farming practice and food production in the light of current and developing knowledge of the biological threat from parasitic helminths. Recently, in response to the lack of concern in the West to the rapidly developing drug-resistant tuberculosis epidemic in the former Soviet Union, a WHO spokesperson put it like this: 'We all live in what could be described as one large forest. A fire is raging at one side and those of us at the other side are unconcerned as we cannot see it or smell it. But sooner or later it will become our problem if we do not take steps to douse the flames'. I think that this accurately reflects our attitudes to parasitic disease – but we in industrialised countries take it one stage further – we are building fire-lighter factories.

Food irradiation

The incidence of food-borne diseases continues to adversely affect the health and productivity of populations in most countries, especially non-industrialised ones. The report of the joint FAO/WHO Expert

Committee on Food Safety stated that: 'illness due to contaminated food is perhaps the most widespread health problem in the contemporary world and an important cause of reduced economic productivity'. Contamination of foods especially those of animal origin with micro-organisms, particularly pathogenic non-sporing bacteria, parasitic helminths and protozoa is among the most important health problem and the most important cause of human suffering world-wide. In addition, many dry ingredients particularly herbs and spices, the major proportion of which are produced in non-industrialised countries giving an important source of their foreign exchange, may be highly contaminated with spoilage organisms.

Considerable data and commercial experience exist which demonstrate that irradiation of foods could play an important role in solving food-borne diseases. At a meeting on the *Use of irradiation to ensure hygienic quality of food* in 1986, it was concluded that no technology was available to produce safe raw foods of animal origin; a situation which poses significant threats to public health. However, where such foods are important in the epidemiology of food-borne diseases, irradiation decontamination/disinfection must be seriously considered[17]. The most apparent health benefit from the use of food irradiation would be: (i) in the treatment of chilled or frozen poultry to destroy Salmonella; (ii) in the treatment of pork, to inactivate *Trichinella* larvae; and (iii) for the decontamination of spices and other dry food ingredients. Very low doses of 0.5–0.6 kGy (1 Gray [Gy] = the energy of 1 Joule absorbed by 1 kg of matter) are sufficient for inactivation of *Taenia saginata* and *Taenia solium* cysticerci in beef and pork, and in the US, irradiation has been approved for raw poultry and meat. However, as the regulations for irradiation of beef products are still being determined, the products are not available in the shops yet. High public awareness of problems caused by pathogens in raw meat means the prospect for the introduction of irradiated meat is favourable in the US. However, in Europe, public acceptance of this technique will be more difficult[18]. An example of successful commercial irradiation has been carried out in Belgium and The Netherlands, where frozen shrimp and frogs' legs for export are dosed with 2–7 kGy. The dose was considered adequate to destroy pathogenic micro-organisms and parasites without causing an adverse effect on the organoleptic properties of the food.

Street-vended food

Street-vended food has an important role in feeding urban populations, particularly the socially disadvantaged. Street food is varied, inexpensive and often nutritious, but has some risk due to inadequate sanitation and waste management. However, authorities charged with the responsibility for food safety have to match risk management action to the level of assessed risk, hence the rigorous codes of practice enforced on larger permanent food service establishments are unlikely to be justifiable for street food vendors. If such rigorous codes of practice were enforced, it would result in the disappearance of the street vendors and result in hunger and malnutrition in those who rely on them for a cheap supply of food. However, WHO encourages the development of regulations that empower vendors to take greater responsibility for the preparation of safe food and codes of practice based on the HACCP system[19].

Conclusions

Food-borne diseases are much more of a concern to governments and the food industry than a few years ago. Some factors which have led to this conclusion are: increasing world trade and travel, migrant populations demanding traditional foods in their country of settlement, the ease of world-wide shipment of fresh and frozen food and the development of new food industries including aquaculture. However, to monitor increases and decreases in food-borne diseases requires an effective surveillance system for which resources have not been available. Initiatives in the US and UK are underway to monitor food-borne diseases. These initiatives should stimulate other countries to conduct similar programmes so the real burden of food-borne disease can be determined. If food-borne disease is recognised as a major concern in industrialised countries, how much more of a problem is it in countries where the urban growth is faster than the public health infrastructure can support and in rural areas where drinking water is frequently contaminated? This issue is becoming increasingly important now that immigration from non-industrialised countries is becoming more frequent, international travel is commonplace and trade barriers between blocks of countries are coming down[20]. Food-borne diseases are for the most part preventable, but food use by Western populations is a dynamic phenomenon responding to fashions, social structure, cultural influences of foreign travel, *etc.*, not to mention the more traditional criteria of suppliers or manufacturers, to provide food with the greatest cost:benefit ratio to their organisation. The risk of parasites entering the food-chain is an ever present threat and public health authorities must be constantly vigilant to meet that threat. Advice to the tourist on reducing the risk of HIV is widely advertised. Vaccination or prophylaxis to prevent infection by the major tropical diseases is often

LIVERPOOL JOHN MOORES UNIVERSITY
LEARNING SERVICES

mandatory, but advice on food use and simple hygienic measures to reduce the risk of food poisoning or parasite infection is rarely seen. More attention by public health authorities to educating the public on how to prevent such organisms entering the food-chain is needed now.

References

1 Whitfield PJ. Parasitic helminths. In: Cox FEG. (Ed) *Modern Parasitology*, 2nd edn. Oxford; Blackwell, 1994; 24–52

2 World Health Organization, Division of Control of Tropical Disease. *Intestinal Parasites Control*, 1998. Available at http://www.who.int/ctd/html/intest.html

3 World Health Organization, Division of Control of Tropical Disease. *Intestinal Parasite Control*, 1995. Available at http://www.who.org/whr/1995/state.html

4 Chan MS. The global burden of intestinal nematode infections – fifty years on. *Parasitol Today* 1997; **13**: 438–43

5 Anderson RM. Epidemiology. In: Cox FEG. (Ed) *Modern Parasitology*, 2nd edn. Oxford; Blackwell, 1994; 75–116

6 Warren KS. The guerrilla worm. *N Engl J Med* 1970; **282**: 810–1

7 Guerrant RL, Blackwood BL. Threats to global health and survival: the growing crises of tropical infectious – our 'unfinished agenda'. *Clin Infect Dis* 1999; **28**: 966–86

8 Eckert J. Workshop summary: 'Food safety: meat-and fish-borne zoonoses'. *Vet Parasitol* 1996; **64**: 143–7

9 Matthews BE. *An Introduction to Parasitology*. Studies in Biology. Cambridge: Cambridge University Press, 1998

10 International Commission on Trichinellosis (ICT). *ICT Country Status Reports 1995–97*. Available at http://www.krenet.it/ict/statusrp.html

11 World Health Organization, Division of Tropical Diseases. *Dracunculiasis eradication,* 1998. Available at http://www.who.int/ctd/html/dracepidat.html

12 Deardorff TL. Epidemiology of marine fish-borne parasitic zoonoses. *SE Asian J Trop Med Public Health* 1991; **22** (**Suppl.**): 146–9

13 Kamiya M, Ooi HK. Current status of food-borne parasitic zoonoses in Japan. *SE Asian J Trop Med Public Health* 1991; **22** (**Suppl.**): 48–53

14 Loaharanu P, Sornmani S. Preliminary estimates of economic impact of liver fluke infection in Thailand and the feasibility of irradiation as a control measure. *SE Asian J Trop Med Public Health* 1991; **22** (**Suppl.**): 384–90

15 *Diphyllobothrium latum*. Available at http://martin.parasitology.mcgill.ca/jimspage/biol/d_latum.htm

16 Food and Agriculture Organization of the United Nations (FAO). *Fish Industry Data/United Kingdom*, February 1997. Available at http://www.fao.org/waicent/faoinfo/fishery/fcp/uke.htm

17 Garrett ES, Lima dos Santos C, Jahncke ML. Public, animal and environmental health implications of aquaculture. In: National Center for Infectious Diseases, Centers for Disease Control and Prevention *Emerging Infect Diseases*. Atlanta, GA: National Center for Infectious Diseases, Centers for Disease Control and Prevention, 1997; 3. Available at http://www.cdc.gov/ncidod/EID/vol3no4/garrett.htm

18 Sigurbjornsson B, Loaharanu P. Irradiation and food processing. In: Somogyi JC, Muller HR. (Eds) *Nutritional Impact of Food Processing*. Bibl Nutr Dieta. Basel: Karger, 1989; **43**: 13–30

19 Moy G, Hazzard A, Kaferstein F. Improving the safety of street-vended food. *World Health Stat Q* 1997; **50**: 124–31

20 Todd ECD. Epidemiology of food-borne diseases: a worldwide review. *Rapp Trimest Statist Sanit Mond* 1997; **50**: 30–50

Food-borne protozoa

Gordon L Nichols

Environmental Surveillance Unit, Communicable Disease Surveillance Centre, London, UK

Pathogenic protozoa are commonly transmitted to food in developing countries, but food-borne outbreaks of infection are relatively rare in developed countries. The main protozoa of concern in developed countries are *Toxoplasma*, *Cryptosporidium* and *Giardia*, and these can be a problem in immunocompromised people. Other protozoa such as *Entamoeba histolytica*, *Cyclospora cayetanensis* and *Sarcocystis* can be a food-borne problem in non-industrialised countries. *C. cayetanensis* has emerged as a food-borne pathogen in foods imported into North America from South America. *Microsporidia* may be food-borne, although evidence for this is not yet available. The measures needed to prevent food-borne protozoa causing disease require clear assessments of the risks of contamination and the effectiveness of processes to inactivate them. The globalisation of food production can allow new routes of transmission, and advances in diagnostic detection methods and surveillance systems have extended the range of protozoa that may be linked to food.

Correspondence to:
Dr Gordon L Nichols,
Environmental
Surveillance Unit,
Communicable Disease
Surveillance Centre, 61
Colindale Avenue,
London NW9 5EQ, UK

Protozoa are a diverse group of organisms that have evolved to occupy a variety of ecological niches. There are over 30 phyla of protozoa, but the enteric ones causing food-borne human disease belong to the phyla Apicomplexa, Rhizopoda, Zoomastigina, Microspora and Ciliophora (Table 1). Most of these have evolved a totally parasitic existence. The enteric protozoa that cause human illness are usually transmitted by the consumption of food and drink, or through environmental contamination and poor hygiene (Table 1). Some of these can cause substantial illness, and have economic consequences[1,2]. Many cause problems in immuno-compromised patients, particularly in HIV-infected people and individuals with T-cell deficiencies. The range of parasitic protozoa present in the human population and agricultural animals is greater in non-industrialised countries than in industrialised ones. There is a greater exposure to infection because food and water distribution systems are poor, and microbial contamination of food and water is common. Toilet facilities in non-industrialised countries are often primitive, and food sold in native markets may be contaminated from hands that have not been washed after defaecation or from flies that land on both food and faeces.

© The British Council 2000

Table 1 Food-borne and water-borne protozoa

Protozoa	Life cycle in a single host	Recognised human pathogen	Host range[a]	Food-borne infections/ outbreaks	Water-borne infections/ outbreaks	Present in animal meat[b]	Present in animal faeces	Present in human faeces
APICOMPLEXA								
Cryptosporidium parvum Type 1	✔	✔	H	✔	✔	✗	✗	✔
Cryptosporidium parvum Type 2	✔	✔	HAW	✔	✔	✗	✔	✔
Cryptosporidium parvum Type 3	✔	S	H	✔c	✔c	✗	?	✔
Cryptosporidium felis	✔	S	HA	✔c	✔c	✗	✔	✔
Cryptosporidium spp. (canine strain)	✔	S	HA	✔c	✔c	✗	✔	✔
Cyclospora cayetanensis	✔	✔	H	✔	✔	✗	✗	✔d
Isospora belli	✔	✔	HA	✗	✗	✗	✗	✔d
Sarcocystis hominis	✗	✔	HAW	✔	✗	✔	✔	✔
Sarcocystis suihominis	✗	✔	HAW	✔	✗	✔	✔	✔
Toxoplasma gondii	✗	✔	HAWB	✔	✔	✔	✔	✗
MASTIGOPHORA								
Chilomastix mesnili	✔	✗	H	✗	✗	✗	✗	✔
Dientamoeba fragilis	✔	✔	H	✗	✗	✗	✗	✔
Enteromonas hominis	✔	✗	H	✗	✗	✗	✗	✔
Giardia lamblia	✔	✔	HAW	✔	✔	✗	✔	✔
Retortomonas intestinalis	✔	✗	H	✗	✗	✗	✗	✔
Trichomonas hominis	✔	✗	H	✗	✗	✗	✗	✔
SARCODINA								
Endolimax nana	✔	✗	H	✗	✗	✗	✗	✔
Entamoeba coli	✔	✗	H	✗	✗	✗	✗	✔
Entamoeba dispar	✔	✗	H	✗	✗	✗	✗	✔
Entamoeba hartmanni	✔	✗	H	✗	✗	✗	✗	✔
Entamoeba histolytica	✔	✔	H	✔	✔	✗	✗	✔
Iodamoeba butschlii	✔	✗	H	✗	✗	✗	✗	✔
Blastocystis hominis	✔	✗	HAWB	?	✔	✗	✔	✔
Acanthamoeba spp.	✔	✔	F	✗	✔	✗	✗	✗
Naegleria fowleri	✔	✔	F	✗	✔	✗	✗	✗
MICROSPORA								
Brachiola vesicularum	?	S	Q	✗	✗	✗	✗	✗
Enterocytozoon bieneusi	✔	✔	HAW	✗	✗	✗	✔	✔
Encephalitozoon cuniculi	?	✔	Q	✗	✗	✗	✗	✗
Encephalitozoon hellem	?	S	Q	✗	✗	✗	✗	✗
Encephalitozoon intestinalis	✔	✔	HAW	✗	✗	✗	✔	✔
Nosema connori	?	S	Q	✗	✗	✗	✗	✗
Pleistophora spp.	?	S	Q	✗	✗	✗	✗	✗
Trachipleistophora anthropophthera	?	S	Q	✗	✗	✗	✗	✗
Trachipleistophora hominis	?	S	Q	✗	✗	✗	✗	✗
Vittaforma corneae	?	S	Q	✗	✗	✗	✗	✗
CILIOPHORA								
Balantidium coli	✔	✔	HAW	✗	✗	✗	✔	✔

A = agricultural animals; H = humans and primates; W = wild animals; B = birds; F = free-living organisms; Q = infects immunocompromised humans rarely, but the main host is unknown; S = has been demonstrated in a small number of patients with disease; ? = not known;

[a]Host range as currently known; the true host range may be greater. [b]It is likely that some of the microsporidia infect man through consuming the infected meat from inadequately cooked birds, mammals or fish but there is no evidence for this.

[c]Information extrapolated from similar species.; [d]Oocysts/sporocysts need to mature in the environment before they are infectious.

Table 1 *(continued)* Food-borne and water-borne protozoa

Protozoa	Transmission stage	Pathogen grows in the environment	Endemic in the UK	Geographic distribution
APICOMPLEXA				
Cryptosporidium parvum Type 1	Oo	✗	✔	World-wide
Cryptosporidium parvum Type 2	Oo	✗	✔	World-wide
Cryptosporidium parvum Type 3	Oo	✗	✔	?
Cryptosporidium felis	Oo	✗	?	?
Cryptosporidium spp. (canine strain)	Oo	✗	?	?
Cyclospora cayetanensis	Oo/Sc	✗	✗	Non-industrialised countries
Isospora belli	Oo/Sc	✗	✗	Non-industrialised countries
Sarcocystis hominis	Oo/Sc/Bz	✗	✗	World-wide
Sarcocystis suihominis	Oo/Sc/Bz	✗	✗	World-wide
Toxoplasma gondii	Oo/Bz	✗	✔	World-wide
MASTIGOPHORA				
Chilomastix mesnili	Cy	✗	✗	Non-industrialised countries
Dientamoeba fragilis	Tr	✗	✗	Non-industrialised countries
Enteromonas hominis	Tr	✗	✗	Non-industrialised countries
Giardia lamblia	Cy	✗	✔	World-wide
Retortomonas intestinalis	Tr	✗	✗	Non-industrialised countries
Trichomonas hominis	Tr	✗	✗	Non-industrialised countries
SARCODINA				
Endolimax nana	Cy	✗	✗	World-wide
Entamoeba coli	Cy	✗	✔	World-wide
Entamoeba dispar	Cy	✗	✗	World-wide
Entamoeba hartmanni	Cy	✗	✗	Non-industrialised countries
Entamoeba histolytica	Cy	✗	✗	Non-industrialised countries
Iodamoeba butschlii	Cy	✗	✗	World-wide
Blastocystis hominis	Cy/Tr	?	✔	World-wide
Acanthamoeba spp.	Cy/Tr	✔	✔	World-wide
Naegleria fowleri	Cy/Tr	✔	✔	World-wide
MICROSPORA				
Brachiola vesicularum	Sp			
Enterocytozoon bieneusi	Sp	✗	✔	?
Encephalitozoon cuniculi	Sp	✗	?	World-wide
Encephalitozoon hellem	Sp	✗	?	?
Encephalitozoon intestinalis	Sp	✗	✔	World-wide
Nosema connori	Sp	✗	?	?
Pleistophora spp.	Sp	✗	?	?
Trachipleistophora anthropophthera	Sp	✗	?	?
Trachipleistophora hominis	Sp	✗	?	?
Vittaforma corneae	Sp	✗	?	?
CILIOPHORA				
Balantidium coli	Cy	✗	✗	Non-industrialised countries

? = not known; Oo = oocyst; Sc = sporocyst; Bz = bradyzoite; Tz = tachyzoite; Cy = cyst; Tr = trophozoite; Sp = spore.

Vegetables and fruit can also be affected by washing with contaminated water.

The protozoa that are of most concern in industrialised countries are *Cryptosporidium*, *Giardia* and *Toxoplasma*, although *Cyclospora* has been identified in a number of outbreaks in the US and Canada in recent years. Food-borne outbreaks of infection with protozoa are not common. This is partly because surveillance systems for detecting outbreaks of protozoan infections are poorly developed in most countries. Pathogens, like *Cryptosporidium* and *Giardia*, can be transmitted by a variety of routes other than food. Some protozoan pathogens, like *Toxoplasma gondii*, cause only mild disease in most people and outbreaks are difficult to detect without mass antibody screening. In industrialised countries, testing for enteric protozoa is often done on patients returning from non-industrialised countries but not on other patients. This results in indigenous infections not being detected. Some protozoa (*Sarcocystis* spp. and *T. gondii*) can be present within meat as part of their normal life-cycle. Others get into food through faecal contamination of the raw materials and inadequate treatment of the food before eating it, or through post-treatment contamination. This is true for the oocysts or sporocysts of *Cryptosporidium* spp., *Cyclospora cayetanensis*, *T. gondii* and *Sarcocystis* spp., and for many of the cysts or spores of other protozoa.

Apicomplexa

Cryptosporidium spp.

Cryptosporidium parvum is a well-recognised cause of large waterborne outbreaks of gastroenteritis[3–7], but can also cause food-borne outbreaks[8–13]. These organisms can cause a chronic life-threatening infection with watery diarrhoea in people with a compromised T-cell condition such as acquired immune deficiency syndrome (AIDS) or severe combined immunodeficiency (SCID). However, in most people, a diarrhoeal episode that can last from a few days to a few weeks is followed by remission of symptoms.

Infection can derive from children, dogs, cats, farm animals and wild animals. Birds are not thought to be infected by human strains, although the oocysts of *C. parvum* can remain viable after passing through their intestines. Water sources are commonly contaminated with oocysts from animal and human faeces, and infection can occur in farmers and veterinarians working with animals.

Work over the last few years[14–24] is indicating that what we currently call *C. parvum* is composed of three or more types that are infectious to humans, and additional isolates from cats and dogs that are regarded as separate species are also infectious to humans. *C. parvum* type 1 is infectious to humans and other primates, but will not infect most agricultural and laboratory animals tested. *C. parvum* type 2 has a wider host range and is infectious to humans, sheep, cattle and laboratory animals. *C. parvum* type 3 has been found in humans, but the animal host range is not known. *C. felis* is infectious to cattle, cats and humans. The main *Cryptosporidium* strains associated with human disease in the UK are *C. parvum* types 1 and 2.

The oocysts of *Cryptosporidium* are infectious when excreted in faeces, and these can pass into rivers and lakes. They are resistant to chlorine and can pass into drinking water when there are failures in filtration or contamination of apparently secure source waters. Food can become contaminated through drinking water at the time of a water contamination incident, and raw products can be contaminated through irrigation or spraying with non-potable water. Outbreaks have been associated with inadequately pasteurised milk[25], apple juice[13], uncooked green onions in salads[8], and chicken salad[26]. Incidents have also been linked to raw milk[27], inadequately pasteurised milk[25], sausage and frozen tripe[9]. *Cryptosporidium* oocysts have a low infectious dose and individual strains have been found to differ in their infectivity, with an LD_{50} for human volunteers varying from 10 to 1000[28]. *Cryptosporidium* oocysts have been found in 14% of raw vegetables in Peru[29]. Foods that are consumed without heat treatment represent an important potential source of infection. Food-handlers who are infected, or are the parents of infected children, can also be a source of infection.

The major identifiable source of human cryptosporidiosis in England and Wales is water supplies that have become contaminated with animal faeces or sewage. During water-borne outbreaks, there is the potential for contaminated water to contaminate food. Special arrangements need to be made by food producers and retailers when the public water supply is thought to be contaminated with *Cryptosporidium* oocysts. Assessments of the risk of oocysts in the water causing infection following food processing need to be made, and depends on the extent of processing. *C. parvum* oocysts are sensitive to drying[30], to moderate heat treatment[31], and are killed by pasteurisation[32]. Oocysts are otherwise quite resistant to most chemical disinfectants and food preservatives, although the biocidal effect of combinations of pH, a_w, temperature, *etc.* have not been fully evaluated. (Water activity value, a_w, is a term that is used to describe the availability of water in a product rather than the total water content. It is taken by measuring the vapour pressure created by a food sample in a head-space of air and values range from 0 to 1 a_w.) Oocysts can survive in water at pH 3–10, and may survive (although in reduced numbers), for more than 24 h in beer, carbonated beverages and orange juice[4].

Cyclospora cayetanensis

Cyclospora is a coccidian parasite that causes protracted watery diarrhoea. It occurs world-wide but is common only in non-industrialised countries. Several recent reviews have summarised the life cycle, clinical manifestations and epidemiology of the parasite[33–40]. In endemic countries, the disease is seasonal with the highest incidence recorded in the late spring and summer months. The incubation period is 7–14 days and the duration of illness is around 7 weeks[34]. In the UK it is normally associated with travel to non-industrialised countries, several cases of cyclosporiosis have been reported in non-travellers in the US and Canada, and imported fruits and vegetables and drinking water have been implicated as vehicles of infection. Person-to-person spread is not thought to occur, because the oocysts need to mature (sporulate) under environmental conditions outside the host for 1–2 weeks before they become infectious[34].

The life cycle of *Cyclospora* is not fully known, but is believed to involve both asexual and sexual stages of proliferation[34]. It appears that *C. cayetanensis* requires only a single host to complete its entire life cycle. The morphology of *Cyclospora* in the intestine is similar to that of *Isospora*. Light microscopy and electron microscopy have been used to identify the asexual stages of *C. cayetanensis* in enterocytes seen in intestinal biopsies, including the sporozoite, trophozoite, schizont, and merozoite[41]. The sexual cycle also takes place in the human host, producing oocysts that are excreted in the faeces. The lamina propria and submucosa are not involved. The oocysts have been reported to be relatively resistant to chlorine[34,42].

Outbreaks of cyclosporiosis in the US and Canada have been associated with raspberries and salad items imported from South America[43–48]. The incidence of this parasite in the population of the UK is thought to be low. There are no known non-primate animal hosts[49], and the *Cyclospora* isolated from baboons differs from human isolates[50]. The numbers of oocysts getting into sewage is likely to be small, and it is unlikely that significant numbers reach source waters. As a consequence, the risk of *Cyclospora* being transmitted via treated mains water in the UK is considered to be low. In non-industrialised countries, transmission is likely to be through sewage contaminated water and the contamination of fruit and vegetables with sewage contaminated water used for irrigation or pesticide application[34].

Although protocols for the detection of *Cyclospora* in food have been used, they are not very sensitive[34]. They involve the use of microscopy or PCR to detect oocysts in washings from foods.

Isospora belli

Human intestinal isosporiasis is caused by *Isospora belli*. Members of the genus *Isospora* cause intestinal disease in several mammalian host species[51]. The symptoms of *I. belli* infection in immunocompetent patients include diarrhoea, vomiting, abdominal pain, dehydration, weight loss, steatorrhoea, headache, fever and malaise. The disease is often chronic, recurrences are common and infections can continue for months to years. Symptoms are more severe in AIDS patients, with the diarrhoea being more watery. In the US, AIDS patients' isosporiasis was more common in people who had travelled abroad and in indigenous Hispanic populations than in the rest of the population[52]. Extra-intestinal stages of *I. belli* have been observed in AIDS' patients but not immunocompetent patients. Asexual and sexual stages grow within intestinal cells of their hosts and produce an environmentally resistant oocyst. Infections are thought to be acquired by the ingestion of sporulated oocysts in contaminated food or water, although good evidence for the source of infection in most infected patients is limited.

Toxoplasma gondii

Toxoplasma gondii and *Sarcocystis* spp. have life cycles involving a sexual cycle with oocyst production in a carnivorous host (*e.g.* cats with *T. gondii*) and an asexual life cycle in other mammals and birds. The parasites form cysts within the secondary host's tissues and the life cycle is completed when the carnivorous primary host consumes the secondary host. Man is infected through consuming inadequately cooked meat from infected secondary host species such as agricultural animals, or from oocysts contaminating food or water.

Toxoplasmosis is common within many countries of the world and is usually a sub-clinical condition. In pregnant women, infection can lead to mental retardation and loss of vision in their congenitally infected children. Intestinal and hepatic toxoplasmosis[53-58], pneumonia[59], disseminated infection[55], cerebral and ocular infection[60] and death can occur in immunosuppressed or immunocompromised patients.

T. gondii is found in the tissues of food animals and is an important cause of abortion and mortality in sheep and goats throughout the world. A live vaccine, using a non-persistent strain of *T. gondii*, is available in New Zealand, the UK and Europe which prevents *T. gondii* abortion in sheep. A live vaccine using a mutant strain of *T. gondii* (T-263) is being developed in the US to reduce oocyst shedding by cats[61]. As yet, there are no drugs that are effective at killing *T. gondii* tissue cysts in human or animal tissues.

Outbreaks of infection have been associated with food[62,63], milk[64-66], water[67,68] and environmental contamination with cat faeces[69,70]. Food-borne infections can arise through the consumption of tissue cysts or trophozoites within meat, offal or unpasteurised milk, or from oocyst contamination. Waterborne infections arise only from the consumption of oocysts[67,68,71,72]. Demonstrating outbreaks is difficult, but common source outbreaks seem to be frequent in the families of patients with acute lymphadenopathic toxoplasmosis[73]. There is some evidence that infections derived from oocysts are more severe than those from tissue cysts[74].

Freezing to −12°C, cooking to an internal temperature of 67°C, or gamma irradiation (0.5 kGy) can kill tissue cysts in meat. The effect of heat on the infectivity of *T. gondii* tissue cysts has been examined using a homogenate of infected mouse brains and pork[75].

A prospective case-control study designed to identify preventable risk factors for *T. gondii* infection in pregnancy was conducted in Norway[76]. A total of 63 of 37,000 women tested in a screening programme for pregnant women had serological evidence of recent primary *T. gondii* infection and 128 seronegative control women were matched by age, stage of pregnancy, expected date of delivery, and geographic area. The factors found to be independently associated with an increased risk of maternal infection included eating raw or under-cooked minced meat products, eating unwashed raw vegetables or fruits, eating raw or under-cooked pork or mutton, cleaning a cat litter box and inadequate washing of kitchen utensils after raw meat preparation.

Recommendations for primary prevention are chiefly designed for 'sero-negative' pregnant women without specific anti-*T. gondii*-IgG and for persons with continuous or temporary immune deficiencies[77,78]. Prevention in this group should focus on meat, and cats. Meat should only be eaten when well cooked or when it has been frozen prior to preparation. There should be no mouth–finger contact while handling raw meat. Raw food that is to be eaten without cooking, including fruit and vegetables, should be carefully washed before consumption. Food should not be prepared in the same place and with the same utensils as raw meat. Household cats should be fed with canned food rather than with raw meat. Contact with cats' faeces, must be strictly avoided (use plastic gloves), and cats' toilets should be disinfected daily with boiling water, and litter discarded daily.

Sarcocystis spp.

Sarcocystis is a tissue coccidian with an obligatory two-host life-cycle, and there are more than 100 *Sarcocystis* species that have life-cycles involving diverse avian, mammalian and reptilian hosts[79]. All have a distinctive life-cycle involving a definitive (usually a carnivore) and an intermediate host (usually a herbivore). The sexual generations of gametogony and sporogony occur in the lamina propria of the small intestine of definitive hosts which shed infective sporocysts in their stools and present with intestinal sarcocystosis[80,81]. Asexual multiplication occurs in the skeletal and cardiac muscles of intermediate hosts which harbour *Sarcocystis* cysts (sarcocysts) in their muscles and present with muscular sarcocystosis. Sarcocysts are long sinuous cylindrical objects and they can be classified by their three dimensional appearance[82]. Humans can get intestinal sarcocystosis through the consumption of raw meat containing sarcocysts and muscular sarcocystosis through the consumption of water or food contaminated with sporocysts. The main species are *S. hominis* acquired from infected beef and *S. suihominis* from pork. Water-borne infection in man has not been reported, but may occur in the same way as water-borne toxoplasmosis (*i.e.* through sporocysts contaminating drinking water). Animal muscular infection is common throughout the world and follows ingestion of food or water contaminated with sporocysts. Monoclonal antibodies against *S. muris* have been used to differentiate different *Sarcocystis* species[81,83]. Experimental studies on human intestinal sarcocystosis showed that a calf could be infected with *S. hominis* sporocysts and developed sarcocysts in cardiac and skeletal muscles. When meat from the calf was fed to rhesus monkeys, they developed intestinal sarcocystosis with sporocyst production[84]. Clinical sarcocystosis is less commonly diagnosed than toxoplasmosis and is not normally associated with fetal infection or abortion in man and only occasionally in animals.

Human *Sarcocystis* infection is probably under-diagnosed, particularly in non-industrialised countries[85-87]. Enzyme-linked immunosorbent assay (ELISA) and indirect fluorescent antibody technique (IFAT) have been used to diagnose extra-intestinal infection[88,89] and muscle biopsy can be used for demonstrating the sarcocysts[90]. In farm labourers in Thailand, where consumption of raw meat is common, intestinal infection with sarcocystis is also common[91]. *Sarcocystis*-like organisms have been demonstrated in immunocompromised patients in Egypt[92]. In non-industrial countries, *Sarcocystis* spp. can be commonly found in the muscles of a range of livestock using haematoxylin-eosin (HE) stained muscle tissue samples[93]. Histological analysis of the tongues of routine autopsy subjects has been used to assess the extent of human infection in non-industrialised countries[86]. Human intestinal infection can be chronic and involve other bacterial pathogens[94,95].

In animals, clinical signs include fever, anaemia, loss of appetite and weight loss or reduced weight gain. Central nervous system signs include hind limb weakness, unsteadiness and partial paralysis, and acute myopathy and death may occur. Diagnosis can be difficult in countries where infection is common because clinical signs can be absent, mild or non-specific. Serology may be useful in some situations and histopathology/immunohistochemistry is valuable for confirming the cause of death. Control of *Sarcocystis* infection in farm animals relies on preventing the contamination of pasture and water with dog and fox faeces and preventing the access of young stock to contaminated land.

Other coccidia

Many coccidia are host specific whereas others have a wide host range. Other coccidia, including *Neospora caninum*, which causes paralysis and abortion in dogs and abortion in cattle[96–98], have not been associated with human disease.

Mastigophora

Giardia lamblia

Giardia spp. are flagellated protozoans that parasitize the small intestines of mammals, birds, reptiles, and amphibians and giardiasis is a common cause of diarrhoea world-wide[99]. Clinical manifestations of *G. lamblia* infection range from asymptomatic to a transient or persistent acute stage, with steatorrhoea, intermittent diarrhoea, and weight loss, or to a subacute or chronic stage that can mimic gallbladder or peptic ulcer disease. Sources of infection in addition to humans include beavers and other wild[100] and domestic animals[101], and carriage in these can be long-term[102]. Experimental inoculation of beavers identified that a dose of 50–500 cysts was required to cause infection with a human strain[103] and similar infectivity studies have been done in gerbils[104]. Experimental human infections have been conducted[105] and a low infecting dose (10–25 cysts) is reported to be sufficient to produce human infection[106].

Giardia species and types have been differentiated using isoenzyme electrophoresis[107–112], phospholipid analysis[113], immunoblotting[114], DNA probes[112,115], RAPD (random amplified polymorphic deoxyribonucleic acid)[111], karyotyping[116,117], DNA fingerprinting with hypervariable minisatellite sequences[118,119] and PCR[120]. *Giardia* species will grow in culture[121] and this makes the application of a variety of typing techniques possible. The antigenic makeup of isolates can change during infection[122].

Outbreaks of infection related to drinking water[123–127], recreational water[128,129] and food[130–133] have been described. Food-borne infections commonly implicate food-handlers in the contamination of prepared foods, often following contact with the faeces of infected young children. The implicated foods have included canned salmon, sandwiches, noodle salad, fruit salad, salad items, raw vegetables and ice. The cysts of G.

lamblia are resistant to chlorine, although less resistant than *Crypto-sporidium* oocysts. Water-borne infection can occur and, although outbreaks have mostly been associated with recreational water use, drinking water related outbreaks can occur[124-126]. The cysts can remain viable in cold water for months.

Dientamoeba fragilis

Dientamoeba fragilis is a protozoan that shares a common evolutionary history with the trichomonads[134]. *D. fragilis* is commonly found among patients with diarrhoea lasting longer than one week[135,136], particularly children[137], and may masquerade as chronic allergic colitis in children[138]. It is common in some non-industrialised countries[139,140] and industrialised ones[135,141]. The importance of stool fixation and staining in diagnosing *D. fragilis* has been emphasised as this pathogen does not produce cysts[142]. The absence of a cyst suggests that it is less likely to survive in the environment than many other protozoa, and its common presentation in children rather than adults suggests a person-to-person mode of transmission. There have been no reports of food or water related infections or outbreaks of *D. fragilis* and infections appear to be sporadic. If food-borne infection does occur, it is likely to be through an infected food-handler.

Other flagellates

Other flagellated organisms that are occasionally demonstrated in the faeces of people with diarrhoea include *Chilomastix mesnili*, *Tricho-monas hominis*, *Retortomonas intestinalis* and *Enteromonas hominis*. These organisms are usually found in non-industrialised countries, but there is no good evidence that any of them cause gastrointestinal disease.

Sarcodina

Entamoeba histolytica

Entamoeba histolytica causes amoebic dysentery and abscesses, particularly in the liver. The motile trophozoites of *E. histolytica* phagocytose erythrocytes and these are diagnostic when seen in fresh faeces. Its cysts cannot be differentiated from those of the non-pathogenic *E. dispar*[143] using conventional microscopic identification and, as a consequence, much of the scientific literature may relate to *E. dispar*. Modern molecular methods can readily differentiate these organisms, but this may not be done routinely[143-146]. Because endemic infection in the UK does not seem to occur, the infection risks are mostly associated with consuming contaminated food or water in countries where it is endemic.

Blastocystis hominis

The significance of *Blastocystis hominis* in diarrhoeal disease has been the subject of much debate. The organism occurs world-wide and appears in both immunocompetent and immunodeficient individuals. The symptoms generally attributed to *B. hominis* infection are non-specific, and the need for treatment is debated[147]. *B. hominis* was detected by faecal examination in 34 of 6,476 healthy people in Japan who visited a health screening centre for a routine medical check-up[148]. *B. hominis* has been associated with development of diarrhoea in travellers to tropical destinations, and concurrent infections with other organisms are common[149]. It occurs as commonly in asymptomatic control populations as in patients with diarrhoea[150]. Serum antibody was detected by fluorescent antibody test in patients with symptomatic *B. hominis* infection[151], and invasive disease has been reported[152]. However, in a group of symptomatic patients with *B. hominis* infection, endoscopy typically did not show evidence of significant intestinal inflammation or impaired intestinal permeability[153]. A study of *B. hominis* in AIDS patients found no association with clinical symptoms[154]. The isolation of *B. hominis* does not justify treatment even in symptomatic, severely immunocompromised patients. Most patients will either have spontaneous resolution of symptoms or successful identification of other infectious or non-infectious aetiologies. *B. hominis* is unlikely to be an important enteric pathogen, and transient symptomatic infection, if it occurs at all, resolves quickly.

Isoenzyme patterns show that *B. hominis* is highly polymorphic, but there is no correlation between isoenzyme patterns and disease[155]. Faecal samples from mammals, birds, reptiles, amphibians, fish, and snails were isolated by culture, put into axenic culture and serogrouped[156]. Most cultures belonged to the four serogroups. Human isolates were mainly serogroups I and II, pigs harboured serogroups III and IV. DNA polymorphisms in *Blastocystis* showed similarities between human and chicken isolates[157]. It was suggested that the genus *Blastocystis* may consist of more than one species.

Colonisation of people with *B. hominis* could well involve transmission via contaminated food or water[158] and it has been isolated from sewage[158,159].

Other amoebae

A number of other amoebae can be found in the faeces of patients with diarrhoea including *Entamoeba coli*, *Iodamoeba butschlii* and *Endolimax nana*, but there is no evidence that these organisms cause diarrhoea in humans. *Acanthamoeba* spp. and *Naegleria fowlerii* can cause water-borne disease but do not infect humans via food.

Microspora

Microsporidia

Microsporidia are a diverse, distinctive and ubiquitous group of protozoa with characteristics including a lack if mitochondria and a distinctive coiled polar tube in the spores[160]. An increasing number of species of microsporidia are being recognised in immunocompromised patients, particularly those with AIDS. Diarrhoea, malabsorption and weight loss are the most common clinical problems, but several other clinical syndromes can affect the eye, kidney, sinuses, lungs, brain, liver, bone and muscle[161]. Even in AIDS patients some infections may be asymptomatic[162]. Their relatively recent emergence as human pathogens and the difficulties in diagnosis mean that food-borne associations have not yet been demonstrated although spores have been demonstrated in water.

Two species, *Enterocytozoon bieneusi* and *Encephalitozoon intestinalis*, commonly cause diarrhoea in AIDS patients throughout the world. Other species cause organ specific or systemic infections and these include *Nosema connori*, *Encephalitozoon hellem*, *E. cuniculi*, *Vittaforma corneae*, *Microsporidium ceylonensis*, *Brachiola vesicularum*, *Pleistophora* spp., *Trachipleistophora anthropophthera* and *T. hominis*.

Enterocytozoon bieneusi

E. bieneusi causes chronic diarrhoea in immunocompromised people and has occasionally been found in people with diarrhoea in the absence of any apparent immune deficiency[163,164]. It is the most common microsporidial cause of intestinal disease. Multi-organ involvement can occur through local extension of the infection to the hepatobiliary tract[165]. Some patients have had respiratory involvement[166,167]. *E. intestinalis* and *E. bieneusi* have been found in stools of more than 40% of AIDS patients with diarrhoea. PCR has been used to examine faecal samples for *E. bieneusi*[168,169]. A study of microsporidiosis in AIDS patients in Tanzania demonstrated *E. bieneusi* in 18% of faeces' samples using modified Trichrome stain and 51% using PCR[170]. Another study, using light microscopy and fluorochrome staining with Uvitex 2B, found 8/104 samples positive compared to 10 positive by PCR[171]. A synthetic, labelled oligonucleotide has been used for the detection and identification of *E. bieneusi* in clinical samples[172].

A variety of methods have been used to detect *E. bieneusi* in water, and PCR approaches seem to be suitable[173,174], and have been used to detect the organism in surface waters[175]. Detection in food remains problematic. This work indicates that *E. bieneusi* may be present in water sources, although there is no evidence to indicate whether the organisms detected are viable.

PCR has been used to detect[176–180] and type[181,182] *E. bieneusi*. *E. bieneusi* has been detected by PCR in 35% of 109 pigs, and the four pig genotypes identified were different from the three human ones from Swiss patients[183]. Isolates have also been detected in cats and dogs[184], and a rhesus monkey[185]. Isolates from humans and macaques with AIDS have been used to infect immunosuppressed gnotobiotic piglets that remained asymptomatic but colonised for up to 50 days[186]. Attempts to culture *E. bieneusi* in tissue culture have so far proved difficult[187,188].

Combination antiretroviral therapy including a protease inhibitor have been shown to restore immunity to *E. bieneusi* and *C. parvum* in HIV-1 infected individuals[189].

Encephalitozoon intestinalis

A second enteric microsporidian, *E. intestinalis* (originally named *Septata intestinalis*) is associated with disseminated as well as acute and chronic intestinal disease[190]. Clinical features of disseminated infection include chronic diarrhoea, fever, cholangitis, sinusitis, bronchitis, or mild bilateral conjunctivitis[191]. The spores of this organism have been differentiated from those of *E. bieneusi* by their smaller size and fluorescence using a specific polyclonal rabbit antiserum[192], but PCR is more definitive[171,178–180,193–195].

E. intestinalis spores have been demonstrated in the faeces of a donkey, dog, pig, cow, and goat using PCR and polyclonal antibody immunofluorescence[196]. These organisms can be grown in tissue culture[197,198]. *E. intestinalis* has been detected in tertiary sewage effluent, surface water, and ground-water using PCR[175].

E. intestinalis was found in two patients who had no obvious immunodeficiency[199]. The pathogenic role of *E. intestinalis* in immunocompetent individuals remains to be demonstrated.

Pleistophora and Trachipleistophora spp. and other microsporidia

These organisms cause disease in immunocompromised patients and are rare. *Pleistophora* spp. have been demonstrated in the muscles of a few patients with myositis, fever and progressive weakness[200,201]. A *Pleistophora* spp.-like microsporidian infection was identified in a patient with progressive severe myosotis associated with fever and weight loss[202]. The organism was demonstrated by light microscopy and electron microscopy in corneal scrapings, skeletal muscle, and nasal discharge and named *Trachipleistophora hominis*. A similar organism *Trachipleistophora anthropophthera* was found at autopsy in the brain of one patient and in the brain, kidneys, pancreas, thyroid, parathyroid, heart, liver, spleen, lymph nodes, and bone marrow of a second patient with AIDS[203]. Two ocular infectious disorders attributed to *Microsporidia* have been observed[204]. One infection involves the corneal stroma leading to corneal ulceration and suppurative keratitis and is caused by *Vittaforma corneae* (synonymous with *Nosema corneum*)[205]. The other infection involves the conjunctival and corneal epithelium and is caused by *Encephalitozoon hellem*[206]. *E. hellem* also causes urogenital and respiratory infections[207]. Identical genotypes of *E. hellem*, determined from the sequence of the rDNA internal transcribed spacer, have been identified from human and bird sources[208]. *Microsporidium ceylonensis* has also caused corneal microsporidiosis[209], as has *E. intestinalis*[191]. A nosema-like microsporidian, *Brachiola vesicularum*, has been identified in biopsied muscle tissue, examined by light and electron microscopy in an AIDS patient with myositis[210]. The organisms develop in direct contact with the muscle cell cytoplasm and fibres.

It is not clear where all these different infections originate from and whether food or water are important in transmission. Most of the microsporidial infections have come to light through the intensive investigation of patients with syndromes associated with an immune deficiency. In most cases, the source of their infections is not known. Limited information on *E. bieneusi* and *E. intestinalis* suggests that agricultural animals may be a source of infection. As viable spores are passed by infected patients, person-to-person transmission and contamination of food and water with human waste remain possible transmission routes. The demonstration of *E. intestinalis* in tertiary sewage effluent, surface water, and ground-water, *E. bieneusi* in surface water and *Vittaforma corneae* in tertiary effluent[175] suggests sewage may be a source of contamination of the environment. Spores of the other microsporidian species have not been found in human faeces. A case-control study of HIV-infected individuals determined risk factors for microsporidiosis[211]. Cases were more likely than controls to have low CD4 cell counts, to be homosexual and to have swum in a pool in the previous 12 months. This suggests faecal–oral transmission through water is possible, but no link was found with treated mains drinking water. The findings were corroborated by a study of HIV positive patients in California[212]. There was no seasonal variation in the prevalence of microsporidiosis. Although a water-borne route of infection with microsporidiosis is possible[213], there is no direct evidence of infection being acquired through the consumption of potable mains water or food.

Ciliophora

Balantidium coli

Balantidium coli causes an ulcerative dysentery in humans. Human infection is sporadic in non-industrialised countries, and very rare in industrialised ones, and seems to occur when there is close contact between people and pigs. Food-borne and water-borne infection have not been well documented, but remain possible. Cysts of *B. coli* from the faeces of infected patients are infectious to piglets and hydrocortisone-treated rhesus monkeys[214]. *B. coli* occurs naturally in wild and domesticated pigs[215], monkeys and apes[216,217], but was not found in wild rodents, dogs or cats[217].

Identifying and managing the risks of protozoan contamination of foods

Within the UK, the main food risks to human health are from *Toxoplasma*, *Cryptosporidium* and *Giardia*. Each protozoan has a different epidemiology and the risks of food-borne transmission are outlined in Table 2. The way foods are produced and distributed can have an important impact on the potential health risks from protozoa. There are specific potential problems associated with the globalization of food production and the import of foods from countries where diarrhoeal disease is more common in the community. This is exemplified by the *Cyclospora* outbreaks in Canada and the US. There are hygiene issues for preventing the contamination of soft fruits and salad items by people employed to pick these crops, by wildlife and from contaminated water used in sprays. There are also potential problems associated with the contamination of potable water with *Cryptosporidium*, and the control measures that are necessary for individual food production processes that use this water. The water industry is tightening its risk assessment and monitoring of drinking water treatment works to satisfy new legislation[218].

Table 2 Identifying and managing the risks of protozoan contamination of foods

Food type	Protozoan risk	Risk management
Raw meat	Intrinsic contamination with *Toxoplasma* or *Sarcocystis* tissue cysts	1 Control the access of cats, foxes and dogs onto pasture 2 Freeze meat 3 Cook meat 4 Determine whether any curing process being used will kill *Toxoplasma* or *Sarcocystis*
	Surface contamination with oocysts and cysts of *Cryptosporidium*, *Toxoplasma* or other protozoa	1 Good abattoir and post processing hygiene 2 Cook meat
Raw fruit and vegetables sold at retail	Surface contamination with oocysts and cysts of *Cryptosporidium*, *Cyclospora*, *Toxoplasma* or other protozoa in foods that are eaten without cooking	1 Prevent faecal contamination by using potable water for spraying, irrigation, *etc.* 2 Wash with potable water containing chlorine 3 Prevent agricultural animals grazing in the vicinity 4 Provide toilet and washing facilities for fruit/vegetable pickers 5 Educate fruit/vegetable pickers 6 Use mechanical picking 7 Control flies and other insects 8 National/international controls
Processed foods	*Cryptosporidium*/other parasites in the water	1 Use a secure supply (deep borehole or surface water with good water treatment process) 2 Determine the risks of water contamination with *Cryptosporidium* from the water provider 3 Determine whether processing will kill the parasites 4 Decide what to do in the event of a boil water notice 5 Install additional water filtration or other treatment if necessary
Retail ready-to-eat foods	*Cryptosporidium*/other parasites causing contamination from food handlers	1 Hygiene training for food handling staff 2 Good washing and toilet facilities 3 Preventing staff with diarrhoea from working
	Cryptosporidium/other parasites causing contamination from pets and other animals	1 Restrict the access of cats, dogs and other pets from the cooking and serving areas
	Cryptosporidium/other parasites in the water	1 Decide what to do in the event of a boil water notice
Unpasteurised milk	*Toxoplasma* or *Cryptosporidium* in milk	1 Pasteurise milk to be used for babies, pregnant women and immunocompromised people 2 Freeze milk

Key points for clinical practice

- Protozoan infections linked to food are not commonly detected
- The main food risks in the UK are *Toxoplasma*, *Cryptosporidium* and *Giardia*
- Many of the protozoa are a particular problem in AIDS patients
- A majority of food-borne protozoan infections are probably acquired abroad
- Protozoa can be transmitted to food through contaminated water
- Imported soft fruit and salad vegetables are a potential risk

References

1   Buzby JC, Roberts T. Economic costs and trade impacts of microbial food-borne illness. *World Health Stat Q* 1997; **50**: 57–66

2   Anon. Issues in pork safety: costs, controls, and incentives. *Agricultural Outlook* 1993; Outlook-32

3   Frisby HR, Addiss DG, Reiser WJ *et al.* Clinical and epidemiologic features of a massive waterborne outbreak of cryptosporidiosis in persons with HIV infection. *J Acquir Immune Defic Syndr Hum Retrovirol* 1997; **16**: 367–73

4   Girdwood RWA, Smith HV. *Cryptosporidium.* In: Robinson RK, Batt CA, Patel PD. (Eds) *Encyclopedia of Food Microbiology.* London: Academic Press, 2000; 487–502

5   MacKenzie WR, Schell WL, Blair KA *et al.* Massive outbreak of waterborne cryptosporidium infection in Milwaukee, Wisconsin: recurrence of illness and risk of secondary transmission [see comments]. *Clin Infect Dis* 1995; **21**: 57–62

6   Richardson AJ, Frankenberg RA, Buck AC *et al.* An outbreak of waterborne cryptosporidiosis in Swindon and Oxfordshire. *Epidemiol Infect* 1991; **107**: 485–95

7   Willocks L, Crampin A, Milne L *et al.* A large outbreak of cryptosporidiosis associated with a public water supply from a deep chalk borehole. Outbreak Investigation Team. *Commun Dis Public Health* 1998; **1**: 239–43

8   Food-borne outbreak of cryptosporidiosis – Spokane, Washington, 1997. *MMWR Morb Mortal Wkly Rep* 1998; **47**: 565–7

9   Smith JL. *Cryptosporidium* and *Giardia* as agents of food-borne disease. *J Food Protect* 1993; **56**: 451–61

10 Djuretic T, Wall PG, Nichols G. General outbreaks of infectious intestinal disease associated with milk and dairy products in England and Wales: 1992 to 1996 [published erratum appears in *Commun Dis Rep CDR Rev* 1997; **7**: R54]. *Commun Dis Rep CDR Rev* 1997; **7**: R41–5

11 Anon. Foodborne outbreak of diarrheal illness associated with *Cryptosporidium parvum* – Minnesota, 1995. *MMWR Morb Mortal Wkly Rep* 1996; **45**: 783–4

12 Laberge I, Griffiths MW, Griffiths MW. Prevalence, detection and control of *Cryptosporidium parvum* in food. *Int J Food Microbiol* 1996; **32**: 1–26

13 Millard PS, Gensheimer KF, Addiss DG *et al.* An outbreak of cryptosporidiosis from fresh-pressed apple cider [published erratum appears in *JAMA* 1995; **273**: 776]. *JAMA* 1994; **272**: 1592–6

14 Nichols GL, McLauchlin J, Samuel D. A technique for typing *Cryptosporidium* isolates. *J Protozool* 1991; **38**: 237S–40S

15 McLauchlin J, Pedraza-Diaz S, Amar-Hoetzeneder C, Nichols GL. Genetic characterization of cryptosporidium strains from 218 patients with diarrhea diagnosed as having sporadic cryptosporidiosis. *J Clin Microbiol* 1999; **37**: 3153–8

16 Awad-El-Kariem FM, Robinson HA, Dyson DA *et al.* Differentiation between human and animal strains of *Cryptosporidium parvum* using isoenzyme typing. *Parasitology* 1995; **110**: 129–32

17 Awad-El-Kariem FM, Robinson HA, Petry F, McDonald V, Evans D, Casemore D. Differentiation between human and animal isolates of *Cryptosporidium parvum* using molecular and biological markers. *Parasitol Res* 1998; **84**: 297–301

18 McLauchlin J, Casemore DP, Moran S, Patel S. The epidemiology of cryptosporidiosis: application of experimental sub-typing and antibody detection systems to the investigation of water-borne outbreaks. *Folia Parasitol (Praha)* 1998; **45**: 83–92

19 Widmer G. Genetic heterogeneity and PCR detection of *Cryptosporidium parvum. Adv Parasitol* 1998; **40**: 223–39

20 Patel S, Pedraza-Diaz S, McLauchlin J, Casemore DP. Molecular characterisation of *Cryptosporidium parvum* from two large suspected waterborne outbreaks. Outbreak Control Team South and West Devon 1995, Incident Management Team and Further Epidemiological and Microbiological Studies Subgroup North Thames 1997. *Commun Dis Public Health* 1998; **1**: 231–3

21 Caccio S, Homan W, van Dijk K, Pozio E. Genetic polymorphism at the beta-tubulin locus among human and animal isolates of *Cryptosporidium parvum* [published erratum appears in *FEMS Microbiol Lett* 1999; **173**: 273]. *FEMS Microbiol Lett* 1999; **170**: 173–9

22 Homan W, van Gorkom T, Kan YY, Hepener J. Characterization of *Cryptosporidium parvum* in human and animal feces by single-tube nested polymerase chain reaction and restriction analysis. *Parasitol Res* 1999; **85**: 707–12

23 Morgan UM, Deplazes P, Forbes DA *et al.* Sequence and PCR-RFLP analysis of the internal transcribed spacers of the rDNA repeat unit in isolates of *Cryptosporidium* from different hosts. *Parasitology* 1999; **118**: 49–58

24 Pieniazek NJ, Bornay-Llinares FJ, Slemenda SB *et al.* New cryptosporidium genotypes in HIV-infected persons. *Emerg Infect Dis* 1999; **5**: 444–9

25 Gelletlie R, Stuart J, Soltanpoor N, Armstrong R, Nichols G. Cryptosporidiosis associated with school milk [letter]. *Lancet* 1997; **350**: 1005–6

26 Besser-Wiek JW, Forfang J, Hedberg CW *et al.* Foodborne outbreak of diarrheal illness associated with *Cryptosporidium parvum* – Minnesota, 1995. *MMWR Morb Mortal Wkly Rep* 1996; **45**: 783–4

27 Casemore DP, Jessop EG, Douce D, Jackson FB. *Cryptosporidium* plus *Campylobacter*: an outbreak in a semi-rural population. *J Hyg* 1986; **96**: 95–105

28 Okhuysen PC, Chappell CL, Crabb JH, Sterling CR, DuPont HL. Virulence of three distinct *Cryptosporidium parvum* isolates for healthy adults. *J Infect Dis* 1999; **180**: 1275–81

29 Ortega YR, Roxas CR, Gilman RH *et al.* Isolation of *Cryptosporidium parvum* and *Cyclospora cayetanensis* from vegetables collected in markets of an endemic region in Peru. *Am J Trop Med Hyg* 1997; **57**: 683–6

30 Anderson BC. Effect of drying on the infectivity of cryptosporidia-laden calf feces for 3- to 7-day-old mice. *Am J Vet Res* 1986; **47**: 2272–3

31 Anderson BC. Moist heat inactivation of *Cryptosporidium* spp. *Am J Public Health* 1985; **75**: 1433–4

32 Harp JA, Fayer R, Pesch BA, Jackson GJ. Effect of pasteurization on infectivity of *Cryptosporidium parvum* oocysts in water and milk. *Appl Environ Microbiol* 1996; **62**: 2866–8

33 Brown GH, Rotschafer JC. *Cyclospora*: review of an emerging parasite. *Pharmacotherapy* 1999; **19**: 70–5

34 Adams AM, Jinneman KC, Ortega YR. *Cyclospora*. In: Robinson RK, Batt CA, Patel PD. (Eds) *Encyclopedia of Food Microbiology*. London: Academic Press, 2000; 502–13

35 Sterling CR, Ortega YR. *Cyclospora*: an enigma worth unraveling. *Emerg Infect Dis* 1999; **5**: 48–53

36 Chalmers RM, Nichols G, Rooney R. Foodborne outbreaks od cyclosporiasis have arisen in North America. Is the United Kingdom at risk? *Commun Dis Public Health* 2000; **3**(1): 50–5.

37 Ortega YR, Sterling CR, Gilman RH. *Cyclospora cayetanensis*. *Adv Parasitol* 1998; **40**: 399–418

38 Soave R, Herwaldt BL, Relman DA. *Cyclospora*. *Infect Dis Clin North Am* 1998; **12**: 1–12

39 Connor BA. *Cyclospora* infection: a review. *Ann Acad Med Singapore* 1997; **26**: 632–6

40 Cann KJ, Chalmers RM, Nichols G, O'Brien SJ. Cyclospora infections in England and Wales: 1993 to 1998. *Commun Dis Public Health* 2000; **3**(1): 46–9

41 Sun T, Ilardi CF, Asnis D *et al.* Light and electron microscopic identification of *Cyclospora* species in the small intestine. Evidence of the presence of asexual life cycle in human host. *Am J Clin Pathol* 1996; **105**: 216–20

42 Wright MS, Collins PA. Waterborne transmission of *Cryptosporidium*, *Cyclospora* and *Giardia*. *Clin Lab Sci* 1997; **10**: 287–90

43 Herwaldt BL, Beach MJ. The return of *Cyclospora* in 1997: another outbreak of cyclosporiasis in North America associated with imported raspberries. Cyclospora Working Group [see comments]. *Ann Intern Med* 1999; **130**: 210–20

44 Koumans EH, Katz DJ, Malecki JM *et al.* An outbreak of cyclosporiasis in Florida in 1995: a harbinger of multistate outbreaks in 1996 and 1997. *Am J Trop Med Hyg* 1998; **59**: 235–42

45 Herwaldt BL, Ackers ML. An outbreak in 1996 of cyclosporiasis associated with imported raspberries. *N Engl J Med* 1997; **336**:1548–56

46 Letendre LJ. Outbreaks of *Cyclospora cayetanensis* infection: United States and Canada 1996. *J Assoc Food Drug Officials* 1997; **61**: 13–7

47 Pritchett R, Gossman C, Radke V *et al.* Outbreak of cyclosporiasis – northern Virginia-

Washington, DC-Baltimore, Maryland, metropolitan area, 1997. *JAMA* 1997; **278**: 538–9

48 Hofmann J, Liu Z, Genese C *et al*. Update: outbreaks of *Cyclospora cayetanensis* infection – United States and Canada, 1996. *MMWR Morb Mortal Wkly Rep* 1996; **45**: 611–2

49 Eberhard ML, Nace EK, Freeman AR. Survey for *Cyclospora cayetanensis* in domestic animals in an endemic area in Haiti. *J Parasitol* 1999; **85**: 562–3

50 Eberhard ML, da Silva AJ, Lilley BG, Pieniazek NJ. Morphologic and molecular characterization of new *Cyclospora* species from Ethiopian monkeys: *C. cercopitheci* sp.n., *C. solobi* sp.n., and *C. papionis* sp.n. *Emerg Infect Dis* 1999; **5**(5): 651–8

51 Lindsay DS, Dubey JP, Blagburn BL. Biology of *Isospora* spp. from humans, nonhuman primates, and domestic animals. *Clin Microbiol Rev* 1997; **10**: 19–34

52 Sorvillo FJ, Lieb LE, Seidel J, Kerndt P, Turner J, Ash LR. Epidemiology of isosporiasis among persons with acquired immunodeficiency syndrome in Los Angeles County. *Am J Trop Med Hyg* 1995; **53**: 656–9

53 Bonacini M, Kanel G, Alamy M. Duodenal and hepatic toxoplasmosis in a patient with HIV infection: review of the literature. *Am J Gastroenterol* 1996; **91**: 1838–40

54 al Kassab AK, Habte-Gabr E, Mueller WF, Azher Q. Fulminant disseminated toxoplasmosis in an HIV patient. *Scand J Infect Dis* 1995; **27**: 183–5

55 Guccion JG, Benator DA, Gibert CL, Dave HP. Disseminated toxoplasmosis and acquired immunodeficiency syndrome: diagnosis by transmission electron microscopy. *Ultrastruct Pathol* 1995; **19**: 95–9

56 Yang M, Perez E. Disseminated toxoplasmosis as a cause of diarrhea. *South Med J* 1995; **88**: 860–1

57 Buhr M, Heise W, Arasteh K, Stratmann M, Grosse M, L'age M. Disseminated toxoplasmosis with sepsis in AIDS. *Clin Invest* 1992; **70**: 1079–81

58 Pauwels A, Meyohas MC, Eliaszewicz M, Legendre C, Mougeot G, Frottier J. *Toxoplasma colitis* in the acquired immunodeficiency syndrome [see comments]. *Am J Gastroenterol* 1992; **87**: 518–9

59 Singh N, Gayowski T, Wagener M, Marino IR, Yu VL. Pulmonary infections in liver transplant recipients receiving tacrolimus. Changing pattern of microbial etiologies. *Transplantation* 1996; **61**: 396–401

60 Park KL, Smith RE, Rao NA. Ocular manifestations of AIDS. *Curr Opin Ophthalmol* 1995; **6**: 82–7

61 Dubey JP. Strategies to reduce transmission of *Toxoplasma gondii* to animals and humans. *Vet Parasitol* 1996; **64**: 65–70

62 Choi WY, Nam HW, Kwak NH *et al*. Foodborne outbreaks of human toxoplasmosis. *J Infect Dis* 1997; **175**: 1280–2

63 Masur H, Jones TC, Lempert JA, Cherubini TD. Outbreak of toxoplasmosis in a family and documentation of acquired retinochoroiditis. *Am J Med* 1978; **64**: 396–402

64 Skinner LJ, Timperley AC, Wightman D, Chatterton JM, Ho-Yen DO. Simultaneous diagnosis of toxoplasmosis in goats and goat owner's family. *Scand J Infect Dis* 1990; **22**: 359–61

65 Chiari CD, Pereira ND. [Human toxoplasmosis acquired through drinking goats' milk.]. *Memorias do Instituto Oswaldo Cruz* 1984; **79**: 337–40

66 Sacks JJ, Roberto RR, Brooks NF. Toxoplasmosis infection associated with raw goat's milk. *JAMA* 1982; **248**:1728–32

67 Bowie WR, King AS, Werker DH *et al*. Outbreak of toxoplasmosis associated with municipal drinking water. The BC Toxoplasma Investigation Team [see comments]. *Lancet* 1997; **350**: 173–7

68 Beneson MW, Takafuji EJ, Lemon SM, Greenup RL, Sultze AJ. Oocyst transmission: toxoplasmosis associated with ingestion of contaminated water. *N Engl J Med* 1982; **307**: 666–9

69 Akstein RB, Wilson LA, Teutsch SM. Acquired toxoplasmosis. *Ophthalmology* 1982; **89**: 1299–302

70 Stagno S, Dykes AC, Amos CS, Head RA, Juranek DD, Walls K. An outbreak of toxoplasmosis linked to cats. *Pediatrics* 1980; **65**: 706–12

71 Aramini JJ, Stephen C, Dubey JP. *Toxoplasma gondii* in Vancouver Island cougars (*Felis concolor vancouverensis*): serology and oocyst shedding. *J Parasitol* 1998; **84**: 438–40

72 Isaac-Renton J, Bowie WR, King A *et al*. Detection of *Toxoplasma gondii* oocysts in drinking water. *Appl Environ Microbiol* 1998; **64**: 2278–80

73 Luft BJ, Remington JS. Acute *Toxoplasma* infection among family members of patients with acute lymphadenopathic toxoplasmosis. *Arch Intern Med* 1984; **144**: 53–6

74 Eckert J. Workshop summary: food safety: meat- and fish-borne zoonoses. *Vet Parasitol* 1996; **64**: 143–7

75 Dubey JP, Kotula AW, Sharar A, Andrews CD, Lindsay DS. Effect of high temperature on infectivity of *Toxoplasma gondii* tissue cysts in pork. *J Parasitol* 1990; **76**: 201–4

76 Kapperud G, Jenum PA, Stray-Pedersen B, Melby KK, Eskild A, Eng J. Risk factors for *Toxoplasma gondii* infection in pregnancy. Results of a prospective case-control study in Norway. *Am J Epidemiol* 1996; **144**: 405–12

77 Jacquier P, Deplazes P, Heimann P, Gottstein B. [Parasitology and human medical preventive importance of *Toxoplasma gondii*] Parasitologie und humanmedizinisch-praventive Bedeutung von *Toxoplasma gondii*. *Schweiz Med Wochenschr Suppl* 1995; **65**: 10S-8S

78 Richards Jr FO, Kovacs JA, Luft BJ. Preventing toxoplasmic encephalitis in persons infected with human immunodeficiency virus. *Clin Infect Dis* 1995; **21 Suppl. 1**: S49-56

79 Rommel M. Recent advances in the knowledge of the biology of the cyst-forming coccidia. *Angew Parasitol* 1989; **30**: 173–83

80 Buxton D. Protozoan infections (*Toxoplasma gondii*, *Neospora caninum* and *Sarcocystis* spp.) in sheep and goats: recent advances. *Vet Res* 1998; **29**: 289–310

81 Kan SP, Pathmanathan R. Review of sarcocystosis in Malaysia. *Southeast Asian J Trop Med Public Health* 1991; **22 Suppl.**: 129–34

82 Wong KT, Clarke G, Pathmanathan R, Hamilton PW. Light microscopic and three-dimensional morphology of the human muscular sarcocyst. *Parasitol Res* 1994; **80**: 138–40

83 Rommel M, Tenter AM, Vietmeyer C, Mencke N. Production and characterisation of monoclonal antibodies for species diagnosis of sarcosporidia. *Rev Sci Tech* 1990; **9**: 235–8

84 Lian Z, Ma J, Wang Z *et al*. [Studies on man-cattle-man infection cycle of *Sarcocystis hominis* in Yunnan]. *Chung Kuo Chi Sheng Chung Hsueh Yu Chi Sheng Chung Ping Tsa Chih* 1990; **8**: 50–3

85 Joubert JJ, Evans AC. Current status of food-borne parasitic zoonoses in South Africa and Namibia. *Southeast Asian J Trop Med Public Health* 1997; **28 Suppl. 1**: 7–10

86 Wong KT, Pathmanathan R. High prevalence of human skeletal muscle sarcocystosis in south-east Asia. *Trans R Soc Trop Med Hyg* 1992; **86**: 631–2

87 Giboda M, Ditrich O, Scholz T, Viengsay T, Bouaphanh S. Current status of food-borne parasitic zoonoses in Laos. *Southeast Asian J Trop Med Public Health* 1991; **22 Suppl.**: 56–61

88 Tadros W, Hazelhoff W, Laarman JJ. The detection of circulating antibodies against *Sarcocystis* in human and bovine sera by the enzyme-linked immunosorbent assay (ELISA) technique. *Acta Leiden* 1979; **47**: 53–63

89 Habeeb YS, Selim MA, Ali MS, Mahmoud LA, Abdel Hadi AM, Shafei A. Serological diagnosis of extraintestinal sarcocystosis. *J Egypt Soc Parasitol* 1996; **26**: 393–400

90 Mehrotra R, Bisht D, Singh PA, Gupta SC, Gupta RK. Diagnosis of human sarcocystis infection from biopsies of the skeletal muscle. *Pathology* 1996; **28**: 281–2

91 Wilairatana P, Radomyos P, Radomyos B *et al*. Intestinal sarcocystosis in Thai laborers. *Southeast Asian J Trop Med Public Health* 1996; **27**: 43–6

92 el Naga IF, Negm AY, Awadalla HN. Preliminary identification of an intestinal coccidian parasite in man. *J Egypt Soc Parasitol* 1998; **28**: 807–14

93 Woldemeskel M, Gebreab F. Prevalence of sarcocysts in livestock of northwest Ethiopia. *Zentralbl Veterinarmed [B]* 1996; **43**: 55–8

94 Bunyaratvej S, Unpunyo P. Combined *Sarcocystis* and Gram-positive bacterial infections. A possible cause of segmental enterocolitis in Thailand. *J Med Assoc Thai* 1992; **75 Suppl. 1**: 38–44

95 Bunyaratvej S, Visalsawadi P, Likitarunrat S. *Sarcocystis* infection and actinomycosis in tumorous eosinophilic enterocolitis. *J Med Assoc Thai* 1992; **75 Suppl. 1**: 71–5

96 Dubey JP. Neosporosis in cattle: biology and economic impact. *J Am Vet Med Assoc* 1999; **214**: 1160–3

97 Dubey JP, Lindsay DS. A review of *Neospora caninum* and neosporosis. *Vet Parasitol* 1996; **67**: 1–59

98 Dubey JP, Carpenter JL, Speer CA, Topper MJ, Uggla A. Newly recognized fatal protozoan disease of dogs. *J Am Vet Med Assoc* 1988; **192**: 1269–85

99 Adam RD. The biology of *Giardia* spp. *Microbiol Rev* 1991; **55**: 706–32

100 Rickard LG, Siefker C, Boyle CR, Gentz EJ. The prevalence of *Cryptosporidium* and *Giardia* spp. in fecal samples from free-ranging white-tailed deer (*Odocoileus virginianus*) in the southeastern United States. *J Vet Diagn Invest* 1999; **11**: 65–72

101 Bednarska M, Bajer A, Sinski E. Calves as a potential reservoir of *Cryptosporidium parvum* and *Giardia* spp. *Ann Agric Environ Med* 1998; **5**: 135–8

102 O'Handley RM, Cockwill C, McAllister TA, Jelinski M, Morck DW, Olson ME. Duration of naturally acquired giardiosis and cryptosporidiosis in dairy calves and their association with diarrhea. *J Am Vet Med Assoc* 1999; **214**: 391–6

103 Erlandsen SL, Sherlock LA, Januschka M *et al.* Cross-species transmission of *Giardia* spp.: inoculation of beavers and muskrats with cysts of human, beaver, mouse, and muskrat origin. *Appl Environ Microbiol* 1988; **54**: 2777–85

104 Schaefer III FW, Johnson CH, Hsu CH, Rice EW. Determination of *Giardia lamblia* cyst infective dose for the Mongolian gerbil (*Meriones unguiculatus*). *Appl Environ Microbiol* 1991; **57**: 2408–9

105 Nash TE, Herrington DA, Levine MM, Conrad JT, Merritt Jr JW. Antigenic variation of *Giardia lamblia* in experimental human infections. *J Immunol* 1990; **144**: 4362–9

106 Wolfe MS. Giardiasis. *Clin Microbiol Rev* 1992; **5**: 93–100

107 De Jonckheere JF, Majewska AC, Kasprzak W. *Giardia* isolates from primates and rodents display the same molecular polymorphism as human isolates. *Mol Biochem Parasitol* 1990; **39**: 23–9

108 Proctor EM, Isaac-Renton JL, Boyd J, Wong Q, Bowie WR. Isoenzyme analysis of human and animal isolates of *Giardia duodenalis* from British Columbia, Canada. *Am J Trop Med Hyg* 1989; **41**: 411–5

109 Stranden AM, Eckert J, Kohler P. Electrophoretic characterization of *Giardia* isolated from humans, cattle, sheep, and a dog in Switzerland. *J Parasitol* 1990; **76**: 660–8

110 Chaudhuri P, De A, Bhattacharya A, Pal SC, Das P. Identification of heterogeneity in human isolates of *Giardia lamblia* by isoenzyme studies. *Zentralbl Bakteriol* 1991; **274**: 490–5

111 Morgan UM, Constantine CC, Greene WK, Thompson RC. RAPD (random amplified polymorphic DNA) analysis of *Giardia* DNA and correlation with isoenzyme data. *Trans R Soc Trop Med Hyg* 1993; **87**: 702–5

112 Homan WL, van Enckevort FH, Limper L *et al.* Comparison of *Giardia* isolates from different laboratories by isoenzyme analysis and recombinant DNA probes. *Parasitol Res* 1992; **78**: 316–23

113 Mohareb EW, Rogers EJ, Weiner EJ, Bruce JI. *Giardia lamblia*: phospholipid analysis of human isolates. *Ann Trop Med Parasitol* 1991; **85**: 591–7

114 Forrest M, Isaac-Renton J, Bowie W. Immunoblot patterns of *Giardia duodenalis* isolates from different hosts and geographical locations. *Can J Microbiol* 1990; **36**: 42–6

115 Archibald SC, Mitchell RW, Upcroft JA, Boreham PF, Upcroft P. Variation between human and animal isolates of *Giardia* as demonstrated by DNA fingerprinting. *Int J Parasitol* 1991; **21**: 123-4

116 Campbell SR, van Keulen H, Erlandsen SL, Senturia JB, Jarroll EL. *Giardia* spp.: comparison of electrophoretic karyotypes. *Exp Parasitol* 1990; **71**: 470–82

117 Upcroft JA, Boreham PF, Upcroft P. Geographic variation in *Giardia* karyotypes. *Int J Parasitol* 1989; **19**: 519–27

118 Upcroft P, Mitchell R, Boreham PF. DNA fingerprinting of the intestinal parasite *Giardia duodenalis* with the M13 phage genome. *Int J Parasitol* 1990; **20**: 319–23

119 Upcroft P. DNA fingerprinting of the human intestinal parasite *Giardia intestinalis* with hypervariable minisatellite sequences. *EXS* 1991; **58**: 70–84

120 Mahbubani MH, Bej AK, Perlin MH, Schaefer III FW, Jakubowski W, Atlas RM. Differentiation of *Giardia duodenalis* from other *Giardia* spp. by using polymerase chain reaction and gene probes. *J Clin Microbiol* 1992; **30**: 74–8

121 Majewska AC, Kasprzak W. Axenic isolation of *Giardia* strains from primates and rodents. *Vet Parasitol* 1990; **35**: 169–74

122 Nash TE, Conrad JT, Merritt Jr JW. Variant specific epitopes of *Giardia lamblia*. *Mol Biochem Parasitol* 1990; **42**: 125–32

123 Hopkins RS, Juranek DD. Acute giardiasis: an improved clinical case definition for epidemiologic studies. *Am J Epidemiol* 1991; **133**: 402–7

124 Rose JB, Haas CN, Regli S. Risk assessment and control of waterborne giardiasis. *Am J Public Health* 1991; **81**: 709–13

125 Moorehead WP, Guasparini R, Donovan CA, Mathias RG, Cottle R, Baytalan G. Giardiasis outbreak from a chlorinated community water supply. *Can J Public Health* 1990; **81**: 358–62

126 Birkhead G, Vogt RL. Epidemiologic surveillance for endemic *Giardia lamblia* infection in Vermont. The roles of waterborne and person-to-person transmission. *Am J Epidemiol* 1989; **129**: 762–8

127 Neringer R, Andersson Y, Eitrem R. A water-borne outbreak of giardiasis in Sweden. *Scand J Infect Dis* 1987; **19**: 85–90

128 Greensmith CT, Stanwick RS, Elliot BE, Fast MV. Giardiasis associated with the use of a water slide. *Pediatr Infect Dis J* 1988; **7**: 91–4

129 Porter JD, Ragazzoni HP, Buchanon JD, Waskin HA, Juranek DD, Parkin WE. *Giardia* transmission in a swimming pool. *Am J Public Health* 1988; **78**: 659–62

130 Porter JD, Gaffney C, Heymann D, Parkin W. Food-borne outbreak of *Giardia lamblia*. *Am J Public Health* 1990; **80**:1259–60

131 White KE, Hedberg CW, Edmonson LM, Jones DB, Osterholm MT, MacDonald KL. An outbreak of giardiasis in a nursing home with evidence for multiple modes of transmission. *J Infect Dis* 1989; **160**: 298–304

132 Anon. Common-source outbreak of giardiasis – New Mexico. *MMWR Morb Mortal Wkly Rep* 1989; **38**: 405–7

133 Petersen LR, Cartter ML, Hadler JL. A food-borne outbreak of *Giardia lamblia*. *J Infect Dis* 1988; **157**: 846–8

134 Silberman JD, Clark CG, Sogin ML. *Dientamoeba fragilis* shares a recent common evolutionary history with the trichomonads. *Mol Biochem Parasitol* 1996; **76**: 311–4

135 van Gool T, Dankert J. [3 emerging protozoal infections in The Netherlands: *Cyclospora*, *Dientamoeba*, and *Microspora* infections] Drie opkomende protozoaire infectieziekten in Nederland: *Cyclospora*-, *Dientamoeba*- en *Microspora*-infecties. *Ned Tijdschr Geneeskd* 1996; **140**: 155–60

136 Shein R, Gelb A. Colitis due to *Dientamoeba fragilis*. *Am J Gastroenterol* 1983; **78**: 634–6

137 Preiss U, Ockert G, Broemme S, Otto A. On the clinical importance of *Dientamoeba fragilis* infections in childhood. *J Hyg Epidemiol Microbiol Immunol* 1991; **35**: 27–34

138 Cuffari C, Oligny L, Seidman EG. *Dientamoeba fragilis* masquerading as allergic colitis. *J Pediatr Gastroenterol Nutr* 1998; **26**: 16–20

139 Windsor JJ, Rafay AM, Shenoy AK, Johnson EH. Incidence of *Dientamoeba fragilis* in faecal samples submitted for routine microbiological analysis. *Br J Biomed Sci* 1998; **55**: 172–5

140 Oyofo BA, Peruski LF, Ismail TF *et al.* Enteropathogens associated with diarrhea among military personnel during Operation Bright Star 96, in Alexandria, Egypt. *Mil Med* 1997; **162**: 396–400

141 Kabani A, Cadrain G, Trevenen C, Jadavji T, Church DL. Practice guidelines for ordering stool ova and parasite testing in a pediatric population. The Alberta Children's Hospital. *Am J Clin Pathol* 1995; **104**: 272–8

142 Grendon JH, DiGiacomo RF, Frost FJ. *Dientamoeba fragilis* detection methods and prevalence: a survey of state public health laboratories. *Public Health Rep* 1991; **106**: 322–5

143 Bruchhaus I, Jacobs T, Leippe M, Tannich E. *Entamoeba histolytica* and *Entamoeba dispar*: differences in numbers and expression of cysteine proteinase genes. *Mol Microbiol* 1996; **22**: 255–63

144 Jacobs T, Bruchhaus I, Dandekar T, Tannich E, Leippe M. Isolation and molecular characterization of a surface-bound proteinase of *Entamoeba histolytica*. *Mol Microbiol* 1998; **27**: 269–76

145 Myjak P, Kur J, Pietkiewicz H. Usefulness of new DNA extraction procedure for PCR technique in species identification of *Entamoeba* isolates. *Wiad Parazytol* 1997; **43**: 163–70

146 Haque R, Neville LM, Hahn P, Petri-WA J. Rapid diagnosis of *Entamoeba* infection by using

Entamoeba and *Entamoeba histolytica* stool antigen detection kits. *J Clin Microbiol* 1995; **33**: 2558–61

147 Stenzel DJ, Boreham PF. *Blastocystis hominis* revisited. *Clin Microbiol Rev* 1996; **9**: 563–84

148 Horiki N, Maruyama M, Fujita Y, Yonekura T, Minato S, Kaneda Y. Epidemiologic survey of *Blastocystis hominis* infection in Japan. *Am J Trop Med Hyg* 1997; **56**: 370–4

149 Jelinek T, Peyerl G, Loscher T, von Sonnenburg F, Nothdurft HD. The role of *Blastocystis hominis* as a possible intestinal pathogen in travellers. *J Infect* 1997; **35**: 63–6

150 Shlim DR, Hoge CW, Rajah R, Rabold JG, Echeverria P. Is *Blastocystis hominis* a cause of diarrhea in travelers? A prospective controlled study in Nepal [see comments]. *Clin Infect Dis* 1995; **21**: 97–101

151 Garavelli PL, Zierdt CH, Fleisher TA, Liss H, Nagy B. Serum antibody detected by fluorescent antibody test in patients with symptomatic *Blastocystis hominis* infection. *Rec Prog Med* 1995; **86**: 398–400

152 al Tawil YS, Gilger MA, Gopalakrishna GS, Langston C, Bommer KE. Invasive *Blastocystis hominis* infection in a child. *Arch Pediatr Adolesc Med* 1994; **148**: 882–5

153 Zuckerman MJ, Watts MT, Ho H, Meriano FV. *Blastocystis hominis* infection and intestinal injury. *Am J Med Sci* 1994; **308**: 96–101

154 Albrecht H, Stellbrink HJ, Koperski K, Greten H. *Blastocystis hominis* in human immunodeficiency virus-related diarrhea. *Scand J Gastroenterol* 1995; **30**: 909–14

155 Gericke AS, Burchard GD, Knobloch J, Walderich B. Isoenzyme patterns of *Blastocystis hominis* patient isolates derived from symptomatic and healthy carriers. *Trop Med Int Health* 1997; **2**: 245–53

156 Konig G, Muller HE. *Blastocystis hominis* in animals: incidence of four serogroups. *Zentralbl Bakteriol* 1997; **286**: 435–40

157 Yoshikawa H, Nagono I, Yap EH, Singh M, Takahashi Y. DNA polymorphism revealed by arbitrary primers polymerase chain reaction among *Blastocystis* strains isolated from humans, a chicken, and a reptile. *J Eukaryot Microbiol* 1996; **43**: 127–30

158 Nimri L, Batchoun R. Intestinal colonization of symptomatic and asymptomatic schoolchildren with *Blastocystis hominis*. *J Clin Microbiol* 1994; **32**: 2865–6

159 Zaman V, Khan KZ, Khan MA, Khan MA. Isolation of *Blastocystis hominis* from sewage. *Southeast Asian J Trop Med Public Health* 1994; **25**: 211

160 Keohane EM, Weiss LM. Characterization and function of the microsporidian polar tube: a review. *Folia Parasitol (Praha)* 1998; **45**: 117–27

161 Kotler DP, Orenstein JM. Clinical syndromes associated with microsporidiosis. *Adv Parasitol* 1998; **40**: 321–49

162 Scaglia M, Gatti S, Sacchi L *et al*. Asymptomatic respiratory tract microsporidiosis due to *Encephalitozoon hellem* in three patients with AIDS. *Clin Infect Dis* 1998; **26**: 174–6

163 Sobottka I, Schwartz DA, Schottelius J *et al*. Prevalence and clinical significance of intestinal microsporidiosis in human immunodeficiency virus-infected patients with and without diarrhea in Germany: a prospective coprodiagnostic study. *Clin Infect Dis* 1998; **26**: 475–80

164 Svenungsson B, Capraru T, Evengard B, Larsson R, Lebbad M. Intestinal microsporidiosis in a HIV-seronegative patient. *Scand J Infect Dis* 1998; **30**: 314–6

165 Gunnarsson G, Hurlbut D, DeGirolami PC, Federman M, Wanke C. Multiorgan microsporidiosis: report of five cases and review. *Clin Infect Dis* 1995; **21**: 37–44

166 Georges E, Rabaud C, Amiel C *et al*. *Enterocytozoon bieneusi* multiorgan microsporidiosis in a HIV-infected patient. *J Infect* 1998; **36**: 223–5

167 del Aguila C, Lopez-Velez R, Fenoy S *et al*. Identification of *Enterocytozoon bieneusi* spores in respiratory samples from an AIDS patient with a 2-year history of intestinal microsporidiosis. *J Clin Microbiol* 1997; **35**: 1862–6

168 Franzen C, Muller A, Hartmann P *et al*. Polymerase chain reaction for diagnosis and species differentiation of microsporidia. *Folia Parasitol (Praha)* 1998; **45**: 140–8

169 Gainzarain JC, Canut A, Lozano M *et al*. Detection of *Enterocytozoon bieneusi* in two human immunodeficiency virus-negative patients with chronic diarrhea by polymerase chain reaction in duodenal biopsy specimens and review. *Clin Infect Dis* 1998; **27**: 394–8

170 Gumbo T, Sarbah S, Gangaidzo IT *et al*. Intestinal parasites in patients with diarrhea and human immunodeficiency virus infection in Zimbabwe. *AIDS* 1999; **13**: 819–21

171 Muller A, Stellermann K, Hartmann P *et al*. A powerful DNA extraction method and PCR for detection of microsporidia in clinical stool specimens. *Clin Diagn Lab Immunol* 1999; 6: 243–6

172 Velasquez JN, Carnevale S, Labbe JH, Chertcoff A, Cabrera MG, Oelemann W. *In situ* hybridization: a molecular approach for the diagnosis of the microsporidian parasite *Enterocytozoon bieneusi*. *Hum Pathol* 1999; 30: 54–8

173 Dowd SE, Gerba CP, Kamper M, Pepper IL. Evaluation of methodologies including immunofluorescent assay (IFA) and the polymerase chain reaction (PCR) for detection of human pathogenic microsporidia in water. *J Microbiol Methods* 1999; 35: 43–52

174 Sparfel JM, Sarfati C, Liguory O et al. Detection of microsporidia and identification of *Enterocytozoon bieneusi* in surface water by filtration followed by specific PCR. *J Eukaryot Microbiol* 1997; 44: 78S

175 Dowd SE, Gerba CP, Pepper IL. Confirmation of the human-pathogenic microsporidia *Enterocytozoon bieneusi*, *Encephalitozoon intestinalis*, and *Vittaforma corneae* in water. *Appl Environ Microbiol* 1998; 64: 3332–5

176 Talal AH, Kotler DP, Orenstein JM, Weiss LM. Detection of *Enterocytozoon bieneusi* in fecal specimens by polymerase chain reaction analysis with primers to the small-subunit rRNA. *Clin Infect Dis* 1998; 26: 673–5

177 da Silva AJ, Bornay-Llinares FJ, del Aguila de la Puente *et al*. Diagnosis of *Enterocytozoon bieneusi* (microsporidia) infections by polymerase chain reaction in stool samples using primers based on the region coding for small-subunit ribosomal RNA. *Arch Pathol Lab Med* 1997; 121: 874–9

178 Kock NP, Petersen H, Fenner T *et al*. Species-specific identification of microsporidia in stool and intestinal biopsy specimens by the polymerase chain reaction. *Eur J Clin Microbiol Infect Dis* 1997; 16: 369–76

179 Liguory O, David F, Sarfati C *et al*. Diagnosis of infections caused by *Enterocytozoon bieneusi* and *Encephalitozoon intestinalis* using polymerase chain reaction in stool specimens [see comments]. *AIDS* 1997; 11: 723–6

180 Ombrouck C, Ciceron L, Biligui S *et al*. Specific PCR assay for direct detection of intestinal microsporidia *Enterocytozoon bieneusi* and *Encephalitozoon intestinalis* in fecal specimens from human immunodeficiency virus-infected patients. *J Clin Microbiol* 1997; 35: 652–5

181 Liguory O, David F, Sarfati C, Derouin F, Molina JM. Determination of types of *Enterocytozoon bieneusi* strains isolated from patients with intestinal microsporidiosis. *J Clin Microbiol* 1998; 36: 1882–5

182 Rinder H, Katzwinkel-Wladarsch S, Loscher T. Evidence for the existence of genetically distinct strains of *Enterocytozoon bieneusi*. *Parasitol Res* 1997; 83: 670–2

183 Breitenmoser AC, Mathis A, Burgi E, Weber R, Deplazes P. High prevalence of *Enterocytozoon bieneusi* in swine with four genotypes that differ from those identified in humans. *Parasitology* 1999; 118: 447–53

184 Mathis A, Breitenmoser AC, Deplazes P. Detection of new *Enterocytozoon* genotypes in faecal samples of farm dogs and a cat. *Parasite* 1999; 6: 189–93

185 Chalifoux LV, MacKey J, Carville A *et al*. Ultrastructural morphology of *Enterocytozoon bieneusi* in biliary epithelium of rhesus macaques (*Macaca mulatta*). *Vet Pathol* 1998; 35: 292–6

186 Kondova I, Mansfield K, Buckholt MA *et al*. Transmission and serial propagation of *Enterocytozoon bieneusi* from humans and rhesus macaques in gnotobiotic piglets. *Infect Immun* 1998; 66: 5515–9

187 Snowden KF, Didier ES, Orenstein JM, Shadduck JA. Animal models of human microsporidial infections. *Lab Anim Sci* 1998; 48: 589–92

188 Visvesvara G, Leitch GJ, Pieniazek NJ *et al*. Short-term *in vitro* culture and molecular analysis of the microsporidian, *Enterocytozoon bieneusi*. *J Eukaryot Microbiol* 1995; 42: 506–10

189 Carr A, Marriott D, Field A, Vasak E, Cooper DA. Treatment of HIV-1-associated microsporidiosis and cryptosporidiosis with combination antiretroviral therapy [see comments]. *Lancet* 1998; 351: 256–61

190 Orenstein JM, Dieterich DT, Kotler DP. Systemic dissemination by a newly recognized intestinal microsporidia species in AIDS. *AIDS* 1992; 6: 1143–50

191 Molina JM, Oksenhendler E, Beauvais B *et al*. Disseminated microsporidiosis due to *Septata*

intestinalis in patients with AIDS: clinical features and response to albendazole therapy. *J Infect Dis* 1995; **171**: 245–9

192 Moura H, Sodre FC, Bornay-Llinares FJ *et al.* Detection by an immunofluorescence test of *Encephalitozoon intestinalis* spores in routinely formalin-fixed stool samples stored at room temperature. *J Clin Microbiol* 1999; **37**: 2317–22

193 Boldorini R, Monga G, Tosoni A *et al.* Renal *Encephalitozoon (Septata) intestinalis* infection in a patient with AIDS. Post-mortem identification by means of transmission electron microscopy and PCR. *Virchows Arch* 1998; **432**: 535–9

194 Dowd SE, Gerba CP, Enriquez FJ, Pepper IL. PCR amplification and species determination of microsporidia in formalin-fixed feces after immunomagnetic separation. *Appl Environ Microbiol* 1998; **64**: 333–6

195 Katzwinkel-Wladarsch S, Deplazes P, Weber R, Loscher T, Rinder H. Comparison of polymerase chain reaction with light microscopy for detection of microsporidia in clinical specimens. *Eur J Clin Microbiol Infect Dis* 1997; **16**: 7–10

196 Bornay-Llinares FJ, da Silva AJ, Moura H *et al.* Immunologic, microscopic, and molecular evidence of *Encephalitozoon intestinalis (Septata intestinalis)* infection in mammals other than humans. *J Infect Dis* 1998; **178**: 820–6

197 Croppo GP, Croppo GP, Moura H *et al.* Ultrastructure, immunofluorescence, Western blot, and PCR analysis of eight isolates of *Encephalitozoon (Septata) intestinalis* established in culture from sputum and urine samples and duodenal aspirates of five patients with AIDS. *J Clin Microbiol* 1998; **36**: 1201–8

198 Katiyar SK, Edlind TD. *In vitro* susceptibilities of the AIDS-associated microsporidian *Encephalitozoon intestinalis* to albendazole, its sulfoxide metabolite, and 12 additional benzimidazole derivatives. *Antimicrob Agents Chemother* 1997; **41**: 2729–32

199 Raynaud L, Delbac F, Broussolle V *et al.* Identification of *Encephalitozoon intestinalis* in travelers with chronic diarrhea by specific PCR amplification. *J Clin Microbiol* 1998; **36**: 37–40

200 Grau A, Valls ME, Williams JE, Ellis DS, Muntane MJ, Nadal C. [Myositis caused by *Pleistophora* in a patient with AIDS] Miositis por *Pleistophora* en un paciente con sida. *Med Clin (Barc)* 1996; **107**: 779–81

201 Chupp GL, Alroy J, Adelman LS, Breen JC, Skolnik PR. Myositis due to *Pleistophora (Microsporidia)* in a patient with AIDS. *Clin Infect Dis* 1993; **16**: 15–21

202 Field AS, Marriott DJ, Milliken ST *et al.* Myositis associated with a newly described microsporidian, *Trachipleistophora hominis*, in a patient with AIDS. *J Clin Microbiol* 1996; **34**: 2803–11

203 Vavra J, Yachnis AT, Shadduck JA, Orenstein JM. Microsporidia of the genus *Trachipleistophora* – causative agents of human microsporidiosis: description of *Trachipleistophora anthropophthera* n. sp. (Protozoa: *Microsporidia*). *J Eukaryot Microbiol* 1998; **45**: 273–83

204 Cali A, Meisler DM, Lowder CY *et al.* Corneal microsporidioses: characterization and identification. *J Protozool* 1991; **38**: 215S-7S

205 Silveira H, Canning EU. *Vittaforma corneae* n. comb. for the human microsporidium *Nosema corneum* Shadduck, Meccoli, Davis & Font, 1990, based on its ultrastructure in the liver of experimentally infected athymic mice. *J Eukaryot Microbiol* 1995; **42**: 158–65

206 Didier ES, Didier PJ, Friedberg DN *et al.* Isolation and characterization of a new human microsporidian, *Encephalitozoon hellem* (n. sp.), from three AIDS patients with keratoconjunctivitis. *J Infect Dis* 1991; **163**: 617–21

207 Croppo GP, Visvesvara GS, Leitch GJ, Wallace S, Schwartz DA. Identification of the microsporidian *Encephalitozoon hellem* using immunoglobulin G monoclonal antibodies. *Arch Pathol Lab Med* 1998; **122**: 182–6

208 Mathis A, Tanner I, Weber R, Deplazes P. Genetic and phenotypic intraspecific variation in the microsporidian *Encephalitozoon hellem*. *Int J Parasitol* 1999; **29**: 767–70

209 Canning EU, Curry A, Vavra J, Bonshek RE. Some ultrastructural data on *Microsporidium ceylonensis*, a cause of corneal microsporidiosis. *Parasite* 1998; **5**: 247–54

210 Cali A, Takvorian PM, Lewin S *et al. Brachiola vesicularum*, n. g., n. spp., a new microsporidium associated with AIDS and myositis. *J Eukaryot Microbiol* 1998; **45**: 240–51

211 Hutin YJ, Sombardier MN, Liguory O *et al.* Risk factors for intestinal microsporidiosis in

patients with human immunodeficiency virus infection: a case-control study. *J Infect Dis* 1998; **178**: 904–7

212 Conteas CN, Berlin OG, Lariviere MJ *et al*. Examination of the prevalence and seasonal variation of intestinal microsporidiosis in the stools of persons with chronic diarrhea and human immunodeficiency virus infection. *Am J Trop Med Hyg* 1998; **58**: 559–61

213 Dowd SE, Gerba CP, Pepper IL. Confirmation of the human-pathogenic microsporidia *Enterocytozoon bieneusi*, *Encephalitozoon intestinalis*, and *Vittaforma corneae* in water. *Appl Environ Microbiol* 1998; **64**: 3332–5

214 Yang Y, Zeng L, Li M, Zhou J. Diarrhoea in piglets and monkeys experimentally infected with *Balantidium coli* isolated from human faeces. *J Trop Med Hyg* 1995; **98**: 69–72

215 Pakandl M. The prevalence of intestinal protozoa in wild and domestic pigs. *Vet Med (Praha)* 1994; **39**: 377–80

216 Goldsmid JM, Rogers S. A parasitological study on the chacma baboon (*Papio ursinus*) from the Northern Transvaal. *J S Afr Vet Assoc* 1978; **49**: 109–11

217 Nakauchi K. The prevalence of *Balantidium coli* infection in fifty-six mammalian species. *J Vet Med Sci* 1999; **61**: 63–5

218 DETR. *The Water Supply (Water Quality) (Ammendment) Regulations 1999*. Statutory Instrument 1524 [June 1999]. London: HMSO, 1999

Marine toxins

Kevin Whittle* and **Susan Gallacher†**

*Torry Research Ltd, Aberdeenshire and †Fisheries Research Services, Marine Laboratory, Aberdeen, UK

Seafood products are important both nutritionally and economically. Within Europe, some £12 billion of fishery products are consumed annually and an enormous variety of species are available. Although seafood is rarely implicated in food poisoning, compared to other food sources, it does provide some specific human health hazards unique to this particular resource. Generally, these are toxins from toxic microscopic algae which accumulate through the food-chain. The toxins can cause various neurological and gastrointestinal illnesses and, potentially, consumers are exposed from seafood produced within Europe, from imported products, or from seafood eaten while travelling abroad. The symptoms of illness which may be encountered, the source and mode of action of the toxins, and some emerging problems are described. European legislation aims to ensure the quality and safety of seafood products by prohibiting sale of some toxic species, setting toxin limits, requiring monitoring and controlling imports.

Fish and shellfish are nutritionally and economically valuable. About 16% of all animal protein consumed world-wide comes from the 66 million tonnes of marine species used annually for food. This roughly comprises 75% fish and 25% shellfish, the total value of which, as landed, is estimated to be £40 billion per year, with total international trade in fisheries' products valued at about £68 billion. Within Europe, some £12 billion of fishery end-products are consumed annually, but consumption varies widely among countries, ranging from 13–80 g of edible meat/person/day (average, 31 g/person/day), and most of the northern European countries fall well below the average.

The nutritional value and benefits to health attributed to seafood are well known. Apart from the high quality protein, essential amino acids, vitamin and mineral content, epidemiological studies indicate lower risk for coronary heart disease, hypertension and cancer among populations eating seafood. This is attributed to the long chain, polyunsaturated, n-3

Correspondence to:
Dr Kevin J Whittle,
Cairnview, Old Skene
Road, Westhill,
Aberdeenshire
AB32 6TX, UK

Definitions: 'shellfish' includes bivalve (mussel, scallop, oyster, clam, etc.) and gastropod (whelk, periwinkles, etc.) molluscs, crustaceans (crab, lobster, shrimp, etc.) and cephalopods (octopus, cuttlefish, squid); 'seafood' includes fish and shellfish from sea, coastal and estuarine sources.

British Medical Bulletin 2000;**56** (No. 1): 236–253

© Crown copyright 2000

fatty acids (PUFAs) for which seafood is the only natural dietary source. PUFAs are also essential for normal development of neural, cerebral and visual functions[1]. For these reasons, people have been encouraged to choose seafood as healthy food, particularly important in northern Europe, where deaths from coronary heart disease in 1986 ranged from 245 to 625 annually per 100,000 men.

Compared with other sources of animal protein in the food-chain, an enormous variety of seafood is available. About 150 species are traded at London's Billingsgate market daily, including many imported from around the world. Although seafood is rarely implicated in food poisoning compared to other food sources, it does provide some specific, potential, human, health hazards that are a consequence of the marine environment. These include toxic syndromes[2-5] which may result from spoilage of fish products, or from specific toxins which accumulate in fish and shellfish[6-9], particularly bivalves. With these syndromes, seafood shows no visible sign of contamination and illness is generally characterised by a rapid onset of symptoms within hours (Table 1). Diagnosis may be complicated by the presence of more than one type of toxin. The toxins, the symptoms, mode of action and the incidence of seafood toxin related illnesses are detailed below.

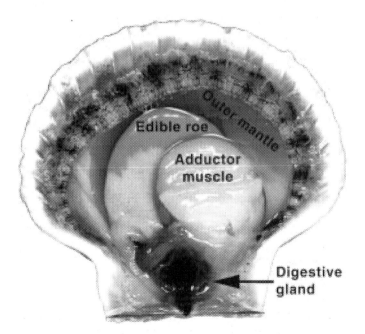

Fig. 1 The soft tissues of an opened bivalve mollusc, the scallop, *Pecten maximus*, showing the digestive gland (hepatopancreas), outer mantle, and the edible roe and adductor muscle. Toxins normally accumulate in the digestive gland, roe and other viscera, but may also be found in the adductor muscle especially when toxin levels are high. Scallops intoxicated with PSP or ASP toxins depurate slowly so that toxic incidents are prolonged.

Table 1 Toxic syndromes associated with seafood, symptoms, mode of action of toxins and regulatory limits

Syndrome/toxin/agent	Range of symptoms	Onset/treatment	Mode of action/regulatory limit in Europe*
Paralytic shellfish poisoning Saxitoxin and derivatives Dinoflagellates	Tingling and burning in face, lips and tongue, peppery taste, paraesthesia and numbness, mild headache and dizziness, muscular weakness, giddiness, incoherent speech, ataxia, motor incoordination, dysmetria, nausea and vomiting, respiratory difficulties and paralysis, hypoxia, hypercapnia, death	Within 30 min to 3–4 h Artificial respiration	Block sodium channels 80 μg/100 g
Diarrhetic shellfish poisoning Okadaic acid and derivatives Dinoflagellates	Acute diarrhoea, nausea, vomiting, abdominal pain, and chills	Within 30 min to 3–12 h Non-specific, supportive	Inhibit essential protein phosphatases Not detected by bioassay
Amnesic shellfish poisoning Domoic acid and analogues Diatoms	Nausea, vomiting, abdominal cramps, diarrhoea, severe headache, dizziness, visual disturbance, weakness, lethargy, mild disorientation, difficulty walking, cranial nerve abnormalities, acute confusion, autonomic nervous system dysfunction, memory loss, deep pain sensation, seizure, coma, death	Gastrointestinal within 24 h Neurological within 48 h Non-specific, supportive	Agonists for glutamate receptors 20 μg/g
Neurotoxic shellfish poisoning Brevetoxins Dinoflagellates	Paraesthesia, dizziness, abdominal pain, nausea, diarrhoea, muscle weakness, unsteady walking, chills, reversal hot/cold sensation, headache, muscle and joint pain, vomiting, double vision, difficulty in breathing. Conjunctivitis and respiratory irritation occur after exposure to sea spray contaminated with lysed, toxic cells	Within 3–6 h Non-specific, supportive	Open sodium channels Not specified
Ciguatera fish poisoning Ciguatoxins, maitotoxin, (possibly others) Dinoflagellates	Prickling of lips, tongue and throat, numbness, headache, arthralgia, erythema, dizziness, cyanosis, insomnia, prostration, ataxia, myalgia, severe pain in arms and legs, visual disturbance and pain, skin disorders and loss of hair and nails, reversal of temperature perception ('dry-ice' sensation), motor incoordination, paralysis, coma, death	Within 3–30 h Symptoms may recur, e.g. after alcohol consumption Mannitol may be effective	Ciguatoxins: open sodium channels Maitotoxin: opens calcium channels Not permitted
Scrombroid fish poisoning Scombroid and clupeoid fish, aetiology unknown	Bright red, sometimes itchy rash on face neck and chest, hot flushing and sweating, tingling of the lips, mouth and tongue, headache, burning in the mouth and peppery taste, swelling or soreness of the tongue, swelling of the face, wheeziness, nausea, abdominal pain, cramps, vomiting, diarrhoea, dizziness, blurred vision, loss of vision, cardiovascular shock, atrial tachycardia	Within a few minutes to a few hours Antihistamines are usually effective	Histamine limits are used as a control measure: 100 ppm (batch mean of 9 samples: 2 samples can be > 100 ppm but < 200 ppm; no sample can be >200 ppm)
Red whelk poisoning Metabolite tetramine	Blurred vision, muscular twitching, tingling of hands and feet, weakness, paralysis and collapse; nausea, vomiting and diarrhoea occur in some cases	Within 30 min to 2 h Non-specific, supportive	Tetramine Not specified
Puffer fish poisoning Tetrodotoxins may be produced by bacteria	Numbness of face and extremities, floating sensation, weakness, ascending paralysis, respiratory failure, cardiovascular collapse, death	Usually within 3 h Artificial respiration	Block sodium channels Not permitted

*Concentrations for the limits in tissues are as specified in the Directives (and amendments) 91/492/EEC and 91/493/EEC.

Toxins produced by phytoplankton

Bivalve molluscs, such as mussels, filter-feed on microscopic algae. About 40 of some 5000 species of these marine phytoplankton, primarily dino-flagellates and diatoms, produce potent toxins[9]. These accumulate in shellfish tissues and are harmful to man when contaminated bivalves are eaten. Other marine animals, such as gastropods, crustaceans and fish, can also accumulate the toxins through the food-chain and pose a threat to seafood consumers. Once contaminated, some shellfish depurate the toxins relatively quickly, whereas others, such as scallops, can retain the toxins for months and even years, particularly in the digestive gland and the gonad (Fig. 1).

Occurrence of these phytoplankton, and shellfish toxins is widespread in both temperate and tropical waters (Fig. 2)[8]. On some occasions, proliferation of certain species of planktonic algae, leads to 'blooms' which discolour the water red, brown, or green, giving rise to the confusing term 'red tide'. Blooms do not have to occur for shellfish to become toxic and phytoplankton normally associated with toxins do not

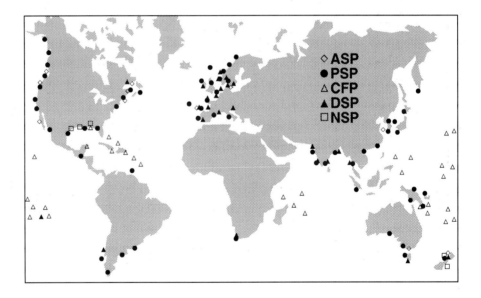

Fig. 2 Current global distribution of the toxins of amnesic shellfish poisoning (ASP), paralytic shellfish poisoning (PSP), ciguatera fish poisoning (CFP), diarrhetic shellfish poisoning (DSP), and neurotoxic shellfish poisoning (NSP) in phytoplankton and seafood. Note the narrow distribution of NSP in the Gulf of Mexico, Florida and New Zealand, CFP in tropical and sub-tropical waters, and the limited distribution of ASP in temperate waters (modified after Leftley and Hannah[8]).

always produce toxins. Indeed, the conditions which trigger the occurrence of toxic phytoplankton species or the production of toxins are not well understood and cannot be predicted accurately. Different species producing different toxins may be present at the same time.

The toxic syndromes which may occur from seafood harvested within Europe are paralytic shellfish poisoning (PSP), diarrhetic shellfish poisoning (DSP) and amnesic shellfish poisoning (ASP). Europeans may also be exposed to two other syndromes through contaminated seafood imports or while eating toxic seafood when travelling abroad. These include neurotoxic shellfish poisoning (NSP) and ciguatera fish poisoning (CFP). All of these toxic syndromes are described in more detail below.

Paralytic shellfish poisoning (PSP)

Illness and death from PSP have been recorded for centuries. Globally (Fig. 2), these toxins are the most common and widespread of the shellfish toxins, and PSP incidents seem to be increasing[10]. Although no outbreaks have been recorded in the UK since 1968[11], toxic shellfish occur frequently.

PSP is a distinctive, neurological illness caused by a group of 20 closely related tetrahydropurine, water soluble, heat stable compounds[8], the paralytic shellfish toxins (PSTs). They vary in potency and are present in toxic shellfish in different concentrations and combinations. They also convert from one form to another[8,10], causing a change in the overall, potential, toxic hazard. Saxitoxin (STX), which was characterised first, is the most potent. In high enough doses, PSP can kill within 2 h and there is no antidote[4]. Exposure is mostly by eating bivalves, such as mussels, scallops and clams, but PSP has also been reported following the consumption of crustacea, gastropods and fish. Generally, dinoflagellates, specifically *Alexandrium* spp. (Fig. 3), are the source of PSTs in Europe; however, zooplankton may act as a vector[10]. PSTs are also produced by several species of cyanobacteria and, more controversially, by marine bacteria[8].

PSTs block neuronal and muscular, voltage-gated, sodium channels, stopping signal transmission[8]. Table 1 lists the symptoms of PSP which generally start with numbness around lips and mouth spreading to face and neck, with prickly sensations in the extremities, followed by impaired muscle contraction. The pulse and heart are not normally affected[10]. In severe cases, symptoms may progress to death, attributed to asphyxiation due to progressive respiratory muscle paralysis. In some instances, death can be prevented by artificial respiration. If the patient survives 18 h, the prognosis is good with rapid and complete recovery[4,10]. Levels at which human intoxification have been reported vary considerably due to

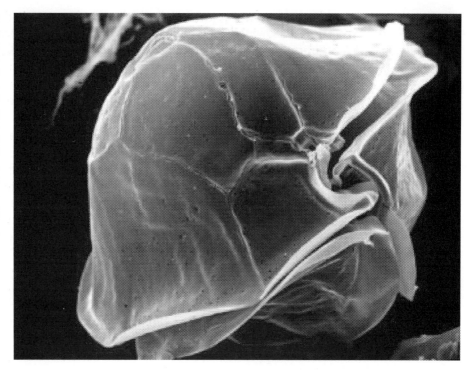

Fig. 3 The dinoflagellate *Alexandrium tamarense* from a water column sample from West Loch Tarbet, Scotland. Cell *circa* 35 μm across. This organism can survive long periods in a dormant, encysted form which can vegetate when conditions are right. (Picture by Jane Lewis, University of Westminster.

differences in individual susceptibility, methods of analysis, and verification of the quantity of material actually consumed. Illness has been reported at doses of 144–1660 μg STX equivalents/person, and fatalities at 300–12,400 μg STX equivalents/person[4].

Diarrhetic shellfish poisoning (DSP)

DSP is primarily a gastrointestinal illness with the first suspected incident occurring in The Netherlands in 1961. After outbreaks in Japan in the late 1970s, the causative agent and toxins involved were identified[12]. DSP is caused primarily by the lipophilic, polyether compound okadaic acid (OA) and derivatives, the dinophysistoxins (DTXs). They inhibit essential serine/threonine protein phosphatases which regulate metabolic processes in eukaryotic cells. Phosphorylated proteins accumulate, leading to calcium influx, cAMP or prostaglandin production, and continued secretion of fluid in gut cells resulting in diarrhoea. Dinoflagellates, particularly species of the genera *Dinophysis* and *Prorocentrum*, are the source[12] and different toxins seem to dominate in shellfish depending on geography, *e.g.* OA in the UK and DTX-2 in Ireland[8].

OA and DTXs are frequently found in European shellfish (Fig. 2) with several food poisoning outbreaks noted. In the UK, DSP toxins were first detected in cockles in 1991, from the Thames estuary. Subsequently, two instances of DSP have occurred in the UK; the first, in 1994, involved imported mussels; the second, in 1997, involved UK mussels harvested from an unauthorised UK site and contained concentrations of 25–36 μg OA/100 g[13].

A mouse bioassay is the principal test for these toxins. Due to its non-specific nature, other compounds lethal to mice were identified in shellfish and named pectenotoxins (PTXs) and yessotoxins (YTXs). Neither PTX nor YTX have been reported to cause human illness. The threat to human health from these compounds and inclusion in the DSP toxin group are debatable; it is a view that they should be excluded[4,8,12]. Evidence for their toxicological effects is based on animal studies which show that PTXs are hepatotoxic. YTX does not cause diarrhoea although signs of cardiac damage have been observed. Some researchers consider that these adverse effects, particularly for YTX, occur only at doses to which humans are unlikely to be exposed.

Symptoms of OA related DSP are listed in Table 1 and diarrhoea is dominant. Although the illness is severe, it is self-limiting. Patients generally recover within 3–4 days and few require hospitalisation[4]. However, since OA and DTX have potent tumour promoting and immunosuppressent activity in animals, the effects of repeated human exposure are a matter of concern[12].

Amnesic shellfish poisoning (ASP)

In Canada, in 1987, 107 people became ill, primarily with gastroenteritis, after eating mussels harvested from Prince Edward Island. Those affected most severely developed neurological symptoms, including memory loss. The toxin was later identified as domoic acid (DA), a water soluble, heat stable, amino acid of molecular mass 111 Da[14]. DA had been identified previously in various red seaweeds but, in this case, the source was a diatom, *Pseudo-nitzschia multiseries*. This was considered unusual, as shellfish toxins were previously only attributed to dinoflagellates. Later studies demonstrated that other *Pseudo-nitzschia* spp. also produced DA[15].

DA is a potent glutamate agonist, disrupting normal neurochemical transmission in the brain. It binds to kainate-type glutamate receptors causing continuous stimulation of neurons, with a subsequent increase in cellular calcium, neuronal swelling and death of nerve cells located in the hippocampus[15]. Several analogues of domoic acid, have been identified but their potency is not well defined[16]. Since the Canadian outbreak, DA has been found in shellfish from a number of countries including the USA, Spain and, most recently, the UK (Fig. 2). In the 1991/92 outbreak in the

US, Californian anchovies *inter alia* were found to be toxic. Anchovy processing was halted until levels of ASP detected fell below the level at which action must be taken and no human cases were reported.

The clinical symptoms of ASP are summarised in Table 1. In Canada, a close association between memory loss and age was noted, with those under 40 years more likely to have diarrhoea, and those over 50 years, short-term memory loss lasting from months to years. Those with the most severe neurological deficits, *e.g.* seizures, were either older than 65 years, or had pre-existing illness, such as diabetes, chronic renal failure or hypertension; three older patients died. The quantity of DA ingested ranged from 15–20 mg for an unaffected person, 60–110 mg produced mild symptoms and levels of 135–295 mg caused serious illness[14]. Based on these data and a series of animal studies, a value of 20 µg DA/g was established as the safety limit for DA concentrations in shellfish[14].

Ciguatera fish poisoning (CFP)

CFP has been known for centuries from eating fish from coral reefs and inshore habitats in subtropical and tropical regions, particularly the Caribbean, South Pacific Islands and Australia, within latitudes 35 degrees north and south (Fig. 2)[5]. World-wide, CFP is considered one of the most common types of poisoning from eating fish[17]. Recent estimates indicate that 20,000 new cases of CFP occur annually[18]. CFP outbreaks are generally sporadic and unpredictable, but may be associated with reef disturbances[17]. Travelling to an endemic area of the Caribbean is estimated to carry a 3% chance of acquiring CFP[5]. In Europe, travellers may present with CFP after visiting endemic areas or it may occur after eating imported fish species.

Ciguatoxins (CTXs), and to a lesser extent maitotoxin (MTX), from the dinoflagellate *Gambierdiscus toxicus* are the cause. CTXs are lipophilic, heat stable, acid resistant polyethers of molecular mass approximately 1110 Da, which selectively open voltage sensitive sodium channels of the neuromuscular junction[8,17]. In contrast, MTX is a water soluble, bisulphated compound of molecular mass 3424 Da, which activates both voltage-sensitive and receptor operated calcium channels in the plasma membrane of cells[8,17]. Other poorly defined toxins may also be involved originating from various epiphytic and benthic dinoflagellates including species of *Ostreopsis*, *Prorocentrum* and *Amphidinium*[19].

Herbivorous fish eat these dinoflagellates and are eaten in turn by larger predatory fish which acquire the toxins. Over 400 species, including groupers, sea basses, snappers, sea perches, emperor fish, Spanish mackerel, jacks, trevallies, carangs, wrasses, surgeon fish, parrot fish, mullet, moray eel and barracuda, reportedly cause CFP[17]. The toxins are so prevalent in barracuda that sale is banned in parts of Florida[5] and the Dominican Republic[14]. The head, liver and gonads are more severely intoxicated than the muscle; eating fillets from large fish also poses higher risk. Curiously, a case has been attributed tentatively to farmed Pacific salmon[20].

CFP is characterised by variable combinations of gastrointestinal, neurological and cardiovascular symptoms, probably because combinations of toxins are involved. Medical diagnosis rests on clinical criteria since there is a lack of specific laboratory tests. Symptoms are listed in Table 1 and vary by location and among individuals. People eating similar portions of the same fish may end up with different symptoms or none at all[5]. The most commonly recognised symptom is reversal of temperature perception in which victims interpret cold as burning or 'dry ice' sensation[17]. Illness is usually short-term and self-limited, and there is no antidote. In most cases, digestive symptoms subside within 1–2 days, cardiovascular within 2–5 days, and neuromotor and neurosensory in 2–3 weeks. In severe attacks, neurological symptoms may last years and recur intermittently, induced by consumption of fish, shellfish, alcohol or nuts, and during periods of overwork and stress[17]. Death may occur in 0.1% cases, but can be as high as 20% in isolated outbreaks[5]. Fatalities have been attributed to direct cardiovascular depression, hypovolaemic shock or respiratory paralysis[5]. CFP may be transmitted by sexual intercourse; in pregnant women it can result in premature labour or harm to the fetus, sometimes causing abortion[5]. Intravenous infusion of mannitol may relieve symptoms if administered soon after intoxification. The danger lies in misdiagnosis of the symptoms which can be confused with organophosphate poisoning, botulism, puffer fish poisoning, or shellfish poisoning[5], and even chronic fatigue syndrome[21].

Neurotoxic shellfish poisoning (NSP)

As with PSP, neurotoxic shellfish poisoning (NSP) has been known for centuries. However, unlike PSP it has only been reported from certain parts of the American continent and New Zealand (Fig. 2)[8,22]. The toxic effects are caused by a group of lipophilic, polyether, compounds named brevetoxins which induce influx of sodium ions into voltage dependent sodium channels and hence have a mode of action similar to ciguatoxins. Although several raphidophytes also produce brevetoxins, the most commonly associated agent is the dinoflagellate *Gymnodinium breve*[8,22] (also known as *Ptychodiscus brevis*[8,9]). The organism is responsible for the infamous Florida red tides and causes NSP through the consumption of contaminated shellfish. Seawater aerosols of lysed dinoflagellate cells also cause eye and respiratory irritation[5]. Adverse effects of *G. breve* are noted more for fish, invertebrate and seabird kills[23] rather than serious effects on human health. The clinical symptoms are listed in (Table 1), no deaths have been reported and a full recovery usually occurs within 48 h[5].

Toxins from other sources

Not all seafood syndromes are necessarily associated with phytoplankton; some may be due to toxins which are indigenous to seafood, such as red whelk poisoning. In others, for example, there are some doubts about the source of the toxins, as in scombroid poisoning and puffer fish poisoning. These syndromes are described in more detail below.

Scombroid fish poisoning (SFP)

The most common cause of seafood poisoning world-wide is thought to be scombroid fish poisoning (SFP)[18]. It is an alarming syndrome, but of short duration, and is sometimes described as 'histamine poisoning'[24] or as a 'pseudo-allergic' reaction[25]. This can occur after eating fresh or processed fatty, dark-fleshed, scombroid fish, *e.g.* tuna, bonito, saury and mackerel and, less frequently, after eating other dark-fleshed, non-scombroid fish, *e.g.* jacks, sardines, anchovies, pilchards, herring and mahi-mahi; even abalone and sockeye salmon have been implicated[18,26,27].

Patients exhibit a range of relatively non-specific symptoms. Most cases are mild, and may show tingling of the lips and mouth, mild gastric discomfort and nausea. More severe cases progress rapidly to nausea, vomiting and/or diarrhoea[28]. In very severe cases, cardiovascular shock associated with subendocardial myocardial infarction or acute pulmonary oedema with myocardial ischaemia can occur (Table 1)[29]. Symptoms usually resolve after a few hours without after effects. Unless complicated by shock or respiratory distress, supportive treatment with antihistamines is usually effective.

Generally, SFP has been associated with fish that contain high levels of the free amino acid histidine which is decarboxylated to histamine by some species of the spoilage flora and can reach high levels in the flesh[27,30]. Indeed, histamine is a useful indicator of time and temperature abuse of the fish *post-mortem*, but low histamine levels do not guarantee safe fish. Although SFP has been reported to be due to histamine[30], the aetiology remains uncertain[28,31,32]. Other factors which support histamine as the cause include: (i) the similarity of symptoms to histamine responses; (ii) the presence of elevated histamine and metabolites in the urine of affected patients; and (iii) the successful alleviation of symptoms with antihistamines[30]. However, of the 440 suspected incidents reported in the UK between 1976 and 1990[11], 60% were associated with histamine below 5 mg/100 g, concentrations unlikely to provoke the observed symptoms[28]. In addition, in controlled, medically supervised, volunteer studies[27,28,31], using fresh mackerel with histamine added to a total concentration of 600 mg histamine/100 g flesh, only mild perioral tingling was observed. Some samples of mackerel, proven to be scombrotoxic but low in histamine, elicited the more severe symptoms of vomiting and/or diarrhoea. Prior administration of antihistamines or a mast cell stabiliser suppressed the symptoms in susceptible subjects. Results were consistent with efficient metabolism of histamine in the normal human gut; but, critically, showed no evidence of a dose-response relationship for histamine, no evidence of potentiation of histamine by other biogenic amines, or that differences in sensitivity between subjects had an allergic basis[27,28,31]. It was concluded that dietary (exogenous) histamine had only a minor role in SFP[28]. It was proposed that an unknown agent was involved (possibly an algal toxin(s)[33]) which was a potent degranulator of mast cells, releasing endogenous histamine. This subsequently caused contraction of smooth muscle and the more severe symptoms of vomiting and/or diarrhoea.

Red whelk poisoning

Food poisoning from eating gastropods is quite common in Japan, but less so in Canada, Norway and the UK. In the UK, red whelks (*Neptunea antiqua*) are sometimes mistaken for the common edible whelk (*Buccinum undatum*)[11,34,35]. Although similar in shape, red whelks are usually larger. The shell is pale yellow/orange and smooth with no ribs, *i.e.* without the characteristic ribs and ridges of the edible whelk. Red whelks contain the heat stable metabolite tetramine in the salivary glands which has a curare-like effect causing the symptoms listed in Table 1; nausea, vomiting and diarrhoea occur in some cases[34]. The symptoms develop rapidly and usually resolve within 24 h. It was estimated that cases in the UK became ill after consuming about 1.75–2.5 mg tetramine[34].

Puffer fish poisoning

This is caused by the water soluble tetrodotoxins (TTXs) which are most commonly found in the puffer fish in the Pacific around China and Japan[2,5,9]. Puffer fish poisoning has also been reported in Mexico. The toxins are concentrated in the liver, gonad, roe and skin, but the flesh can also become toxic. In Japan, puffer fish flesh is a delicacy but, despite government licensed preparation to protect consumers, about 50 deaths are reported each year. Ten deaths were reported in Europe from 1974 to 1979 as a result of eating wrongly labelled toxic puffer fish. Sale is no longer permitted in Europe but European travellers may encounter the toxin abroad. The symptoms are listed in Table 1 and the human lethal dose has been reported to be about 2 mg of TTX[2]. Originally, TTX was thought to be an endogenous icthyosarcotoxin. However, there is evidence that a range of common marine bacteria, particularly vibrios, produce TTX or a derivative[2], and may be the primary source, but this is still a matter of debate.

New and emerging toxins

The occurrence of seafood toxins seems to be increasing and new potential food poisoning hazards are continuously being described[9,36]. This is exemplified by the examples given below which emphasise that it is important to maintain a world-wide watching brief.

Azaspiracid

In The Netherlands, in 1995, 8 people became ill with symptoms similar to DSP after eating mussels originating from Ireland. However, this differed from DSP in that only very low concentrations of OA and DTXs were present and mice reacted differently in the bioassay[37]. Research identified the toxic agent as a lipophilic, highly oxygenated, polyether, containing an unusual azaspiro ring structure, azaspiracid. However, the primary source of the toxin[38] and the mode of action are unknown, but animal experiments suggest that the main target organs are the liver and the pancreas[39]. The extent of the risk to public health has yet to be established.

Cyanobacteria toxins

Several cyanobacteria species produce toxins that cause illness. These include the hepatotoxins (microcystins and nodularin), and the neurotoxins (anatoxins and PSTs). Health risks from these sources are generally associated with drinking water, but they have been detected in both freshwater and marine shellfish, although no cases of illness from this source have been reported[8].

Pfiesteria toxins

In the US in 1991, *Pfiesteria piscicida* was identified as a dinoflagellate that produced a definite chemosensory response towards targeted fish, which it killed within minutes. Researchers exposed to cultures of this toxic alga suffered recurrent skin lesions, memory problems, emotional changes and asthenia; residual symptoms lasted at least 6 years[40]. Users of contaminated waterways became ill before and during fish kills caused by this dinoflagellate. *Pfiesteria* was shown to produce two toxins, one of which is a neurotoxin but, to date, they have not been fully characterised. The potential for shellfish to accumulate these toxins and the human health hazard to seafood consumers is currently the topic of further research[41].

Other compounds

Many other compounds associated with marine microalgae are lethal to mice, but are thought to be unlikely to be a health hazard consumers to seafood, *e.g.* gymnodinine and prorocentrolide[8].

Incidence of illness

For the period 1980–1990 in the UK, there were 390 recorded incidents of suspected SFP, 4 incidents of red whelk poisoning and 2 incidents of CFP[11]. Information reported to the WHO Surveillance Programme for Control of Foodborne Infections in Europe, for 1995–1998 lists some 3000 cases of illness attributed to seafood from the 9 countries issuing data, including the UK. These consisted of 275 outbreaks: 26 were due to SFP; 14 viral; 4 bacterial; one DSP; and 230 of unknown origin. These statistics give some idea of the relatively small scale of the problem within Europe, but should be viewed cautiously. Reporting to the WHO Surveillance Programme is patchy and incomplete and it is thought that a significant degree of under-reporting exists. Significantly, the implementation of comprehensive monitoring programmes, particularly in relation to shellfish toxins, prevents a large quantity of contaminated seafood from reaching the market.

Monitoring, control and depuration

Legislation

The EU has defined minimum requirements to ensure that fishery products are not harmful to health by issuing Directives which also require countries exporting to the EU to meet the same standards as the internal market. Council Directive 91/492/EEC and subsequent amendments lay down the health conditions for producing and marketing live bivalve molluscs and include shellfish toxin standards for PSP, DSP and ASP. Authorities in Member States are required to monitor shellfish harvesting areas for the occurrence of toxic phytoplankton, and shellfish flesh for the presence of toxins; producers are also expected to meet end-product standards. Areas are closed when toxins in shellfish exceed the limits (Table 1) and closures are frequent. National Reference Laboratories (NRL) have been established (Council Decision 93/383/EEC) and a Community Reference Laboratory co-ordinates NRL activities, which include exchange of information, promotion of the harmonisation of regulations and improvement of monitoring and management of shellfish toxins[42].

Council Directive 91/493/EEC lays down the health conditions for producing and marketing fishery products. The placing on the market of certain families of poisonous fish is not permitted, and fishery products containing biotoxins such as ciguatera toxins or muscle paralysing toxins are not permitted. The problem here is that there are no reliable methods available for routine detection of ciguatoxins, for example, in a monitoring situation[43]. Commission Decision 95/149/EC stipulates sampling schemes and histamine limits for the flesh of scombroid and clupeoid fish. Fish that have undergone ripening processes in brine may have higher levels, but should not exceed twice the values quoted in Table 1.

Methods of detection[9]

Mouse bioassays are the official procedures for the analysis of shellfish for PSP and DSP, and these have been used effectively in monitoring programmes world-wide for many years. However, these techniques have limitations in terms of specificity and accuracy, and the use of animals for such purposes is becoming increasingly unacceptable for ethical reasons. This has resulted in the development of alternative techniques such as cell culture assays, ELISAs, HPLC, CE-MS and LC-MS[8], but none are validated yet for monitoring purposes. For ASP, the mouse bioassay was deemed too insensitive during the Canadian outbreak, and HPLC methodology was adopted[16]. Histamine can be assayed by a variety of methods including ion exchange chromatography and capillary zone electrophoresis, tetramine by high voltage electrophoresis[34], and tetrodotoxin primarily by HPLC.

Detoxification of shellfish[43]

All of the toxins are heat stable and survive normal cooking, canning, smoking, pickling, marinating and freezing. No useful economic processing method has been validated that eliminates toxins to yield a safe, palatable product. This includes the purification systems which are generally used to cleanse pathogenic bacteria from live bivalves. Therefore, in most cases, natural depuration is the only safe option, although in some instances this can take years.

Future perspectives

Occurrence of toxins which threaten valuable seafood resources seem to be increasing in frequency, intensity and geographic distribution[9]. In the last 30 years, a new toxin group has been discovered almost each decade, generally through food poisoning outbreaks. In all probability, this trend will persist and so, on occasion, consumers are likely to continue to present with seafood related illness of unknown nature. Increasingly, patients may present with symptoms complicated by the presence of multiple toxins with different effects. The novel toxins will generate needs for identification of source and toxin(s), an understanding of the mode(s) of action, and decisions on methodology and action limits. Overall, there are needs to develop and validate diagnostic methods for illness, remedial treatments, and antidotes where appropriate.

Regulatory authorities will be faced with new demands to minimise the impact of these toxins on both the consumer and the industry. Increasing seafood poisoning may result in more stringent EU legislation. However, there is an urgent need to undertake appropriate risk assessments for marine toxins which take into account all relevant factors. These include: (i) effects from constant sub-acute exposure; and (ii) realistic evaluations of the hazard to consumers from compounds that, so far, have shown damage only in animal models at high concentrations.

More research is required to gain a better understanding of the factors that determine seafood toxicity, and to develop processes by which intoxicated seafood can be detoxified and remain palatable. Improved detection methods are also urgently required to replace mouse bioassays, and to develop and validate effective, rapid, low-cost screening methods for monitoring purposes.

Overall, the low incidence of some of these seafood syndromes within Europe can be attributed to the efficiency of the monitoring regimens implemented; but these are likely to come under increasing pressure to meet new demands. New legislation will have important economic implications for national and international trade and a balance must be maintained which minimises these effects while protecting public health.

Acknowledgements

The authors gratefully acknowledge the assistance of Dr Jane Lewis (University of Westminster) who provided the photomicrograph for Figure 3, Dr Katrin Schmidt (BgVV, FAO/WHO Collaborating Centre Research and Training in Food Hygiene and Zoonoses) for the data for Europe on Foodborne Disease Outbreaks Associated with Seafood, 1995 to 1998, Ms Maria Calvo (Sea Fish Industry Authority) for European trade statistics, and Mr Tom McInnes and Mr Keith Mutch (Fisheries Research Services) who produced the illustrations for Figures 1 and 2.

References

1   Simopoulos AP. Nutritional aspects of fish. In: Luten JB, Børresen J, Oehlenschläger J. (Eds) *Seafood from Producer to Consumer, Integrated Approach to Quality.* Amsterdam: Elsevier, 1997; 589–607

2   Motohiro T. Biotoxins in seafood. In: Huss HH, Jakobsen M, Liston J. (Eds) *Quality Assurance in the Fish Industry.* Amsterdam: Elsevier, 1992; 243–58

3   Falconer IR. (Ed). *Algal Toxins in Seafood and Drinking Water.* London: Academic Press, 1993

4   van Egmond HP, Aune T, Lassus P, Speijers GJA, Waldock M. Paralytic and diarrhoeic shellfish poisons: occurrence in Europe, toxicity, analysis and regulation. *J Nat Tox* 1993; 2: 41–83

5   Mines D, Stahmer S, Shepherd SM. Poisonings food, fish, shellfish. *Emerg Med Clin North Am* 1997; 15: 157–77

6   Aune T. Health effects associated with algal toxins from seafood. *Arch Toxicol* 1997; 19 (Suppl.): 389–97

7   Anderson DM, Cembella AD, Hallegraeff GM. (Eds) *Physiological Ecology of Harmful Algal Blooms.* Berlin: Springer, NATO ASI Series, 1998

8   Leftley JW, Hannah F. Phycotoxins in seafood. In: Watson DH. (Ed) *Natural Toxicants in Food.* Sheffield: Sheffield Academic 1998; 182–224

9   Park DL, Guzman-Perez SE, Lopez-Garcia R. Aquatic biotoxins: design and implementation of seafood safety monitoring programs. *Rev Environ Contam Toxicol* 1999; 161: 157–200

10 Kao CY. Paralytic shellfish poisoning. In: Falconer IR. (Ed) *Algal Toxins in Seafood and Drinking Water.* London: Academic Press, 1993; 75–86

11 Scoging AC. Illness associated with seafood. *Communicable Dis Rep* 1991; 1: R117–22

12 Aune T, Yndestad M. Diarrhetic shellfish poisoning. In: Falconer IR. (Ed) *Algal Toxins in Seafood and Drinking Water.* London: Academic Press, 1993; 87–104

13 Scoging A, Bahl M. Diarrhetic shellfish poisoning in the UK. *Lancet* 1998; 352: 117

14 Todd ECD. Domoic acid and amnesic shellfish poisoning – a review. *J Food Protect* 1993; 56: 69–83

15 Bates SS, Garrison DL, Horner RA. Bloom dynamics and physiology of domoic acid producing *Pseudo-nitzschia* species. In: Anderson DM, Cembella AD, Hallegraeff GM. (Eds) *Physiological Ecology of Harmful Algal Blooms.* Berlin: Springer, NATO ASI Series, 1998; 267–92

16 Wright JLC, Quilliam MA. Methods for domoic acid and the amnesic shellfish poisons. In: Hallegraeff GM, Anderson DM, Cembella AD, Enevoldsen HO. (Eds) *Manual on Harmful Marine Microalgae.* IOC Manuals and Guides No 33. UNESCO, 1995; 113–33

17 Bagnis R. Ciguatera fish poisoning. In: Falconer IR. (Ed) *Algal Toxins in Seafood and Drinking Water.* London: Academic Press, 1993; 105–15

18 Lipp EK, Rose JB. The role of seafood in food borne diseases in the United States of America. *Rev Sci Tech Off Int Epiz* 1997; **16**: 620–40

19 Tindall DR, Morton SL. Community dynamics and physiology of epiphytic/benthic dinoflagellates associated with ciguatera. In: Anderson DM, Cembella AD, Hallegraeff GM. (Eds) *Physiological Ecology of Harmful Algal Blooms*. Berlin: Springer, NATO ASI Series, 1998; 293–313

20 Ebesu JSM, Nagai H, Hokama Y. The first reported case of human ciguatera possibly due to a farm-cultured salmon. *Toxicon* 1994; **32**: 1282–6

21 Pearn JH. Chronic fatigue syndrome: chronic ciguatera poisoning as a differential diagnosis. *Med J Aust* 1997; **166**: 309–10

22 Steidinger KA, Vargo GA, Tester PA, Tomas CR. Bloom dynamics and physiology of *Gymnodinium breve* with emphasis on the Gulf of Mexico. In: In: Anderson DM, Cembella AD, Hallegraeff GM. (Eds) *Physiological Ecology of Harmful Algal Blooms*. Berlin: Springer, NATO ASI Series, 1998; 133–53

23 Steidinger KA. Some taxonomic and biologic aspects of toxic dinoflagellates. In: Falconer IR. (Ed) *Algal Toxins in Seafood and Drinking Water*. London: Academic Press, 1993; 1–28

24 Taylor SL. Histamine food poisoning: toxicology and clinical aspects. *CRC Crit Rev Toxicol* 1986; **17**: 91–128

25 Kerr GW, Parke TR. Scombroid poisoning – a pseudoallergic syndrome. *J R Soc Med* 1998; **91**: 83–4

26 Gessner BD, Hokama Y, Isto S. Scombrotoxicosis-like illness following the ingestion of smoked salmon. *Clin Infect Dis* 1996; **23**: 1315–8

27 Clifford MN, Walker J, Wright J, Hardy R, Murray CK. Studies with volunteers on the role of histamine in suspected scombrotoxicosis. *J Sci Food Agric* 1989; **47**: 365–75

28 Ijomah P, Clifford MN, Walker J, Wright J, Hardy R, Murray CK. The importance of endogenous histamine relative to dietary histamine in the aetiology of scombrotoxicosis. *Food Additives Contaminants* 1991; **8**: 531–42

29 Ascione A, Barresi LS, Sarullo FM, De Silvestre G. Two cases of 'scombroid syndrome' with severe cardiovascular compromise. *Cardiologia* 1997; **42**: 1285–8

30 Morrow JD, Margolis GR, Rowland J, Roberts LJ. Evidence that histamine is the causative toxin of scombroid fish poisoning. *N Engl J Med* 1991; **324**: 716–20

31 Clifford MN, Walker R, Ijomah P, Wright J, Murray CK, Hardy R. Is there a role for amines other than histamines in the aetiology of scombrotoxicosis? *Food Additives Contaminants* 1991; **8**: 641–52

32 Rawles DD, Flick GJ, Martin RE. Biogenic amines in fish and shellfish. *Adv Food Nutr Res* 1996; **39**: 329–65

33 Clifford MN, Walker R, Ijomah P *et al.* Do saxitoxin-like substances have a role in scombrotoxicosis? *Food Additives Contaminants* 1993; **9**: 657–67

34 Reid TMS, Gould IM, Mackie IM, Ritchie AH, Hobbs G. Food poisoning due to the consumption of red whelks (*Neptunea antiqua*). *Epidemiol Infect* 1988; **101**: 419–24

35 Black NMI. Red spells danger for whelk eaters. *Communicable Dis Rep* 1991; **1**: R125

36 Yasumoto T, Satake M. New toxins and their toxicological evaluations. In: Reguera B, Blanco J, Fernandez M, Wyatt T. (Eds) *Harmful Algae*. Xunta de Galicia and Intergovernmental Oceanographic Commission of UNESCO, 1998; 461–4

37 Satake M, Ofuji K, James K J, Furey A, Yasumoto T. New toxic event caused by Irish mussels. In: Reguera B, Blanco J, Fernandez M, Wyatt T. (Eds) *Harmful Algae*. Xunta de Galicia and Intergovernmental Oceanographic Commission of UNESCO, 1998; 469

38 Satake M, Ofuji K, Naoki H *et al.* Azaspiracid, a new marine toxin having unique spiro ring assemblies isolated from Irish mussels *Mytilus edulis*. *J Am Chem Soc* 1998; **120**: 9967–8

39 Ito E, Terao K, McMahon T, Silke J, Yasumoto T. Pathological changes in mice caused by crude extracts of novel toxins isolated from Irish mussels. In: Reguera B, Blanco J, Fernandez M, Wyatt

T. (Eds) *Harmful Algae*. Xunta de Galicia and Intergovernmental Oceanographic Commission of UNESCO, 1998; 588–9

40 Glasgow HB, Burkholder JM, Schmechel DE, Tester PA, Rublee PA. Insidious effects of a toxic estuarine dinoflagellate on fish survival and human health. *J Toxicol Environ Health* 1995; **46**: 501–22

41 Greer J, Leffler M, Belas R, Kramer J, Place A. Molecular technologies and *Pfiesteria* research a scientific synthesis. *Maryland Sea Grant Publication* UM-SG-TS-98-01, 1998, 21

42 Fernandez ML. Phycotoxins: regulatory limits and effects on trade. In: Miraglia M, van Egmond H, Brera C, Gilbert J. (Eds) *Mycotoxins and Phycotoxins – Developments in Chemistry, Toxicology and Food Safety*. Fort Collins: Alaken, 1998; 503–16

43 ICMSF (International Commission on Microbiological Specifications for Foods). *Microorganisms in Foods 5: Characteristics of Microbial Pathogens*. ICMSF. Blackie Academic & Professional, London, UK. 1996; 265–79

The future relationship between the media, the food industry and the consumer

W A Anderson

Food Safety Authority of Ireland, Dublin, Ireland

The relationship between the media, the food industry and the consumer is probably at its lowest point as we start the new millennium. The frequency of food scares appears to be increasing and news reports sometimes seem both sensational and polarised. High profile issues like the development of bovine spongiform encephalopathy in the UK and the dioxin contamination of poultry products in Belgium have undermined consumer confidence in the food industry. The recent genetically modified foods' debate has served to demonstrate the gulf that has grown between the food industry, food safety experts and the public. This is a rift that has been exploited by environmental pressure groups and fuelled by the media.

This paper examines some of the underlying causes of the current air of mistrust that seems to exist between the media, the food industry and the consumer. Also, by examining the projected trends in these root causes, it draws some conclusions for the future relationship between the parties involved and suggests some changes that may improve the present situation.

Food safety was once a topic debated exclusively by the food industry and the regulatory authorities. Consumers accepted that food was safe. It was not something to be worried about. It was not something that would determine what was eaten or by whom it would be eaten. The media rarely saw the issue of food safety as a news-worthy topic and few, if any, reports on food safety ever found their way into the popular press. That was the relationship between the food industry, the consumer and the media less than 30 years ago.

In the late 1960s and early 1970s, few people could have predicted that food safety would become the major world issue it is today. Even fewer people could have foreseen the part that the media might play in this. Today, food safety is rarely out of the media spotlight. The consumer is now lobbied constantly by pressure groups, the food industry and the government via the media. Debates are public and polarised and increasingly it seems that those who adopt the middle ground are marginalised.

In the industrialised world, food safety has become a global issue that influences political careers and policy, sells television air time, newspapers

Correspondence to:
Dr W A Anderson, Food
Safety Authority of
Ireland, Abbey Court,
Lower Abbey Street,
Dublin 1, Ireland

British Medical Bulletin 2000;**56** (No. 1): 254–268

© The British Council 2000

and magazines and frightens the majority of consumers. The relationship that has developed between the food industry, the media and the consumer is one of suspicion and mistrust. This chapter will endeavour to examine some of the issues surrounding the development of this relationship by analysing some of the external and internal influences on the three groups involved. The immediate future development of the relationship between the food industry, the consumer and the media into the new millennium will be shaped by factors at work today.

Consumers

A consistent supply of good quality and safe food is the major requirement of any consumer. In the non-industrialised world this is still the consumers' main goal and, understandably, it overshadows other considerations. However, in the industrialised world where this goal has been achieved, the consumer can now focus on less fundamental aspects of food supply.

In the industrialised world, the present-day consumer is a very different creature to the consumer of 30 years ago. Today, the consumer perception of food safety has been influenced by many factors and this has shaped their relationship with the food industry. Eating is a fundamental and personal activity that cannot be avoided. Therefore, food influences all our lives and may be it is this shared reality that makes food safety such an emotive issue with universal interest.

Consumer perception of risk

Risk is an unavoidable element of living, it enters every facet of our lives. One of the most difficult messages that the consumer has been asked to accept is that eating food involves an element of risk. Risk, meaning the risk of food-borne illness and, in a small number of cases, illness that can be fatal. Consumers want to know that their food is safe, not that their food is as safe as possible. If society is to halt the cycle of food scares that exemplifies the relationship between the food industry, the consumer and the media then this is a fundamental message that needs to be understood by the consumer. Currently, this is not the case and the food industry, national governments and the media must all accept partial responsibility for this failure. Most communication from these sources is aimed at 'educating' the public, as if a simple statement of the facts is all that is required to get them to see the scientific point of view. All parties will only understand the concept of risk if they enter into dialogue with each other and participate in the risk evaluation process.

Research has shown that there are many factors that modulate the consumers perception of risk (adapted from Covello & Merkhofer[1]):

- Trust (did this person tell the truth the last time?)

- Receptivity (it happens to other people but not to me!)

- Familiarity (the risk of *Escherichia coli* O157 infection versus the risk of slipping on ice)

- Understanding (the risk of genetically modified foods versus the risk of sunburn)

- Scientific uncertainty (the risk of Creutzfeldt-Jakob disease from beef versus the risk of crashing the car)

- Controllability (exposure to antibiotic residues in meat versus the risk of flying)

- How voluntary (exposure to pesticides in food versus contracting cancer from smoking)

- Impact on children (risk perceived greater if children affected)

- Dread (a slow death from Creutzfeldt-Jakob disease versus a quick death from a plane crash)

- Media (source of popular understanding influences risk perception)

- Benefits (risk versus benefit: the risks involved with taking the contraceptive pill versus the benefit of preventing unwanted pregnancy)

Many of these factors are understood either consciously or unconsciously by the food industry, the media and pressure groups that may wish to pursue a particular agenda. Most, if not all, of the recent food scares reported in the media have exploited one or more of the factors aimed at increasing or decreasing the fears of the consumer in the fight to influence food consumption patterns.

Environmental awareness

One of the major changes that has occurred in recent years giving rise to the publicity surrounding the food supply is the rise of environmental awareness in the industrialised world. This has resulted in an increase in the strength and size of the environmental lobby, particularly from those who wish to move away from intensive farming systems to organic food production. The food industry is no longer able to move in the direction it would like without meeting stiff resistance from environmental pressure groups. This has led to some well-publicised clashes, where both parties have attempted to gain the support of consumers by manipulating the factors that modulate consumer perception of food safety and risk. The recent opposition to genetically modified foods in Europe is without doubt the best example of this new phenomenon.

To cite the rise of environmental awareness as the sole reason for the change in consumer perception of food safety would be to over simplify the current situation. Environmental pressure groups have existed for many years and have been active in their opposition to issues like intensive farming techniques. Yet these techniques have proliferated and expanded with little regard to their opposition. The major change would seem to be that consumer has only recently woken from a long and complacent sleep. The reason for this sudden awareness of food safety is undoubtedly due to a few monumental and catastrophic mistakes by the food industry. The trust of the consumer in the food industry has vanished over the last 10 years and trust is a key factor in the modulation of risk perception. Environmental groups have been able to exploit the distrust that now exists between the food industry and the consumer and hence they have gained a major victory. This may or may not prove a benefit for the consumer in the long-term, only time will tell. However, the food industry can certainly no longer ignore the environmental lobby and the relationship between the two groups that finally emerges will undoubtedly effect the future relationship between the food industry and the consumer.

Life-style changes

Life-style changes over the past 30 years have affected two of the other main factors that modulate the perception of risk. In one version of an ideal world, consumers would be able to produce, process and eat their own food, thus taking control of its safety. However, an increasing proportion of the world population has abandoned this life-style for urban living. In 1955, 32% of the world's population lived urban life-styles. By 1995 this had risen to 45% and by 2025 it is estimated that this figure will grow to 59%[2]. If the rise in world population figures is taken into account, then this would mean that approximately 4.7 billion people will live in cities and towns far removed from the source of food production. For the majority of these people, the ability to control the safety of their own food will be lost and, with the loss of controllability, the fear of a food safety incident is likely to increase.

Urbanisation and an increasing reliance on others to supply wholesome food will also increase the sense of fear because exposure to the risk of food poisoning is not voluntary. This factor can easily be illustrated. According to the World Health Organization, there are currently 4 million deaths per year from smoking-related illness and this is estimated to rise to 10 million deaths per year by 2030[3]. From a scientific perspective, it is completely illogical for smokers to be concerned about the risk of food poisoning. However, in reality, they are as concerned as any other group and one of the reasons is their voluntary exposure to risk. Smokers know the risks of smoking, but have chosen to continue; in contrast, they have not chosen to suffer from food poisoning. As urbanisation increases, the perception of food safety as a risk factor in life will also increase. Thus, to a certain extent, consumers may feel that they are in a more vulnerable situation than they were and hence they are more susceptible to the influence of the food industry or the media and pressure groups.

The changes in life-style patterns within urban life in recent years may have also contributed to the current climate of distrust and vulnerability. In the UK, for example, the number of women in employment rose from 9.9 million in 1984 to 12 million in 1997 whilst the number of men in employment remained relatively static[4]. The number of families where both parents go out to work has risen dramatically. Families are, therefore, less likely to prepare their own food from basic ingredients. Current trends in eating away from the home are arguably the ultimate expression of the consumers' increasing reliance on the food industry. The level and pattern of employment is not only just exerting time constraints on families but it is increasing affluence. In the US this trend has been at work for longer than in Europe. The average US household spent $4411 on food in 1994 with 38% being spent away from home. Consumers are now reliant on the food industry from farm-to-fork and have little control over the safety of the food they eat. It is not surprising that fears have intensified as a result of our modern life-styles. In some cases these fears are justified, eating away from home appears to carry with it a greater risk of food poisoning. Analysis of the causes of 42 food poisoning outbreaks in Ireland between 1996 and 1999 showed that 90% of outbreaks occurred outside of the home in institutions and organised functions[5].

Consumer summary

Consumers are increasingly aware of environmental issues and their life-styles are changing rapidly. Both these trends have eroded some of the social factors that affect perception of risk. It is likely, therefore, that the consumer in the late 1990s is more susceptible to fears about food-borne illness. An increasing reliance on the food industry to supply wholesome food is coupled to an increasing distrust amongst consumers. It is unlikely that this distrust would have materialised without some foundation and clearly the number of incidents of food-borne illness is increasing at an alarming rate. Therefore, decreasing consumer confidence is only part of the background to the current relationship between the consumer, the food industry and the media.

The food industry

The food industry, like any other industry, supplies the demand from consumers. If consumers demand low cost food then the industry will supply it. If consumers demand more convenience foods then they will be supplied with those as well. Trends in consumer purchasing drive changes in the food industry. However, the food industry also exists for profit and commercial considerations dictate the approach the industry takes to supply demand. Developments in food science and technology have managed to supply consumer demands, but occasional failures have fuelled current concerns.

Intensive agriculture

The number of people in the world is increasing. Table 1 shows that there is likely to be an extra 2 billion mouths to feed by 2025. In the industrialised world, the population increase will be slower adding 38 million consumers to the burden of food supply. However, with an increase in the number of people comes a decrease in the amount of agricultural land available to produce food. Therefore, each area of land will have to produce more food. For example, in the UK wheat yields increased from 5.9 tonne/hectare in 1980 to 8.1 tonne/hectare in 1996. Similarly, barley yields increased from 4.4 tonne/hectare in 1980 to 6.1 tonne/hectare in 1996[6]. In another development, aquaculture is now the fastest growing food production system in the world expanding at an average of 9.2% over the last decade. At this growth rate, aquaculture will produce more fish for human consumption than capture fisheries by 2007[7]. This pattern is repeated throughout the industrialised world in

Table 1 Population trends (000s)

Area	1998 Total population	2025 Total population
World	5,926,062	7,919,803
Less industrialised countries	4,750,551	6,708,592
More industrialised countries	1,175,511	1,213,211

Data from Bureau of the Census USA[19].

both crop and animal production. Intensive agriculture has increased food supply, decreased costs and increased profits. In France, for instance, only 15% of the household budget goes towards food compared to 40% in 1940[8]. Based on the projected population increase and the demand for cheap food, the food production process is unlikely to become less intensive in the future.

The cost of this solution to the demand for plentiful cheap food has been several major and minor food scares. The arrival of bovine spongiform encephalopathy (BSE) in the UK during the late 1980s was a turning point in the relationship between the consumer and the food industry. The link between BSE and new variant Creutzfeldt-Jakob disease (CJD) a few years later was merely confirmation of what the majority of consumers already suspected. Few urbanised consumers realised that intensive agricultural practice involved using animal derivatives in feeds for herbivores. For many consumers this may have been the first time that they had considered the ethics and manner that their food was produced in, despite the work of environmental pressure groups. As consumers themselves, the media were not slow to develop the story and explore the ethical angles. The last decade has, therefore, seen the rise of consumer awareness of the ethical considerations of food production and this has lasted through into the more recent debates surrounding genetically modified foods and biotechnology. However, with the rise in world population and the increase in urbanisation, food production cannot revert to the practices of the 1940s; but, in Europe at least, there is likely to be a growing trend against the increase in the intensity of agricultural practices. With an increase in consumer affluence, the size of the niche market for organic produce will grow. Thus, in the future, we may witness the growth of 'food elitism' where one sector of the population can, in monetary terms, afford ethically-produced food with a perceived image of increased safety. It is important that the food industry and governments ensure that this remains a perception and that mass-produced, cheap food is also safe. If this does not happen, then it is likely that consumers will be justified in feeling that the food industry is letting them down which would put further pressure on the relationship between the two groups.

Globalisation of the food supply

Food is no longer produced and consumed in the same locality. World trade in food is a feature of the late 20th century. Produce is imported from around the world leading to year-round supply of certain fruits and vegetables that in past years would have only been available during a short season. Similarly, the origins of processed foods have become equally diverse. To illustrate this, Figure 1 shows some of the potential

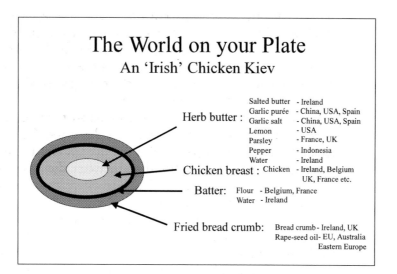

The World on your Plate

An 'Irish' Chicken Kiev

Herb butter :	Salted butter	- Ireland
	Garlic purée	- China, USA, Spain
	Garlic salt	- China, USA, Spain
	Lemon	- USA
	Parsley	- France, UK
	Pepper	- Indonesia
	Water	- Ireland
Chicken breast :	Chicken	- Ireland, Belgium
		UK, France etc.
Batter:	Flour	- Belgium, France
	Water	- Ireland
Fried bread crumb:	Bread crumb	- Ireland, UK
	Rape-seed oil	- EU, Australia
		Eastern Europe

Fig. 1 An example of processed food origins

origins of a chicken Kiev manufactured in Ireland. Ingredients are imported from many countries and thus a food safety problem in one country can easily find ramifications around the world. Recently, in Belgium, dioxin contaminated fat found its way into animal feeds and contaminated farm animals and products derived from them. Although the full history of this food safety incident may well be clarified in the future, it appears that contamination from one animal feed factory in one country resulted in a massive product recall in all 15 European Union Member States and other countries. In Ireland, a relatively small importer of Belgian produce, over 200 product lines were recalled. Elsewhere, the recall was much larger and affected farms as well as retail product. This amply demonstrates the potential dangers of the globalisation of food supply. The food industry is no longer national; it is international and, hence, food safety problems have become international. They are more frequent and more widespread than ever before increasing the consumers perception of the risk.

International food safety standards

For some consumers, trusting a national food industry is difficult, but trusting the industry in a totally different country with different perceived standards can be almost impossible. The food industry will not stop the globalisation trend, in fact it cannot; it can, however, disseminate food safety practices and hence international organisations like the Codex Alimentarius Commission (CAC) will play an increasing role in the harmonisation of food safety standards. The work of these organisations should help to protect public health across the world and increase trade in safe foodstuffs. In recent years, the formation of the World Trade Organization and two agreements on Sanitary and Phytosanitary Measures and Technical Barriers to Trade should speed up the standardisation process in the long-term. However, in the short-term, it seems that trade arguments over different interpretations of food safety can serve to increase the perceived risk by the consumer. It is often difficult for consumers to believe what experts say is safe when often they cannot agree what is safe amongst themselves. Opposition groups and the media seeking to influence the choice of consumers often exploit the different opinions held by different sectors of the food industry. International, independent, expert consultations on food safety issues, such as those convened by CAC, may well serve to harmonise scientific opinion in different countries and increase consumer confidence.

The adaptation of bacteria and susceptibility of humans

Bacterial populations can double every 20 min under optimum conditions. Although these simple organisms benefit from only limited heterogenetic diversity, other mechanisms exist which alter the genetic information such as natural mutation and plasmid transfer. When these mechanisms are coupled with the exceptionally fast reproduction rate, the genetic diversity of bacteria is far greater than that found in humans, up to 5 times greater in fact when subjected to similar measures[9]. It is no surprise, therefore, that bacteria can adapt rapidly to their surroundings.

In some instances, bacteria have adapted to modern food production practices. For example, it is no coincidence that the increase in listeriosis in the industrialised world has mirrored the increase in the preservation of food by the use of chill storage temperatures. In the 1980s, consumers began to demand fresher, less preserved food and this demand was supplied by the food industry by the use of chill storage and distribution. *Listeria monocytogenes* is a bacterium that has been known since the early decades of the 20th century, but it was not known to cause food-borne disease. In England and Wales, figures on cases of listeriosis were first collected in 1983 and 111 cases were diagnosed. By 1988, this had peaked at 278 cases falling back to 115 cases by 1996 probably as a result of the recognition, research and control of the organism in the food factory[10]. In another example of adaptation, some bacteria have developed resistance to antibiotics. In the UK, *Salmonella typhimurium* DT104 has been the most common antibiotic resistant strain in humans since 1992 and it is resistant to 5 antibiotics[11]. There is evidence to suggest that some antibiotic-resistant bacteria are transmitted to humans from animals via food, but the extent of the problem remains to be established[18]. Equally, there is some evidence that these organisms cause illness in humans. It seems likely that resistance has been caused by the selective pressures exerted on enteric bacteria in the guts of farm animals due to the use/mis-use of some antibiotics required by intensive farming methods. By nature of their antibiotic resistance, these bacteria are much more difficult to remove from the food-chain; research/surveillance is being funded to establish more clearly carriage of antibiotic-resistant microbes and their importance.

In other instances, bacteria have emerged that were not present 30 years ago. For example, *E. coli* O157:H7 and related strains cause critical food-borne illness and seem to have emerged from normal gastrointestinal *E. coli* in cattle. Unlike their harmless ancestors, these organisms have acquired a series of virulence factors that have made them into the serious threat they are today. Cases in the England and Wales have risen from 470 in 1992 to 1087 in 1997[10]. World-wide, the pattern is repeated.

Food-borne pathogenic bacteria present a greater hazard to immuno-compromised groups than to the general healthy population. These vulnerable groups are the very young, the elderly, pregnant women and people with immune systems weakened by diseases like cancer and AIDS. Although, in industrialised countries, population growth will be slower than in non-industrialised ones, the population will age faster. It is predicted that, in 2025, approximately 21% of people will be older than 65 years. This represents over 900 million more people. The ageing patterns are shown in Table 2. In addition, it is estimated that 30.6 million people world-wide were living with HIV/AIDS at the end of 1997, with figures expected to rise well into the 21st century[12]. Essentially, the population is set to become more vulnerable to food-borne disease.

Food industry summary

Manufacturing practices shaped by consumer demand and profit margins have increased the risk of delivering new bacteria to vulnerable people. It is inevitable that this has added to the growth in the number

Table 2 Population trends (000s)

Area	1998		2025	
	Total population	Population aged over 65 years (% total)	Total population	Population aged over 65 years (% total)
World	5,926,062	400,672 (6.8%)	7,919,803	821,096 (10.4%)
Less industrialised countries	4,750,551	234,141 (4.9%)	6,708,592	563,950 (8.4%)
More industrialised countries	1,175,511	166,562 (14.2%)	1,213,211	257,146 (21.2%)

Data from Bureau of the Census USA[19].

of cases of food-borne illness in the past 20 years in particular. The food industry is faced with a growing challenge to the safety of the food supply and, unless it can redress the balance in the next few years, it is unlikely that its relationship with consumers and the media will improve.

The media

There can be no doubt that currently food is news. A study commissioned by the International Food Information Council and carried out by The Centre for Media & Public Affairs in the US analysed 3 months' of news coverage from May to July in 1995. There were 979 food and nutrition reports from 37 news outlets in that period, covering newspapers to television. This accounted for 10,000 column inches and 11 h of broadcasting[13].

The food industry has often charged the media with biased reporting of food safety issues. It is difficult to look into the reality of these claims because surveys of reporting bias are lacking or not publicly available. The IFIC study provided a rare opportunity to test this accusation. It was found that, in the area of food safety, stories covered additives, contaminants, food labelling and causes of food-borne illness. In the case of additives and contaminants, they found that the negative effects of these issues were highlighted twice as often than the positive effects and that environmental and health activists were quoted 5 times as often as industry sources. This would, at first sight, appear to lend support to the claims of the food industry. However, a repeat of the survey in 1997 found that this trend had disappeared and activists were no longer the major group quoted.

Quality of reporting

Perhaps the most interesting result of both IFIC studies was the finding that most reports lacked the information required to communicate the context of the topic being reported. Essentially reports were too brief and focussed on black and white issues. Perhaps here lies the problem in the relationship between the media, the food industry and the consumer. The media are often viewed with suspicion by scientists who complain that they have been quoted out of context or even misquoted completely. In reality this does happen, but it can be due to both parties. The media have been known to sacrifice reality for a news angle on occasions, but it occurs far less than some would suspect. Often misquotes and context problems are simply a reflection that the two parties to the interview speak different languages. Not in the literal sense of course, but the language of science is very different from the language of the media. Few reporters have science training and many scientists, after years of science training, have forgotten how to communicate a simple, clear and unambiguous message. Under such circumstances, the context of reports is often difficult to express and often dropped when there is pressure on column space or broadcast time.

Media competition

Global communications are expanding and the newspaper or television is no longer the sole source of information. However, for the majority of consumers, these traditional forms of reporting are still their sole 'window on the world'. Competition in the media has increased dramatically over the past 30 years. Television has moved from terrestrial-based stations to satellite stations and is now moving into digital format. For example, in 1980, the American cable network CNN was founded and broadcast 24 h news to 1.7 million American cable households. However, in 1998 CNN and CNN International broadcast news to 190 million households in 210 countries around the world via satellite and international broadcast stations[14]. The number of stations available is expanding at an exponential rate and, in addition, people also have access to television stations outside national boundaries. Food safety stories in one part of the world are now rapidly transmitted across the globe raising the awareness of the consumer to the issue.

Newspapers are under stiff competition as well, from new newspapers, magazines and alternative publishing formats like the internet. According to the *American Journalism Review*, on-line newspapers have grown from just 20 in 1994 to 3622 in 1997[15]. Many are traditional newspapers expanding their publishing format, but some are new competitors. The fight for a share of the lucrative world wide web advertising market fuels the fight for readership but now on a global scale. Even so-called 'local' newspapers publishing on the internet no longer have a local readership. In addition, as if the media world were not complex enough, traditional radio and TV news broadcasters have also started multimedia sites on the world wide web consisting of written news, and live TV and radio broadcasts. These sites are becoming increasingly popular, for example, by March 1999, monthly page impressions at BBC On-line had reached over 80 million[16].

Media summary

It is not surprising that with the proliferation and globalisation of the media, the food industry and consumer believe that they have lost control of the food safety agenda. This trend is unlikely to change in the foreseeable future and, therefore, it is essential that the food industry learns to communicate clearly and truthfully with the media. A relationship needs to be generated where journalists respect and trust the information disseminated by scientists and scientists need to recognise the constraints and pressures that competition has placed on the journalists. Food-related stories will always interest consumers, but the media has a duty to restrain itself from sensationalist reporting where facts and context are abandoned in the quest for a eye-catching headline. It is important that both parties work to ensure the context to food safety stories is included and, in this way, both their relationships with consumers should improve.

Conclusions

As we enter the new millennium, the stage is set for further deterioration in the relationship between the media, the food industry and the consumer unless action is taken. The factors that influence consumer acceptance of risk are changing and are likely to ensure that consumers perceive a greater risk involved with their food supply. The intensity of food production and the global supply chain are likely to increase the number of large-scale food safety incidents. As will emerging bacterial pathogens and the increase in the numbers of vulnerable people. There is undoubtedly a greater burden on the food industry to get it right first time and every time. The move towards risk analysis and hazard and critical control point systems is essential to meet this challenge.

The risk analysis approach proposed by the Codex Alimentarius Commission is important for the future of food safety[17]. This approach requires that all interested parties become involved in a transparent risk analysis process. However, for the system to work to the benefit of consumers, two problems must be overcome. Currently, risk analysis exercises are dominated by science based decisions. The 'value' judgements of consumers that include environmental and ethical views do not receive enough consideration either during the risk assessment or risk management procedure. The recent GM foods' debate has demonstrated the need for a broader base to risk analysis than science alone if consumers are to be re-assured. The second problem lies with the independence of experts. Today, the relationship between the scientific community and the public has never been worse. Most industrialised nations have adopted a policy of privatisation of science leaving experts to rely less on public money and more on corporate sponsorship of research. The concept of independent expertise within this framework is difficult for the public to accept and it exposes scientists to conflicting interests. The risk analysis model should help to repair the relationship between the media, the food industry and the consumer but only if the public can be re-assured that experts are truly independent and that 'value' judgements have been considered.

A transparent risk analysis system also has implications for the media. Faced with intense competition, the media must still adopt a responsible approach to reporting. It is important that the context of the food safety risk is communicated and not lost in the battle for column inches or broadcast time. The media could ensure this approach via a code of practice that could offset any need for national intervention along the lines of existing legislation in the US. Food scientists must work with journalists and strive to convey their message clearly in non-scientific language. A better relationship between the media and the food industry would benefit consumers who rely on the two parties to supply information that influences purchase decisions.

Everybody involved in food, whether they buy it, report about it, make money from it or research into it, should work to repair the relationship that has served only to damage consumer confidence over the past 30 years.

Acknowledgements

I would like to thank Dr Patrick Wall and Mr Alan Reilly for their insight into the subject of this paper and Ms Christina Tlustos for her help in finding suitable sources of statistics.

References

1 Covello, Merkhofer. *Risk Assessment Methods*. New York: Plenum, 1994
2 United Nations. *World Population Prospects 1996 Revision*. ISBN 92 11 513162; 1996
3 World Health Organization. *Ageing and Tobacco Use*. www.who.int, 1999
4 Government Statistics Service, UK. *UK in Figures*. www.statistics.gov.uk/ststs/ukinfigs/employ.htm, 1999
5 Food Safety Authority of Ireland. Unpublished figures, 1999
6 Ministry of Agriculture, Fisheries and Food, UK. *UK Food and Farming in Figures*. www.maff.gov.uk/esg/miscpdf/ukfff.pdf, 1997
7 Reilly A, Kaferstein F. Food safety and products from aquaculture. *J Appl Microbiol Symp Suppl* 1999; **85**, 249S–57S
8 Usher R. Hard to swallow. *Time* 1999; **154**: 30–9
9 Feng P, Lampel KA, Karch H, Whittam TS. Genotypic and phenotypic changes in the emergence of *Escherichia coli* O157:H7. *J Infect Dis* 1998; **177**: 1750–3
10 Public Health Laboratory Service, UK. *Disease Facts*. www.phls.co.uk/facts/, 1998

11 MAFF. *A Review of Antimicrobial Resistance in the Food Chain.* www.maff.gov.uk, 1998

12 McDevitt. *World Health Report. Life in the 21st Century — A Vision for All.* ISBN 92 4 156189 0. Geneva: World Health Organization, 1998

13 Lichter SR, Amundson D. *Food for Thought — Reporting of Diet, Nutrition and Food Safety.* International Food Information Council Foundation. http://ificinfo.health.org, 1996

14 Anon. CNN: charting a new frontier for news gathering. *Broadcast Engineering,* November 1998

15 Meyer EK. An unexpectedly wider web for the world's newspapers. *Am Journalism Rev* http://ajr.newslink.org, 21–27 September 1999

16 British Broadcasting Corporation. *BBC Annual Report - Review of the Year 1998/1999* http://www.bbc.co.uk/info/report99/review2f.shtml

17 World Health Organization. *Application of Risk Analysis to Food Standards Issues.* Report of the joint FAO/WHO expert consultation 13–17 March 1995. Geneva: WHO, 1995

18 ACMSF (Advisory Committee on Microbiological Safety of Food). *Report on Microbial Antibiotic Resistance in Relation to Food Safety.* London: The Stationery Office, 1999

19 Data from US Department of Commerce, Economics and Statistics Administration. Bureau of the Census United States of America. March 1, 1999

Index

© The British Council 1999

Stroke

Scientific Editor: Martin M Brown

LIVERPOOL
JOHN MOORES UNIVERSITY
AVRIL ROBARTS LRC
TITHEBARN STREET
LIVERPOOL L2 2ER
TEL. 0151 231 4022